A
Kinesthetic
Legacy

The Life and
Works of
Barbara Clark

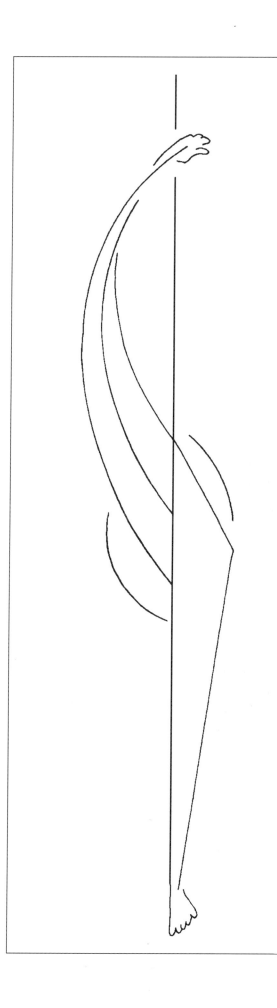

A Kinesthetic Legacy

The Life and Works of Barbara Clark

By Pamela Matt

CMT PRESS

Copyright © 1993 Pamela Matt

Anatomical illustrations in Part II reprinted with permission of Bohn Strafleu Van Loghum, Houten, The Netherlands from Spalteholz-Spanner: *Handatlas der Anatomie des Menschen (Atlas of Human Anatomy)* 16th ed., 1967.

Part III of the book includes an expansion and revision of the following works previously published by Barbara Clark: *Let's Enjoy Sitting, Standing and Walking,* © 1963; *How to Live in Your Axis – Your Vertical Line,* © 1968; *Body Proportion Needs Depth,* © 1973.

ISBN: 1-881914-25-9

Cover Design
    by Jeanne Smith, Tempe, Arizona
Typography and Book Production
    by Walsh and Associates, Tempe, Arizona

Printed in the United States of America

To J.D.M.

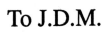

TABLE OF CONTENTS

> *Introduction • Rolling • Crawling • Sitting • Standing •*
> *Jumping • Resting • Sequencing Basic Movements*

> *General Introduction and Spinal Construction • Spinal*
> *Awareness • Thigh Fulcrum Awareness • Psoas Action*
> *Awareness • Rib Fulcrum Awareness • Thigh Action • Atlanto-*
> *Axial Socket • Shoulder Action • Thigh Movement • Spinal*
> *Axis Movement • Shoulder Movement • Foot Awareness •*
> *Diaphragm Action – Inhalation • Abdominal Action • Foot*
> *Movement • Lengthening the Spine • Shoulder Movement •*
> *Centering to Move • Axes of Thigh Movement • Sternal*
> *Suspension • Pubic Fulcrum Awareness • Spinal-Rib Thrust*
> *Diagonals*

> *How Do We Sit? Touching the Spots • How Do We Stand?*
> *Feeling the Action • The Cat's Center Line – Tracing It Out •*
> *Your Own Center Line – Tracing It Out • Your Leg Lines*
> *Come from the Center Line • Your Own Center Line –*
> *Breathing With It • Your Toe Lines Lead to the Center of the*
> *Body • Stand and Walk – Tall*

> *Introduction • How Imagery Works • Sitting with a Center*
> *Line • Rest as You Sit • Standing with a Center Line • Rest as*
> *You Stand • Walking from Your Axis is a Game • The Secret of*
> *Breathing • Sitting Down and Getting Up • Ankle Action • The*
> *Dance Plié • Circling the Axis–The Vertical Position •*
> *Circling the Axis–The Horizontal Position • More Sitting and*

Standing Exercises • More Walking Exercises • More Sitting Down–Getting Up Exercises • More Breathing Exercises • More Exercises for Foot and Ankle Action • More Plié Exercises

How To Live In Your Axis – Your Vertical Line

Introduction • Balancing Down the Back of the Cycle–The Plié • Exhalation Count Strengthens Down the Back Action • Rhythm Continues Through Your Lower Back and Thighs • Balancing Through Your Axis • Walking Into Yourself–Action in the Psoas Muscles • The Center of Your Foot • The Outside of the Arm Falls Away • The Shoulder Blades Steer the Collar Bones Into Their Sternal Sockets • Raising An Arm Begins Along the Side of Your Axis • The Shoulders Aid the Weight Transfer • Raise the Top of the Sternum in the Front to Lower the Shoulder Blades in the Back • The Shoulder Blades Serve as Floating Rafts • Lower Your Sacrum in the Back to Raise the Front of the Pelvis • Balancing the Body Alternately on the Top of Either Thigh • Cross Patterning–The Oblique Lines Involved • Cross Patterning Using An Arm with the Opposite Leg • Following the Hand Path to the Shoulder and Lower Back • Inhalation–Up the Front Follows Exhalation –Down the Back • Lower Your Heels in the Back Line –Come Up from Your Toes in the Front Line • The Body Cycle–Suggestions for Further Practice

Body Proportion Needs Depth – Front to Back

Introduction • Body Proportion Needs Depth • Streamline Your Structure in Sitting and Standing • How Alive Are Your Feet? Being Alive Means Action in the Joints • Toe to Heel – Heel to Toe Action • A Mound Makes a Base for the Body and Heightens Long Arches • Don't Crowd Your Vertebrae – Hold Each Bone Loosely Between the Disks • How Alive Is Your Spinal Column? Being Alive Means Action in its Joints • The Thigh Heads Swing In and Up as the Knees Bend • The Little Trochanters Are More Important than the Large • Your Rectus Abdominis Muscles Narrow in Moving Up Your Front Line • Your Sternum Leads Up in Your Mid-Front Line • Balance Your Body on the Tops of Your Thigh Heads – Walk High • The Heels of the Pelvis Are Behind the Thigh Sockets • Your Hand Belongs to Your Radial Bone • Come Up On Your Radial Joint – Go Down On Your Elbow • Center Your Arms In Their Sockets by Letting Your Shoulder Blades Float • Your Floating Ribs Slide Down to Work with Your 13th Ribs • Allow Space Between Your Shoulder Frame and Ribs • The Bone and Muscle Design in Your Back Floats Your Shoulder Blades Back and Down • Your Head is a part of Your Vertebral Column • Rhythm Flows Easily as You Slide Down Your Spinal Heels on Exhalation • Rhythm Plays Through Muscle Activity When Harmony Plays Through All Your Joints

PREFACE AND ACKNOWLEDGMENTS

WHEN BARBARA CLARK DIED IN 1982, she left the records of her lifetime of research and writing in my safekeeping. Knowing the material should be made available to the growing number of students and teachers interested in her ideas, I attempted to organize her work in various ways as I personally explored its meaning. Aligning the development of her writing with the story of her life gradually emerged as the most fitting and comprehensive means of presentation.

For the biographical aspects of this book presented in Part I, Barbara herself was of great assistance. She frequently reminisced about the childhood influences which shaped her avid interest in an approach to kinesthetic education which was begun by Mabel Todd. Soon after she met Miss Todd in 1923, she began to keep notes on her lessons at Todd's Boston studio, as well as all she could glean of the historical development of the approach. Later, as a teacher of young children, Barbara carefully recorded her own experimentation with Todd's ideas and the progress of the youngsters in her care. Her record keeping became less diligent as her attention turned from teaching to drawing and writing. However, her appointment books and correspondence continued to provide a log of her work with actors and dancers, along with occasional commentary. Since most of this source material was recorded without attention to dates or locations, specific documentation of Clark's historical narrative could not be completed in the *Notes*. Therefore, the reader can assume that most of Clark's quotations were taken from one of the many diaries and notebooks found in her papers, or remembered from the life stories which she frequently retold.

Part II presents two groups of lesson plans originally prepared for individuals who expressed interest in sharing Barbara Clark's teaching techniques with their own students. The first group of lesson plans, *Posture Plays*, developed in the early 1930s, was designed for use by parents and teachers of preschool children. Classic nursery rhymes and songs were suggested as accompaniment for many of the movement activities which were described. In most instances, the words for the rhymes, or the variations Barbara created, were included in the lessons; sometimes only the titles were cited. Hopefully, the melodies and words for less well-known selections can be accessed through other sources. In the 1950s, Barbara trained several students to teach her approach to a growing clientele of performing artists in New York. A second collection of lesson plans, the *Technique for Movement Lessons*, was prepared for their use. Bohn Stafleu Van Loghum, Houten, The Netherlands must be thanked for their generous permission to reproduce illustrations for these lessons from the 16th edition of the *Spalteholz-Spanner Handatlas der Anatomie des Menchen (Atlas of Human Anatomy)*. This book, first published in 1895, was a reference for teachers in Todd's Boston studio and used extensively by Clark in her own teaching. Many of the drawings which accompany her later writing were inspired by the illustrations in this classic work.

Barbara Clark's previously published and unpublished educational "manuals" have been organized and edited for Part III. Only one manuscript was discovered in Clark's papers for *The Children's Book*, which was probably written in the 1940s. Although unfinished, several lessons for this manual are presented largely as they were found. Clark saved many drafts of her subsequent published works as well the sketches and phrases which must have served as the raw material for their development. Perhaps she recognized her own inclination to retreat from some of her boldest ideas as she grappled with the finality of placing her work into published form. André Bernard and Joanne Emmons, her long-time students and colleagues, later explained this tendency grew out of Barbara's concern that she had gone beyond what "the public" could easily accept and understand. They both provided invaluable assistance in the process of identifying and editing material which was excluded from the published versions of *Let's Enjoy Sitting – Standing – Walking* (1963) and *How to Live in Your Axis – Your Vertical Line* (1968). As witness to the influence of Barbara's inner critic in the development of *Body Proportion Needs Depth – Front to Back*, I reinstated several lessons and drawings which were deleted from the version published in 1975.

At first, in the editorial process, I endeavored to carefully document each instance in which unpublished material was incorporated into the formerly published versions of the manuals. However, I quickly found the proliferation of notes, brackets and parentheses becoming a serious impediment to the readability of the lessons. With the advice and encouragement of her longstanding students and my growing confidence in my understanding of her ideas, I gradually became less concerned with scholarly accuracy and more committed to Barbara's charge to simply "redo all the manuals."

The Body is Round – Use All the Radii, a manual which Barbara named but did not complete, serves as a repository for other drawings and lessons she judged "too advanced," as well as material from her notebooks which supports those themes. The process of serving as editor (or perhaps ghost writer) for Barbara Clark's final manual was the most time consuming, difficult and yet, personally gratifying aspect of my work on this project. Sifting through her papers, I often found myself hopelessly intrigued by an image hastily sketched on the margin of a church circular or a line of body poetry jotted down on the back of a shopping list. Often these posthumous messages from my teacher would sustain me in kinesthetic exploration for a matter of weeks. Finally, after years incubation with these gems of imagery, passing many of them through the filter of my own teaching, I felt able to organize the material for Clark's final manual around the themes she revisited most frequently and developed to the fullest extent. In the process of drawing together the various threads of her conceptual tapestry, I became particularly grateful to the inventor of the personal computer. The capacity to sort the material in a variety of ways, recalling linkages through the identification of key words and phrases, truly saved me from being overwhelmed by the scope and complexity of Barbara Clark's prolific genius. Although liberties were taken with this writing in order to smooth transitions between concepts, clarify directions or improve sentence structure, critically important facets of Clark's style and values in instructional writing have been carefully preserved.

In reviewing the manuals readers should be aware of Clark's deliberate use of repetition as a means of instruction. Rather than describing all she knew about the alignment of a certain area of the body in one lesson or chapter, Barbara preferred to develop kinesthetic understanding of its balance in smaller increments over time. Thus, she repeated various anatomical concepts several times throughout the manuals, offering new more sophisticated insights into old material as her readers progressed. Because the repetition of some concepts becomes more obvious when considering the manuals as a group of works, it must be noted that Barbara never planned for her pamphlets to be read at one sitting or published together as a book. By developing her manuals over several years and printing them separately, she planned to focus on discrete aspects of awareness, moving from one theme to the next as her readers were "ready" for more material. The choice to combine Barbara Clark's writings with her biography and other elements of her work, was made to facilitate a more complete appreciation of the development of her unique point of view. Teachers interested in using the manuals separately as Barbara intended, should contact the publisher regarding availability for classroom use.

Clark's commitment to draw students into an interactive process of learning through her manuals was also respected in the editing of the material. Although she appreciated the importance of scholarly efforts to gain scientific acceptance for Todd's work, she was philosophically opposed to the objectification of the material in teaching or educational writing. Instead, in order to appeal directly to the student's imaginative capacity to transform the body, Barbara's goal was to personalize and subjectify. The light, sometimes child-like quality this gives to her writing may distract some readers expecting something more serious. Students engaged in the fun of learning through her lessons may be startled by the gravity of their effect.

Throughout this project, the task of making editorial improvements to Clark's writing was also tempered by a commitment to retain the charm of her personality and the flavor of her times. When points of clarification were absolutely necessary to shed contemporary light upon dated concepts or terms, they have been inserted within brackets [ ]. In view of the historical context, readers should understand Clark's exclusive use of masculine pronouns was typical of the conventions of her era. With the masculine gender firmly established in Barbara's works and quotations, my own use of "he or she," "she/he," or "s/he" in the biographical section seemed awkward and incongruous. With apologies to those with feminist linguistic sensitivities, I am confident that analysis of the content of Clark's work will reveal a larger more egalitarian perspective which was, and perhaps still is, well ahead of its time.

Without the guidance and support of Barbara Clark's former students, André Bernard and Joanne Emmons, I would have been unable to complete this project. The memories and perspectives of John Hawkes, Anthony Mannino, and Nancy Udow were also very helpful. The teachers and mentors from my student days, Margaret Erlanger, Laura Huelster, Marsha Paludan and Joan Skinner, must be recognized for courageously standing up for this point of view long before education had realized its value. I would also like to extend appreciation to Beth Lessard and my colleagues in the Department of Dance at Arizona State University for their acceptance of my teaching and their support of the unusual nature of my research. Megan Morris of the Arizona State University Institute for Studies in the Arts must be thanked for her editorial endurance and the organizational improvements she suggested for the work. Rosemary Walsh of Walsh and Associates should be acknowledged for her work in typesetting and her many helpful insights into the self-publishing process. Jeanne Smith should also be thanked for her creative work on the cover design. Bill Packard lent his special expertise to the restoration of the photographs. The staff of the Arizona State University Microcomputer Resource Facility supported my work on the illustrations. Several special students, Joanna Cashman, Kelly Corder, Barbara Gilson and Katherine Longstreth, assisted me with facets of my research and writing. Their energetic efforts, and the encouragement of all of my students, often bolstered my enthusiasm when the joy of writing was inevitably overtaken by the drudgery of getting the project out. Finally, I must lovingly acknowledge the assistance of my husband, whose steadfast support of my interest in this work has made everything possible.

Part I

Do
Thou
Thy
Work

INTRODUCTION

I MET BARBARA CLARK IN 1971 when I was graduate student in dance at the University of Illinois. My undergraduate study with Joan Skinner really paved the way to finding Barbara. Skinner's *Release Technique* exposed me to the power of the imagination as an avenue for learning. Visualization became the means I relied on for my personal exploration of kinesthesia and my creative arousal in dance.

Because Miss Skinner often referred to Mabel Elsworth Todd as one of the early thinkers who gave credibility to our point of view, I found a copy of *The Thinking Body* and attempted to understand Todd's ideas. I remember being intrigued by the juxtaposition of anatomical facts and principles of engineering with simple suggestions for mental picturing. I was amazed that Todd had set forth such a vital and contemporary philosophy of movement so many years ago. Realizing the study of mind/body integration would continue to be the focus of my graduate studies in dance, I became interested in attending a conference on the subject sponsored by the Menninger Foundation. When I learned that Barbara Clark, an 82-year-old teacher of Todd's principles, would be speaking and teaching there, I jumped at the chance to learn more first-hand.[1]

Several like-minded graduate students made the trip to Kansas. When we arrived, Barbara was in the middle of our hosts' living room floor, sitting like a child on her heels. She greeted us with a broad, open grin and immediately urged us to join her for our first "body alignment" lesson. After removing our shoes and "balancing our heads between our sitting bones" for a moment, we began to imitate her massage of the feet. She said this "kneading" of the bottoms of the feet was the best way to recover from the strains of our day of travel—making the soles of the feet "softer, more like the palms of the hands." Barbara went on to explain the importance of relating the heels of the feet to the "heels of the pelvis," and the "heels of the vertebrae." I did not completely understand these concepts, nor did my companions, but we were carried along by Barbara's enthusiasm, her interest in her subject and in us. Gradually, the imagery eased us into a state of enhanced kinesthesia. We rested, centered, and absorbed the feeling of buoyancy Barbara's body so clearly expressed.

Throughout the course of our visit, Barbara dominated conversation with reminiscences of her fifty-year involvement with "the work."[2] As a nurse, her early career had been devoted to applying Todd's ideas to the motor development of infants. Later, she became involved with teaching young children in Boston's nursery schools. For the last twenty years, she lived in New York City where she studied drawing and taught many prominent actors and dancers. Now, since organizing her ideas into educational "manuals," she was free to travel and perhaps begin a biography of Miss Todd.

Imbedded in her stories were subtle indications that Barbara might also be looking for a new home. There were hardships in living alone in New York City on a modest Social Security pension; I sensed a yearning for a slower, more natural life. I urged Barbara to move to Illinois, where life was certainly much simpler and many young dance students could help with her writing and research.

Barbara arrived several weeks later with a leather suitcase and three cardboard boxes, the sum total of all of her worldly possessions. She had given almost everything else away. This was easy for Barbara; she relieved herself of things with impunity. To give "the old" away was part of starting something new, which gave her great pleasure. As she settled into a small apartment near the university, she assured me that it was the best possible place for her. She loved being around the students and laughed to herself as she told me that even at her age, she felt herself to be one of them.

Barbara's rather unconventional lifestyle fit right into the university environment. Her simple, stylish wardrobe of skirts, blouses and dresses was remade from fashions friends handed down. She loved the process of hand-tailoring these clothes to fit or adding a scarf for a splash of color; it was economical and it was fun. When it came to the selection of footwear however, expense could not be spared. Her sensible Dr. Scholl's Roundabouts were precisely sized to her foot dimensions and special-ordered from her "shoe man" in New York. Her thick, brown cotton stockings were only available through the Sears catalog, along with the "union suits" she wore in the winter. She donned gloves and a beret for formal occasions, but ignored the tradition of using a handbag whenever she could. Barbara said men had an advantage in this regard; filling pockets with the essential keys, change and checkbook distributed the load evenly around the body and allowed the arms to swing free.

Barbara furnished her rooms rather sparsely to leave plenty of space for movement practice. Her guests were accommodated with light-weight aluminum garden chairs which could be folded when not in use. Paperwork was accomplished on card tables that she moved from place to place, depending on the position of the natural light. Barbara slept on an unfinished wooden platform padded with spare blankets and sheets. A similarly styled bench in one corner was her favorite spot for sewing, eating or reading her mail. Thus, Barbara's apartment became a movement studio and office, unencumbered by the clutter of the usual household accoutrements. Her sense of "home" was cultivated in the view from her window and the many memories evoked by her gaze.

When Barbara was settled, we began to go through her boxes, searching out drawings and lesson ideas for her next body alignment "manual." Much of the material was carefully organized in spiral notebooks and diaries; but some of what she called her "best imagery" was found on the backs of envelopes and church bulletins, or in the margins of letters long ago received. Somehow all this material had to be sorted, typed, redrawn and organized into a format which would be similar to her earlier works.

My friends and fellow dance majors, John Rolland and Nancy Udow offered to help with this process and the three of us performed various tasks for Barbara in exchange for our weekly lessons. Barbara welcomed our novice interest in the content of the work as if we would soon be teaching it. In her thinking, all of the dancers who would visit, and their friends and family members were potential teachers, too. She used the phrase "each one—teach one," to urge us to take charge of the work and pass it on.

Over the next six years, as I gathered my own groups of children and dancers to teach, Barbara's tutelage evolved into a dialogue. Our time together passed very quickly, without pause for reflection or synthesis. There was certainly no way of predicting how important her friendship would become to me, both personally and professionally. I simply immersed myself in Barbara's wisdom and resilient dignity, and vowed to continue her unique approach to kinesthetic education.

The Early Years

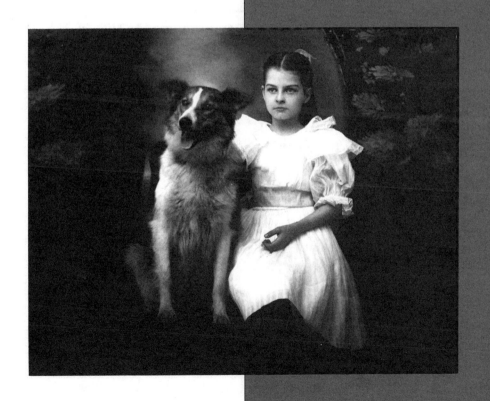

A LETTER WRITTEN ON THE EVENT OF Barbara Clark's birth in 1889, by her father, included this verse:

> Do thou thy work
> It shall succeed
> In thine or in another's day
> And if thou fail the victor's mead
> Thou shalt receive the toiler's pay.

Barbara often said this poem was strangely appropriate to the events of her life.

> I was born in Vermont, of parents whose forebearers had lived there since the early beginnings of the state. Independence was woven into the warp of my being. My father was Marion Wright Clark, a prominent dairy farmer, and my mother was Mary Elisa Tracy. We lived with my grandmother, and my aunts and uncles were always coming and going. I don't think of myself as 'I' or 'me'. I am a product of those people. They put themselves into me. They loved me, taught me, showed me how to do things on my own.

When Barbara spoke of her childhood, she referred to herself as "the weakest of seven children." From this vantage point, it seems likely that some of the frailty she remembered was the result of a slight neurological impairment. Initially, Barbara's family worried because she was slow to develop. As an infant, she "hopped like a bunny" rather than moving through the usual stages of rolling and crawling. The Clarks agonized over Barbara's habit of sucking her own tongue which continued, despite all of their efforts, until the age of eight. Barbara also remembered being hypersensitive to touch as a child. The feeling of a cat rubbing against her legs, an experience which most children find quite pleasurable, was intolerable for her. The rough and tumble play enjoyed so freely by her siblings frightened and bewildered Barbara. Knowing, even at four years of age, that she was somehow different from her brothers and sisters, Barbara asked her mother, "'What makes Philena [a sister] wiggle so much?' Mother's smile as she looked at me seemed to say, 'I wish you wiggled more.' "

At five years of age, Barbara contracted rheumatic fever. Her joints were so swollen and painful that she was unable to walk for several weeks. At the age of eight, another illness occurred which tightened the muscles on the right side of her body in a temporary paralysis. This episode, which doctors later concluded was a mild case of polio, rendered her right leg somewhat shorter than the left. Although she regained normal function in most ways, the tendency to pronate and a painful hammer toe persisted as troublesome reminders of the affliction. Her coordination was also affected and it was apparent to the family that the illness had diminished her self-confidence. Even the simple task of standing on one leg to put on a pair of pants was physically challenging. Keeping up with her brothers and sisters as they worked on the farm was almost impossible. Her occasional efforts to join the pace of their raucous play must have been very awkward. Sensing Barbara's self-consciousness, the children teased and humiliated her.

Barbara turned to the adults of the family for acceptance and understanding and they searched for ways of helping her adapt and improve. Her grandmother was especially concerned.

> I slept with my grandmother and she would straighten me out in bed at night, as she was evidently not satisfied with my position. She was very relaxed, a deep breather, and I was very tense.

Barbara's mother also became "interested in teaching me how to conserve my strength, to not attempt too much, to keep my aspirations within my performance level." Her father however, "gave me the opposite slant—to fix my sights as high as I could reach and then get there some way." Other relatives offered commentary, as relatives will do, which sometimes discouraged Barbara, but also challenged her to improve. "I can remember Aunt Flora saying, 'That child will never be able to do anything but wash and wipe silver.'"

Barbara enjoyed the companionship of her elders: making social calls with her mother and grandmother, taking trips to town with her father to conduct the business of the family farm. As she grew older, her parents relied on Barbara to manage the activities of the younger children. Taking on the role of the "most grown-up" of the youngsters, Barbara mimicked mature behavior and began to espouse the traditional New England values which would sustain her for the rest of her life.

> My parents were extremely practical, and they also had lofty ideals which they reached inch by inch. They were not impressed by money or the accent on get-rich-quick success. There was a lot of teamwork in the family, making beds, clearing the table and doing dishes, wiping them and putting them in cupboards. My family were like what was usual in Vermont, they only spoke when there was something valuable to say and there were long silences. They liked to use the quotable sayings from the old English and Ben Franklin like, 'better to be ready and not go than to go and not be ready,' or 'a stitch in time saves nine.' They were people with common sense.

Barbara's special interest in the accounts of the farm kept by her father, led to her official appointment as his secretary. She took pride in this position, enjoying the envy of her brothers who must have also desired responsibility in matters of importance on the farm. Barbara loved working closely with her father and like him, she became quite serious and a great reader.

> I read all that came into the house. I played with the imagery. I was always identifying myself with a character in a book I was reading. The

Dutch boy with his hand in the dike made a terrific image for me. Prevention while the matter is small.

Barbara's favorite aunt, a painter, nurtured her artistic bent. Barbara loved to visit Aunt Sadie's studio, but her own attempts to draw or paint often ended in considerable frustration.

> I was held up as a child in expressing myself in drawing. My designs were stiff and rigid and the pictures were tiny. My coordination was not too good and my back tired easily.

When she was not visiting relatives and neighbors, or occupied with her many responsibilities, Barbara continued to play in movement. When she was inevitably alone, or when the others were not aware of it, Barbara experimented with the coordination she did have, endeavoring to understand her body and extend its range. The physicality of the other children and the rhythms of the natural world around her provided imagery of the pleasure and ease which was possible in movement. The monotonous chores of the household supplied the means for practice and a way to improve.

> In the first place I was interested in movement. I loved to watch clouds floating along over head—animal movement of which I saw much since I grew up on a dairy farm—the flight of birds which intrigued me greatly— the running of water in brooks from the overflow of the springs high on the hills to the mouth of the river. Movement is like a well spring. It moves through you, it moves out of you and into you. The boggy ground as frost comes out of it in the spring—as the sun melts the ice, the water is restored to the soil and it becomes springy. You can feel its springiness as you plié. It lets you down and springs you up. It is one of nature's trampolines. One finds these areas in the grassy places too, as well as in the roadways. The clay soil is the foundation under each. Where the soil is more sandy, the bogginess is not as evident. I used to go around in different places to test the springiness and that nearest like the trampoline was the most gratifying in its response to the pressure of my body.

> I can still remember the awareness of feeling those mattress shavings. They curled somewhat and this lent a springiness to the foundation they gave to the mattress. I did not talk about these thoughts. They just seeped through my mind for a moment or moments at a time. The person making the other side of the bed was desirous of getting on to her next job of the morning.

Barbara's mother was also quite sensitive to touch and kinesthesia. Their times together in gentle play were calming and centering for Barbara.

> Mother used body movement in relaxation or centering—she did not realize that what she was doing then, I would be active about now. It is the awareness of touching a part of the body with the fingers or combining the

hands by putting one fist in the hollow of the other hand interchangeably. She did not do the wrong things or what I now term wrong, such as putting the hands on the hips, called the washerwoman's stance in that day. She made much of pat-a-cake with the children. And she never seemed to be effected by monotony. I think her rhythm was so natural that all of this was enjoyment to her. She frequently would start to skip, but for only a few steps as though she recalled something that she should be doing and quickly sacrificed enjoyment for duty.

Barbara often recalled these memories of "the natural" in her family and farming life when she worked with her students many years later. Disturbed by our preoccupation with progress and achievement, she encouraged us to develop a larger awareness of our bodies as part of the natural world. For her, the work was much more than a movement technique; it was a philosophy for living. When one of us would ask too many questions or demonstrate impatience with our limited understanding, Barbara would remind us:

> We would hurry the process, but patience seems to be a part of the process, as is the breath. Picking the lettuce, pulling the radishes and carrots. Waiting and watching for the corn, the melons and tomatoes to ripen. Planting and transplanting the seeds and small plants. Starting them in the house, watching the roots develop, made me realize later on in life how the human body muscles do something similar for the body in making the balance firm. How slow growth seems when it is being closely observed. The Eternal seems to prefer this inching growth in all areas.

In her teenage years, Barbara began to excel in school. Doing well academically became a way to assert herself among the older children in the family.

> I loved a heavy school assignment. I can remember one instance of how I could really breathe as a reaction to the feeling of challenge it gave me.

Barbara's elder brother took particular notice of her academic talent and a jovial sense of competition evolved into a closeness that Barbara had not known before. Her success in school and the friendship of her brother inspired Barbara to take more risks, as if her new confidence demanded physical expression. She found it in the thrill of driving a horse-drawn buggy to school and around the family farm.

> Driving horses was the joy of my life, although Aunt Flora would warn, 'You know you shouldn't be doing this.' The power and speed of the animals drawing the wagon gave me a sense of power. Not having it in my own body, driving horses let me feel it through the reins.

Unfortunately, a serious back injury was the consequence of Barbara's equestrian adventures. Upon his examination the doctor proclaimed to the family, "Barbara has no development of her lower back muscles." He advised osteopathy and although the treatments provided some relief, cycles of pain recurred with increasing frequency.

> I was never right to begin with and everything I did made me worse. When Dr. Maynard said to me at sixteen, 'Barbara whatever you do, don't be a neurotic,' I had no idea of what he was speaking. How to avoid being a neurotic was something totally out of my power of understanding. Gradually, I grew to realize that it had something to do with self-discipline, but that just made me feel guilty and resulted in greater tension.

At the age of nineteen, with a new determination to "be more normal," Barbara applied for admission to the Physical Education program at Oberlin College. Naively, she assumed such a department would be the place to become "physically educated"—to learn to understand and overcome her physical limitations. However, the athletic faculty were rather impatient with her efforts in their classes. They urged Barbara to find another course of study and advised that her interest in exercise should be limited to a daily walk. She tried other college course work but realized, "using my mind tensed my body. I could only do a little at a time and so I had to drop out of college work."

There was a change in Barbara when she returned home from Oberlin that worried the family. She refused to see old chums she had known in high school, particularly if they were men. She was detached and disapproving of her younger brothers and sisters as they occupied themselves in the spirited fun of school dances and parties. Spending long periods alone in her room, she insisted that she was quite busy with "more serious pursuits such as reading and church work." Cloaked in a mantle of maturity far beyond her years, Barbara "shrank, fearing critical analysis and humiliation, taking everything too seriously."

Concerned over the situation, Barbara's father arranged a tour of Europe for her. In celebration of her twenty-first birthday, Barbara and her Aunt Sadie were to spend five months together touring museums and churches in Germany, Switzerland, Belgium, England and Ireland. Planning the trip rejuvenated Barbara's interest in life and learning, particularly about art. Her adventuresome spirit returned as she prepared to be the first of her siblings to undertake such a journey. But, when they arrived in 1910, they found Europe preparing for war. Barbara and her aunt felt the apprehension of the people wherever they went. They were frightened by soldiers who inspected their baggage when they boarded trains, and officials who scrutinized their travel plans at the borders. Although many of their experiences in the museums and churches were inspiring and remarkable, Barbara and her aunt decided to return home much earlier than they had planned.

Almost immediately, Barbara became very ill. The family doctor suspected a festering appendix and advised an operation. The appendix was removed along with an ovarian cyst. The surgeon remarked to the family that Barbara's was the "worst case of abdominal ptosis I have ever seen," redoubling their concern over her poor state of health. With the order of extended rest, Barbara was confined to her bed for several weeks to recover from the operation. As the family went about their work on the farm, Barbara was again alone with her thoughts of the impending war and preoccupation with her physical difficulties. As spring approached, she became completely despondent, the victim of what doctors then called "a nervous breakdown."

No one except her mother was allowed to see Barbara the summer of the breakdown. She was kept away from the others, living outside the house in a large tent. Such isolation could only have been the result of the prevalent misunderstanding of mental illness during that period and the fear of association with it. Later, Barbara still hesitated to discuss this period of her life saying only, "that was when I hit rock bottom."

Some traveling evangelistic preachers helped Barbara pull out of her depression. In ministering to what they said were "ills of the spirit," they encouraged her away from her dependence on family, toward a life of devotion to the church. Over the next few years, although she continued to live on the farm, Barbara became almost fanatically involved in church work and found a measure of self-reliance and happiness there. Through her church school teaching, Barbara discovered an outlet for her interest in art and genuine appreciation for her special talent in working with children. Engrossed in the development of the youngsters at the school, she grew stronger in a life of teaching and service to others.

At the age of twenty-nine, Barbara announced to the family, "the balance between the physical and mental is what I need." In February of 1919, she left the family farm and enrolled in a two-year nurse's training program at Faulkner Hospital in Cambridge, Massachusetts. She was completely determined to make a success of it.

> I had the desire for independence, to be of use, to be part of the group, and the ambition to accomplish. But before Miss Todd, I was always affected by mechanical factors which caused emotional strain. The doctors said my philosophy of life was good. It got me on my feet when ill and kept me going until mechanical factors would block me again.

At Faulkner, there were new physical challenges for Barbara. Student nurses were charged with cleaning and maintaining the hospital. This sort of activity felt quite familiar, much like the work on the farm. However, the amount of work the student nurses were expected to complete each day aggravated Barbara's back problem.

> Dr. Perrin T. Wilson was an osteopath whom my aunt and uncle employed when he first started working in Cambridge during the First World War. As I entered the hospital for training, they referred me to him. It was through his treatments that I was able to stand up under the nurse's training of that day—the long hours, making beds, turning mattresses as well as patients, heavy trays to carry, stairs to climb, operating room floors to mop.

As the training progressed, Barbara became very interested in her course work in science, although she recoiled at first from the study of human anatomy. During lectures in which human cadavers were used for demonstration, Barbara would position herself in the top row of the lecture hall or behind a column to obstruct the view. Although she was curious about the workings of the human body, the appearance and smell of the cadavers repulsed her. As she explained, "I couldn't watch the anatomy lectures. They were such poor imagery."

Barbara also enjoyed the practical courses at the school and the insight into touch and kinesthesia the more experienced nurses provided. From them she absorbed elements of the art of nursing: how pillows could be positioned to comfort the body and simple techniques of relaxing massage. Barbara tried to internalize this knowledge as she coped with the long hours of work in the hospital. However, even with these new insights and the help of osteopathy, periods of illness and physical exhaustion interrupted Barbara's progress through the training program.

The physical toll involved in caring for adults eventually convinced Barbara it would be best to specialize in nursing children, toddlers and infants. Concerned over her physical limitations, the hospital staff agreed and encouraged her to continue training in this direction. Finally, after nearly four years of tenacious effort, Barbara Clark graduated as a Registered Nurse from Faulkner Hospital Training School. It was a personal triumph and a source of tremendous pride for the rest of her life.

In 1923, toward the end of her nurse's training, Barbara found Mabel Elsworth Todd. Todd had been working in Boston for some years with a form of therapeutic physical re-education called, "Natural Posture." In the early 1920s, Todd's work was receiving attention and approval from several spheres. Many prominent Boston orthopedists and osteopaths knew of her approach and were sending their patients to Todd's studio. Professional athletes, dancers, actors and musicians were among them, as well as several wealthy society matrons suffering from the strain of supporting the war effort. The enthusiasm of the latter group brought Todd into vogue in Boston's social circles and thus to the attention of Barbara's Aunt Sadie. By the time Barbara learned of the approach, there was so much interest that several of Todd's more experienced students had been enlisted as assistant teachers.

In the course of her first few lessons, Barbara learned that Miss Todd had developed her work from several sources. First, her interest in the sciences had developed early and energetically. As a teenager in an exclusive girl's school, Todd was so eager to learn about the physical and biological sciences, that a special teacher was hired for her private instruction. Then, just before her graduation, Mabel sustained a back injury resulting from a fall. The doctors were unclear about the exact nature of the injury but were quite pessimistic when Todd initially was unable to walk. With little help from anyone but her mother, Todd taught herself to move again, using concepts learned from biology and physics to guide the development of her own rehabilitation.

The Early Years   15

In 1906, Todd enrolled in the Emerson College of Oratory with the intention of becoming a teacher of voice. Through her study there, Todd began to think that problems with the vocal apparatus, in singing and public speaking, might be the result of poor habits of posture and general coordination. As she prepared herself to teach, she became interested in the problems of the worst students and how their skeletal alignment and basic movement patterning might be improved.

Todd became convinced that a new concept of posture was needed, not only for those practicing oratory but for the public at large. As she familiarized herself with the research in the field, she learned to apply the principles of mechanics to the analysis of posture and movement. However, she was unique in concluding that this information meant that the condition of mechanical balance of the skeletal structure, "implies freedom from strains, absence from stress, a readiness for action, a mobility —the opposite of fixity." [3] Her emphasis on finding **balance** rather than "imposing upon our bodies a fixed position of any part, which we feel to be the 'right', 'correct', or 'ideal' one," [4] was unusual and separated Todd's from other concepts of posture.

The accepted view was influenced more by notions of morality than by body mechanics. The Victorian notion of maintaining rigid verticality as a sign of uprightness of spirit was still prevalent. Physical education further reinforced this concept of posture during exercise classes which were conducted much like military drills. The liberal thinking of the twenties did generate a more fashionable body image which proclaimed freedom from the Victorian physical concept. However, it was really only its opposite—an equally self-conscious positioning into a coy and slightly sexy slouch. In this climate, Todd argued for a vastly different postural premise in which, as she described for Barbara, "you don't hold anything, everything is in flux."

In discovering a finely tuned balance of the structure, one would also be returning to what Todd considered to be a more natural use of the body. It was this aspect of Todd's approach which initially attracted Barbara. Todd confirmed that nature provided excellent imagery for movement. Further, she insisted, it was critical to maintain awareness of natural rhythms, as the faster pace of industrialized life in the twenties threatened to confuse the kinesthetic sense. About this Barbara wrote:

> Mabel Elsworth Todd helped to develop and keep alive the idea that the human body is a vertebrate and needs to follow through on it's inheritance. The individual was not being given the education necessary in making the change from the horse-and-buggy era to the more mechanical one. Education for more scientifically designed equipment zoomed ahead but it did not catch on too readily to what effect unnatural movement or the lack of movement might have upon the human structure. For instance, you could go farther and do more in a shorter period of time. It became more fun to ride than to walk. Breathing became shorter and more rapid. The diaphragm and heart began to get lazy as the legs went on strike. Vision had to jump fast to observe what was passing before it instead of moving more slowly from one object to another.

Along with her unique ideas about the attributes of good posture, Todd challenged the accepted notions of how to change posture. Todd believed improvement could be made, "by thinking continuously of a familiar motivating picture," [5] or visualizing images.

> Concentrating upon a picture involving movement results in such responses in the neuro-musculature as are necessary to carry out specific movements with the least effort. In playing a part, the actor first forms a picture in his own mind of the character he is to depict and creates the impressions he wishes to give of that character largely through his bodily attitudes reacting automatically to the mental picture through the central reflexes. . . . In postural education we can take advantage of this fact. This psycho-physiological process operates unerringly in forming better postural patterns in response to a concept of good anatomical adjustment based on clearly-defined mechanical principles. [6]

Todd's process of postural education took place through a procedure she called the "table work." In a typical lesson, the "pupil" dressed in a loose-fitting kimono. The skeleton or pictures from an anatomy book were shown to illustrate how an aspect of skeletal balance could be related to a law of mechanics. The pupil was taught to locate the area being discussed in his own body or helped to understand the principle through practice of an appropriate exercise. An image would then be suggested as a simple metaphor for the ideas which had been explored. Finally, the pupil reclined on the table and was guided by the teacher's touch to concentrate more precisely upon the location of the image and its action.

> Miss Todd placed students precisely in the rest position, to lengthen the little toe and get the thigh muscles to fall up the front—although she didn't tell you the reasons behind the positioning. Miss Todd's hands were so well centered, they did exactly as she wanted them to, in giving exact sensations of pressure and direction to the student. At the same time she gave directions describing an image for the student to think about or practice. This allowed both treating and teaching. It gave the students a sense of cooperating in the procedure and helped them to become independent. There were areas of concentration for each lesson but ultimately the whole body was affected.

As the lesson concluded, the results were discussed or considered before a mirror. Sometimes photographs were taken of the student in various positions, which the teachers later analyzed. Finally, imagery was suggested for practice in rest or in simple movement, as a way of maintaining the new awareness of better balance in daily life.

Barbara did not know exactly how Todd's table work had developed. She did say that some doctors and nurses in Boston medical circles belittled it as "glorified osteopathy." Because Todd knew and worked with many osteopaths, it seems logical that some aspects of her approach could have been influenced by that therapeutic tradition. However, the use of the teacher's touch in the table work was always considered supplementary to the student's own involvement with the mental image. Thus, the students at Todd's studio had "lessons" rather than treatments, and teachers who tended to be heavy handed in promoting the progress of their pupils were dismissed. In discussing the table work with Barbara, Miss Todd explained, "This work is not manipulation. The purpose of the finger touch is to bring consciousness to the pupil, to make him respond and become active in readjusting the structure."

To work correctly with the visualization process was a challenge for many of the students. Guided by the teacher's touch, the pupil was simply to concentrate upon the image, without voluntarily directing the musculature toward any preconceived realization of the goal the image described. Relaxing on the table during the sessions encouraged the student's physical detachment from the process. However, there was a discipline to be mastered in learning to allow, rather than force, a neuromuscular response. Barbara related how Todd often used a statement made by a child during one of his lessons to help others understand the nature of the process: "Now I understand. First you think it, then you see it, then you forget it, and then it happens."

It was probably difficult for some of Todd's students to accept her view that a process of picturing images would be sufficient to produce an observable improvement in posture and movement. Those that did found that taking charge of the disciplined direction of the imagination and the growth of kinesthetic awareness was not easy. This may have been why the number of lessons taken by students varied widely. Some remained for only for a brief period, while others worked with Todd indefinitely and whenever they could. Irrespective of the extent of their mastery of her approach, almost everyone who was touched by Miss Todd was drawn to her as an appealing, if not charismatic figure.

> When anyone said 'Miss Todd' the inflection in his voice stayed high. It brought an image to mind of great pleasure such as having a lesson or hearing her talk about one. Her touch, her voice, her glance all carried a feeling of particular concern. Her body was buoyant and she was light on her feet, about average in height and a few pounds overweight. Miss Todd was a handsome woman with color in her cheeks, laughing blue eyes and brown hair that was beautifully dyed for several years. She was a grand exponent of her principles; not perfect, but in command of more of them than any other teacher. She had the build of an athlete, without the corners. It gave her the appearance of great supple strength that simply oozed over you. Her touch was light, yet penetrating. There was a firmness and balance with gentle fingers centered through her back. Her strength went into you. Not one of the teachers had the personality that Miss Todd did. Her personality was so electrifying that it struck sparks in many people. They became enthused about her and the ideas that she put forth. Once in a while when she was tired she would stay with an idea too long. But most people excused her I thought, the same as I, because they were so fond of her.

Miss Todd's ideas brought glamour and enthusiasm to perplexed and discouraged minds, to weary and aching bodies. She put hope in their souls that there was a way of thinking and feeling on their own that could take the place of their uncertain attitude toward their condition.

Mabel Todd certainly inspired such hopefulness in Barbara. Despite her optimism, however, Barbara's first few lessons were rather discouraging. She described one of her early lesson experiences:

With me, Todd concentrated on the table work—my body was so bad she probably thought the educational work would not penetrate. I couldn't comprehend what she wanted when I was standing. My body was so tense and out of line in so many respects that I felt very conscious when I first tried to do what she asked.

Initially, Barbara was reluctant to discuss her problems with Todd or any of the teachers.

I had to avoid discussions relating to my body. It made me more tense and uncomfortable. The nervous breakdown had taught me to stay away from conscious thinking about myself—it tired me. Thinking of something outside myself relaxed me and I enjoyed it. That was why I had to drop out of college work—using my mind tensed my body. With Todd, I could only do a little at a time.

Miss Todd and the other teachers were also concerned about Barbara's slow rate of progress. In a monthly meeting of the teachers, Barbara overheard their discussion.

The teachers, Miss Todd, Miss Galbraith, Miss Colwell and Mrs. Lawson, were in consultation about the pupils one day and my name came up. They were speaking about how bad a body I had. After a bit one of them said, 'Well, we don't need to take the time thinking about her. She is so in need of help and it will take so long to get results that she won't have the courage, patience or money to stay with us.' Miss Colwell said that I should be given the chance and was particularly helpful for many years.

Barbara's interest would not be daunted. Supporting herself with her work in nursing and some secretarial work in Todd's studio, Barbara began to devote as much time as possible to her lessons with Miss Todd and the other teachers.

In the mid 1920s, Todd left Boston to begin work on a Bachelor of Science degree in Physical Education at Columbia University. Dr. Jesse Feiring Williams, head of the Physical Education curriculum at the time, became interested in Todd's approach and paved the way for her to begin teaching at the institution while she pursued her degree. Williams, inspired by the leadership of John Dewey at Teachers College, was involved in the progressive ideas which were developing in education at that time. In Todd's work, he saw an approach which bridged the gap between mind and body and supported his notion of a new physical education. In his classic work, *The Principles of Physical Education*, he wrote:

> Physical education must study the human motor mechanism with reference to body control, strains and expenditure of energy. It is a mistake to regard parts of the body as isolated and unrelated mechanisms. Integration of the entire mechanism as a mechanical instrument is just as important for success in the correction of defect or education in use, as integration with reference to physical, mental and social aspects of life. [7]

Todd began to teach formal course work in Columbia's Department of Physical Education in 1928. The catalog description of her course, *Basic Principles of Posture*, read:

> This course presents for practical application in teaching, the fundamentals of bodily dynamics with particular reference to the thinking processes involved in kinesthetic development. The following will be considered: (a) methods of discovering, analyzing and cultivating bodily attitudes of mechanical advantage and free somatic and visceral functioning; (b) psychological aspects of posture education with attention to methods of facilitating visualization as a motivating factor in muscular coordination. [8]

The university work exposed Todd to a wide variety of students, with academic as well as personal interest in the field. [9] Todd's classes were popular and her ideas about imagery were quite controversial. Eventually, a series of debates took place at Columbia between John Dewey, a devoté of the Alexander Technique, and James Harvey Robinson, a prominent professor of history, who studied with Todd. Most of the discussion focused on Todd's use of visualization as a corrective method. As Barbara wrote:

> It was extremely important that attention be called to the fact that natural body movement is under the guidance of the unconscious. Physical education was over-directing movement in too conscious a way. But in those days the idea of working with mental imagery was very new and not very well accepted. In that age most people felt that imagery was esoteric, if not pure craziness.

As her professional activities expanded in New York City, Todd opened a second private studio there. Although she occasionally returned to Boston to teach private pupils and advise her assistants, it was clear to Barbara that Todd's approach to the work and perhaps her values were changing. Some of the teachers who had been with Todd from the beginning, feared that she was growing away from her original dedication and idealism.

> Miss Todd got more interested in the science of the work, than in teaching individuals how to use their minds in it. You felt the accent was on the lesson from the teacher rather than on what one had to do for oneself.

In Todd's absence, the work in Boston became less monolithic and the other teachers began to develop reputations of their own.

> I was always amazed at the wide range of backgrounds that the teachers came from. They were teachers of other subjects in colleges and schools and there were a few graduate nurses. They had learned of Miss Todd through friends and practically all of them had serious health difficulties that her approach relieved and gradually improved. This gave them sufficient time to really know and understand her principles. Then, they wanted to share their experiences with others, and so they became teachers. Naturally, this brought in the less fitted for the teaching as well as the best. Not all who taught stayed on long as teachers of body movement and alignment. The ones who did were well enough organized in themselves to carry out good business practices. Those who left went into more lucrative work, which appealed to them now that they had better health.

All the teachers in the Boston studio continued the principles and goals that Todd had established as necessities in the postural reeducation of any student. Certainly, they all promoted Todd's unique focus upon the use of visualization as the means for correcting poor neuromuscular habits. However, several variations of her method became evident as unique expressions of the values and personalities of each individual. Barbara described one of the teachers who, "slanted her work toward the joints, centering the student's body with both hands, adjusting and freeing the muscle patterns." Notes from her work with another teacher describe lessons which seem to have been primarily devoted to exercises, with titles indicative of an interest in animal movement such as, "the bear walk," "the robin hop," "the chicken" and "the kangaroo." Although Barbara felt that she benefited from all of the teachers at the Boston studio, Miss Galbraith and Miss Colwell were the two women she mentioned most frequently.

> Beatrice P. Galbraith R.N. was a grad of Massachusetts General. She was in her seventies through the years that I knew her. Miss Galbraith was very devoted to Miss Todd and a very good example of Todd's principles. Her figure was like a young woman's. Her rib cage was very relaxed and easy and she used the pelvic muscles extremely well. Her shoulder action was beautiful for a woman of her age and her spine was beautifully aligned. She could walk very easily like a bear as she demonstrated it for me. It involves stepping the feet almost into the hands as one walks on all fours. Miss Galbraith was an exceptional example of what the alignment could do. She was an inspiration to younger teachers, very patient and eager to help them.

> Elizabeth W. Colwell M.A. was a teacher of French at Radcliffe. She too, had been ill and did not have robust physique. But she built amazing endurance during the years of her teaching. Her posture remained excellent in spite of the fact that working in therapy over a pupil was very fatiguing. As Miss Whitman (a secretary), who knocked at teacher's door ten minutes before the lesson was to be over remarked, 'When she comes

to the door in response to a knock, you would never think she was doing a thing. She was so nonchalant about it.'

> Miss Colwell was better at the organization of material for student grasp and assimilation. Miss Galbraith's body was so far in advance that it was hard for her to remember the first steps. She had too much massage technique. So she resorted to that to help my body, rather than being creative in direction I needed. Miss Colwell was very helpful for several years. She taught in 'crumbs of knowledge,' which is an excellent way for establishing new patterns and replacing old ones gradually. I had to think it out for myself.

Barbara kept notes from her lessons with Miss Todd, Miss Colwell and Miss Galbraith at the Boston studio (see *Appendix A*). From these notes, it is clear that Miss Todd was the authority who supplied the theory of the work. The subtle nature of Miss Colwell's use of imagery, in contrast to Miss Galbraith's emphasis on exercise and massage, is also apparent. Because the notes were taken for Barbara's reference after her lessons, not all the procedures which took place were recorded. Many one or two-word references to imagery were sprinkled throughout the original manuscript. Intriguing pictures such as, "kite's tails," "heavy cobwebs," "frog shrinking," "piling stones," "poking tail through hole in egg," "slip covers," "paper cutters," "digging clay out of sea shells," "curtain rods" or "depth of biscuits—not top crust," appeared in the notes without accompanying explanation. When Barbara was asked about any of this material, she would emphatically put an end to our curiosity, insisting that the new images she was currently developing were really much better than most of those she had learned at the studio. Caught up in the excitement of getting her own ideas down on paper, there was no need to try to remember "the old."

The more obvious imagery and lesson procedures provide a glimpse of the character of the early teaching. Often Barbara's notes were well delineated, with directions related to imagery which must have been used many times with various pupils. Other ideas seem to have been improvised on the spot to quickly communicate the quality of weight or suspension the teacher was encouraging Barbara to experience. From this vantage point, approaching the beginning of the twenty-first century, many of the old images seem quite silly and childish. Barbara said she had the desire to "remake all Todd's imagery" from the start. Even in this early stage of her education in the work, Barbara realized that the images she preferred imbued the body itself—the muscles and bones—with a liveliness and qualitative nature she could think about as she moved. If the imagery from one of the teachers displeased Barbara, she ignored it, translating the implied meaning into her own terms.

Barbara's need to become "physically educated" was finally satisfied by Mabel Todd. As Todd and the other teachers presented objective anatomical information and provided an environment in which students were not compelled to conform but encouraged to explore, Barbara began to change. Although dependent at first upon the table lessons, Barbara's emerging kinesthetic sense of what balanced, efficient movement could be like became her internal teacher. Engrossed in Todd's imagery, Barbara rebuilt her body, from the inside, socket by socket. She said it was simply a matter of "learning to center," finding balance through the centers of the joints and using muscles at the center of the body. In the process she began to "let go of the old"—old habits of moving, old ways of thinking and old emotions.

The Children's Teaching

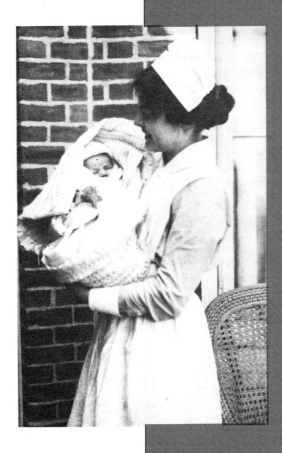

FOR TODD'S MOST SERIOUS STUDENTS, teaching was the natural outcome of learning the work as pupils. Giving the lessons to beginners provided new opportunities for deepening understanding of the material at all levels. The demands of the table work compelled the teachers to continue to improve their own alignment. Explaining Todd's principles to students with diverse backgrounds enlarged their comprehension of her ideas. Striving to appeal to a wide range of imaginative sensibilities spawned new ideas for the imagery. Instilling confidence in the approach and then witnessing improvement confirmed their faith in the process. Thus, each lesson given was also a lesson received. Immersed in kinesthetic awareness and speaking a language of imagery, the Boston studio teachers became living examples of Todd's principles. Reflecting on the development of the teachers over several years, Todd's secretary said, "The teachers have the best of this." As part of her growing commitment to the approach, Barbara planned to become one of them.

Sometimes children were brought to the studio for lessons, usually by parents who were already studying there. Although Barbara knew she wanted to work with these children, Miss Todd was skeptical about her chances for success.

> Miss Todd had started a nursery school for the small children of her pupils the year before I began with her. It had not gone over, and she had spent a lot of money equipping it. Balsa wood furniture was one of the expenditures. Mabel was still so disappointed about this that she laughed at me when I said I planned to work with children of that age. But I understood why she laughed. She did not have what I considered the right attitude. She tended to be a silly adult with children, from my point of view, and so I would not expect her to reach them. I did not say anything, but my subsequent success proved my theories were better than hers and more in line with the beginning of the nursery school movement.

By the mid-1920s, most of the infants and children who came to the studio were referred to Miss Clark for their lessons. Many of those children suffered muscle weakness or some form of spasticity. Some had breathing problems associated with asthmatic conditions. Others came because suspected "mental retardation" interfered with the normal progression of physical development.

As she worked with these children, Barbara carefully followed the instructions of the more experienced teachers and absorbed their philosophy. From them, Barbara learned a natural progression of developmental movement activities was the foundation of ideal postural patterns. Sucking, crying, squirming and wriggling were the first steps in the development of a baby's strength and physical integration at center. Rolling, pushing up to balance on the hands, and rocking between elbows and knees were the next important experiments in coordination. Sitting and crawling were the last major milestones, strengthening the use of the deep pelvic and spinal muscles, which prepared the child to stand and walk. If this developmental process was interrupted by some circumstance of illness or accident, Todd's teachers utilized table work techniques to help the child return to a more normal sequence of development. With the youngest children verbal directions and images were used sparingly. Touch alone was sufficient to convey the critical directions for the release of muscular tension and the key locations of bony support.

As she gathered experience, Barbara began to work not only at the studio, but also in the homes of many prominent Boston families. With the assurance of her qualifications as a Registered Nurse, several physicians referred their cases to her. Officially, her help was enlisted as a "baby nurse," to serve children with special developmental needs. Pleased parents spread the word about Miss Clark to other families facing similar problems, and her reputation grew.

Initially, Barbara felt she learned more from the children than they did from her.

> I had trouble at first in the work because my mental rhythm was speeded up way beyond the body rhythm. The rhythm of early development is much slower. I tuned in to that with the children. It helped me to move in my axis. Touching their bodies gave me the feeling of elasticity and suppleness. I sensed this in all of their joints. It began releasing me in mine. Working on older bodies was so fatiguing, I knew I did not want to go in that direction.

As she gained more assurance, Barbara refined her technique for teaching her tiny pupils through the tactile sense. Touching the child's body and watching him move, she perceived the tension and weakness which interfered with normal development. Then, she traced along the outside of the baby's body the directions she wished the child to internalize. Using a circular massage on the tense areas, Barbara freed the baby of muscular holding patterns. With gentle pressure directed to the centers of his joints, she encouraged exploration of new neuromuscular pathways. Barbara's tactile guidance was intended, through frequent repetition, to "teach the child a more balanced use of the body." Recognizing the importance of "working with the baby," her tactile messages simply nudged the child back toward nature's plan for achieving strength and security in movement.

Many of Barbara's table lessons began with work on the rib cage. Placing her fingertips into the intercostal spaces along the lateral aspects of the ribs, she traced upward between each pair of ribs toward the sternum. This was repeated as the baby's pattern of breathing was observed. As the child let go of muscular holding in the thorax, the diaphragm released into a fuller excursion, resulting in a deep yawn or sigh. Barbara watched for these signs of freer breathing before going on to other aspects of the lesson.

Typically, attention to the feet and legs followed the work on the ribs. "Centering the foot into the thigh socket," began by tracing the "axes of the toes" back from the tips of the toes toward the ankle joint. While giving a gentle thrust at the center of the foot, just forward of the heel, Barbara traced up the center front of the leg toward the thigh crease area, directing the line of thrust to the iliofemoral joint.

Often this patterning stimulated the baby to kick. As he moved against the light resistance she provided, Barbara observed the baby's muscular balance in movement. To help the baby improve his coordination she used touch to encourage tense muscles to release and weak muscles to become more active. To assess the relative strength between the two legs, Barbara had the baby kick both feet against her own abdomen. Feeling for which was the stronger side of the body, she pressed her fingertip into the center of the foot on the weaker side, encouraging that leg into more vigorous action.

Watching her young pupils at play or being handled by their parents, Barbara observed that babies who were encouraged to walk early were often poorly coordinated. The muscles on the outside of their legs were quite tense, while the muscles on the inside were somewhat underdeveloped. Barbara attempted to counteract this tendency by "snugging the great toe inward," [10] toward the center of the foot. From there, the "inner lines of the legs" were drawn upward toward the center of the body to "stimulate the adductors and psoas into greater action." In an attempt to relax the superficial muscles which had become tense in the premature standing effort, lines of relaxation were lightly traced downward along the lateral aspect of the leg from the greater trochanter toward the little toe.

Usually, the shoulders, arms, and hands were not emphasized in Barbara's table lessons. She thought that parents, who eagerly encouraged their infants to manipulate toys and rattles, made babies overly aware of those parts of the body. Thus, most of Barbara's attention was given to the lower half of the body to offset the effects of parents tending to play too much with the upper half. In some instances however, problems in the neck and shoulders demanded the most attention, as described by a mother whose infant son was diagnosed as suffering from severe scoliosis:

> Soon after his birth I noticed that Chucky could not turn his head to one side, but that he turned it on the other side almost around to the back. It was grotesque! His left side was very inactive and the right side was over active. A specialist said that the sternocleidomastoid would have to be cut at the age of three, and a rod would have to be inserted into his spine or he would surely be a hunchback. That never happened thanks to Miss Clark.

> When he was about two months, we worked out that in all of his waking hours I would hold his spine toward straight. It was grueling, but I could see his movement changing. When I positioned him well, both his right and left arms and legs would be in motion. I learned to relax his right side and massage the left to get it into action. Every day I would write down for Miss Clark, everything that he did. Then, at four months, he turned his head on his own to the bad side, and Miss Clark said we were 'out of the woods.' After that he was really good actually and he is straight to this day. The doctors had to change the scoliosis diagnosis because his was supposed to be incurable. [11]

Usually, the progress of Barbara's pupils was somewhat less dramatic than this example, but often equally poignant. The records Barbara kept on her cases were fascinating, detailed accounts of the physical and emotional behavior of her young pupils. Noting how they were progressing along the continuum of postural development, Barbara carefully documented their habits of eating, sleeping, elimination and play. The procedures used in the table session for each child were recorded along with comments parents made about the child's activities between the lessons. Usually, improvement was noticed first by the parents. Better appetite, sleeping habits and less irritability led to increased stamina for more normal patterns of movement. Eventually, the child's physician also became aware of the improvement, noting stronger muscle tone, less spasticity, better color, weight gain, and other indications of enhanced development and general health.

Appendix B presents a particularly complete teaching record of a tiny 19-month-old boy. Tom McEvoy was referred to Barbara by the family doctor because of poor weight gain and the inability to sit up. The physician's evaluation revealed no medical explanation for the lack of development and "mental deficiency" was suspected. Barbara's involvement in this case lasted less than four months, and in this time the baby learned to stand and walk.

Barbara's teaching records for Tom McEvoy and many other children demonstrate that she worked holistically with her young students. She knew, from the experience of learning to align her own body, that movement habits were subtly influenced by everything an individual encountered. Nutrition and environmental factors, the nature of social interactions and the daily rhythms of rest and activity, all had an impact on learning. To make a real difference often meant going beyond the table lessons for the baby, to find ways of teaching the parents and other adults involved in the care of the child.

Working in the homes of her infant pupils in the twenties and thirties, Barbara began to see trends in handling children which she felt were quite detrimental to the natural course of physical development. In following the fashion of "modern baby care," nursemaids and housekeepers, as well as parents themselves, made mistakes which exacerbated the problems of Barbara's little pupils. Lacking understanding of the importance of the developmental movement patterns, adults ignored the baby's large movement patterns and became preoccupied with his efforts to control the face and hands. Without awareness of the infant's need for proper support under the head, spine and pelvis, adults picked up their babies by the arms and carried them carelessly. Babies were propped up with pillows in vertical postures, well before they had achieved the strength to assume such positions on their own. Confinement in a playpen almost always followed the child's first attempts to crawl. Unaware of the value of crawling as a form of coordination which prepared the body for upright locomotion, the newly mobile baby was quickly "caged." Ostensibly, this was done for the child's protection. Barbara suspected it was more a matter of adult convenience. Ultimately, it robbed the baby of opportunities to engage in essential exercise and to learn by exploring the environment.

The design of playpens also encouraged the child to pull himself up to standing quite early. The importance of being vertical was underscored by adults who showered praise on the child in this effort, as if early standing was an indication of superior intelligence. Clumsy, rigid shoes were immediately imposed on the baby to support the arches and celebrate the accomplishment. The excitement continued in exhausting sessions in which the child, hanging from well-meaning adult fingers, was taught to walk. The natural urge to return to the floor, as a relief from the strain of maintaining balance while standing, was then thwarted with warnings not to get dirty or the notion that "only babies need to crawl." Thus, in Barbara's opinion, adult ignorance of the importance of early, horizontal movement activities compromised the child's ability to develop strength and ease in the vertical. Misunderstanding the role of each step along the spectrum of motor development, adults rushed and then subverted the development of ideal postural patterns.

Using bottled formula at an early age to free the mother from the confinement of breast-feeding, was also beginning to be accepted in that era. Solid foods were introduced early, and in some cases the child was rushed into toilet training. Barbara wrote of the young nurse of one of her infant pupils who placed the baby on a potty chair for toilet training and in a high chair for feeding at the age of three months. The notion that nurses' training schools lent credibility to such practices absolutely dismayed Barbara. As she worked with these children, she could feel the resulting muscular tension, and sense the kinesthetic confusion such practices caused. Clearly, modern mishandling of the baby threatened to undermine all she was trying to achieve through the table lessons. To help the children, Barbara knew she must begin to educate their parents.

Barbara's guidance of the families of her pupils was offered through casual hints rather than anything resembling formal instruction. Barbara knew that child rearing was a delicate matter and took care not to presume too much or appear officious. Following her example, parents learned better ways to hold and carry their infants. Barbara's focus on the strength of the core of the baby's body encouraged them to be less concerned about busying the child with the manipulation of toys. Instead, parents learned that the supporting surface beneath the baby was his most important plaything. A firm, open and interesting supporting environment allowed free experimentation with the neuromuscular pathways which would serve to control upright balance and body movement. Barbara helped parents understand that although the baby might not be completely content or socially interactive as he moved through these developmental activities, wriggling, kicking, rolling and crawling were the baby's best means of preparing for the milestones of learning to come. Finally, Barbara showed parents that their own tension and anxiety could result in more stress for their babies. Perhaps the most challenging lesson for these troubled parents was to detach from their concerns and learn to relax with their child.

Barbara's work, helpful advice and attentiveness were deeply appreciated in these families. Some parents were so grateful to Miss Clark that they paid far more than her usual fee. Others went to great lengths to bring her to their vacation homes so the lessons could continue without interruption. With a few, Barbara's visits were the beginning of longstanding bonds of friendship which continued after the children were grown. In those households, Barbara came to be regarded not so much as a nurse or teacher, but loved and respected as a member of the family. Thus, from her cautious beginnings as a pupil in the Boston studio, Barbara grew into a teacher with a special cause. Her task was not only to help children develop through Todd's principles, but also to educate a whole generation of adults.

Gradually, Barbara began to seek other ways of reaching the public with her message. She talked to women's clubs and church groups about the necessities of motor development and, in 1927, she wrote a small pamphlet called *Structural Hygiene for the Preschool Child* (see *Appendix C*). Designed to accompany her talks on child development, Barbara supplied these booklets to members of her audiences, to the families of her young pupils and to the pediatricians and baby nurses she knew.

Eventually, Barbara's work with families and her reputation as a lecturer led to the opportunity to influence Boston's emerging nursery schools. She began by associating with several of the schools as a visiting nurse. In this position, Barbara took charge of the physical examinations of the children at the beginning and end of each year. She was also consulted to insure that the school environment was safe and fostered optimum physical development.

Barbara found many like-minded individuals working in these schools; women who shared her belief that the child's spirit and intelligence should be given the freedom to unfold according to its own nature. There was great interest during this period in a form of naturalistic observational research Barbara called "child study." Such studies concluded that play was inherently educational: mentally, physically, socially and emotionally. Nursery schools evolved as "play schools," where teachers provided for a wide range of age-appropriate educational play. In contrast to elementary schools, the teachers taught indirectly in the nurseries, observing the activity of the children and restructuring the environment when needed to offer new opportunities for growth. In this atmosphere, Barbara's interest in observing the movement patterns of young children seemed to fit right in. Barbara's ideas about the importance of early movement experiences and her sensitivity to children's behavior intrigued her colleagues. Known as a child development specialist throughout the local nursery school scene, Barbara was hired as a master teacher in Boston's first nursery teacher training school, Ruggles Street Nursery School.

At Ruggles Street, Barbara enlarged the typical school medical examination to include an evaluation of the child's posture, movement habits and preferences. Her purpose was to assess physical development and identify those children who might need remedial help. Barbara developed a form called the "Physical Action Record" (see facing page) to record data from her observations. Typical attributes of posture and movement behavior for the age group were listed on the form which made the observations simple to conduct and compare. Aspects of the child's "emotional response" as well as his choices of favorite movements were also recorded. With this information, Barbara tracked the motor development of each of the children. Along with the observations made by the other teachers in other areas, Barbara's records were used to evaluate and promote the total learning process.

In the margins of the Physical Action Records, Barbara also made notes to herself about each child. These notes disclose the particular facets of a child's movement behavior which gave Barbara some cause for concern. Generalized neuromuscular tension could be seen in fast, jerky movement, excitability and the habit of tensing the eyelids in rest. Shortened quadriceps muscles were indicated by the inability to sit on the heels or squat fully to the floor in play. Tense hamstrings and calf muscles showed up in the tendency to walk on the toes or bounce up rapidly from the heel after heel strike. Barbara also became concerned if a child lost control or seemed to "flop over" while rolling. In crawling, "cross patterning," or using the arms and legs alternately, indicated full maturation; less sophisticated homologous or homolateral patterning was a sign of arrested development. In all of their movement, Barbara hoped to see equal development of the right and left sides of the body and neutral, rather than outwardly rotated, positioning of the arms and legs. Barbara was also sensitive to signs of immature balance such as bracing the legs in upright positions by locking the knee joints. Poor balance was indicated if shoulder, arm, hand or tongue tension was exhibited as the child hopped or balanced on one leg.

With the permission of their parents, Barbara gave table lessons to the children with poor movement habits. As part of her role as school nurse, she took on the responsibility of helping such children to improve. The work was quite different from what she had done previously in the quiet, calm atmosphere of private homes. With a new age group, in a new environment, Barbara encountered a new set of challenges.

> To help the nursery child to improve his movement is a matter that calls for thought and ingenuity. An exercise for the adult, who can think of the benefit to be derived from it, and therefore accepts it gladly, is one thing. But to the young child, without future vision, it is most likely to come as an imposition on his good nature and helplessness.

The high energy level of the children was another problem.

CRAWLING

	Head	Hands/Feet	Speed	Emotional Response
	in line / with back	fingers in / fingers out	fast	excited
	held up / drops down	toes in / toes out	slow	calm

STANDING

	Abdomen	Feet	Arms	Emotional Response
unoccupied	ahead of feet / behind feet	parallel / toes in / toes out	rigid / relaxed	calm / excited
walking	ahead of feet / behind feet	parallel / toes in / toes out	rigid / relaxed	calm / excited
jumping	used well / used poorly	rigid / relaxed	rigid / relaxed	calm / excited

CLIMBING STAIRS

	Holding Rail	Alternate Feet	Leading Foot	Emotional Response
up	yes no	yes no	right / left	calm / fearful
down	yes no	yes no	right / left	calm / fearful

Desire expressed for which movements	rolling	jumping	crawling	skipping	running	squat	walk
Dramatization of what animal desired	horse	elephant	pig	rabbit	cow	duck	cat dog

RESTING

	Legs	Feet	Arms	Emotional Response
on back	flexed / straight		over head / under head	rigid / relaxed
on side	flexed / straight	toes in / toes out	over head / under head	rigid / relaxed
on abdomen	flexed / straight	toes in / toes out	over head / under head	rigid / relaxed
on abdomen head raised	flexed / straight		on elbows / on hands	rigid / relaxed

ROLLING

	Legs	Speed	Arms	Emotional Response
	flexed	fast	over head	rigid
	straight	slow	under head	relaxed
			one to side, one overhead	

SITTING

	Legs	Feet	Arms	Hands
on floor	straight / flexed / crossed	toes in / toes out	around knees / elbows/knees	in lap / on floor
on feet	on heels / between heels	toes in / toes out		in lap / on floor
squat	r knee up / l knee up / even	heels up / heels down		
on chair		front of chair / under chair		on table / in lap

To the child, lying down is very apt to mean a cessation of activity. The average child hates to go to bed or to have a rest. To him it means restriction of movement, physically and mentally. Lying on the table for a lesson then is a reminder of something unpleasant. For most children it is necessary to form a new association with lying down before asking them to do it.

If the child has seen an older child on the table for a lesson, he will want to imitate him and this is perhaps the most natural way of all. Imitating a teacher very seldom works. At school I have used a stool and a hassock to make the steps to the table and they love this idea. My usual method is to have some object with me that can be used to advantage in conveying some idea of the principles of the teaching. With this in their hands, they climb to the table and I allow them to keep the object until they become more interested in the movement of their bodies than in the toy. When the child is finally on the table, the first few minutes of finger touch are very important psychologically. Until he finds that your touch makes him feel more comfortable, he merely tolerates you for various reasons. The teacher's personality could dominate the child but this would not be positive for the learning that he needs to do. The ideal teaching I carry in mind for myself is the gradual opening of a door, letting in the light for the child's own vision of his individual development.

Barbara was also challenged by the problem of sustaining the interest of the youngsters in the table procedures. She wrote that often they were, " . . . so full of energy that attention changed rapidly from one thing to the next. Minute suggestions are all that succeed; but with lots of repetition they will stick." The children were also becoming quite verbal and therefore reliance upon touch alone to communicate the teaching was no longer sufficient. Although they needed the same tactile directions as the infants, their interest in language mandated that the imagination be engaged to achieve the desired results. Barbara began to find ways of accompanying the table work with playful images, presented through stories and games. In this way, she began to teach the children, "consciously, as well as unconsciously."

One of the most important concepts for the children to understand was relaxation. Youngsters with poor movement habits were often very tense children. Habits of holding had been substituted for the strength that should have been attained through a normal sequence of motor development. Before she could teach better coordination, Barbara first had to relax these patterns of tension. This was not an easy task as the kinesthesia of a tense body felt natural to the child and the experience of relaxation was foreign. Such children might resist Barbara's efforts by fidgeting, trying to divert her attention through conversation or reacting emotionally. However, with patience, understanding and many repeated sessions, even the most difficult children began to learn to let go and accept the teaching.

To teach relaxation, Barbara often began a session with the "bran dolly." This doll, like our present-day rag doll, was soft and heavy. Barbara gently shook the child's legs and arms as she suggested the image of shaking all of the bran in the dolly's limbs down into its torso. Imagining the doll, the child was helped to relax the tension that collects in the hands and feet, and made more aware of the center of the body. To promote deeper breathing, a dressmaker's tape was used to "measure the length of the exhalation." Barbara challenged the child to let the exhalation reach the shoulders, then the middle of the back, the backs of the thighs, and finally the heels. Barbara found, as the child worked with this simple imagery for lengthening exhalation, he released the diaphragm for deeper inhalation. A small sponge was used to facilitate the understanding of relaxation in the rib cage. The child held the dry sponge and felt its texture change when Barbara poured warm water over it. As Barbara worked to free the ribs through the intercostal spaces, she called upon the child's memory of the experience. "Oh, I won't make it be so hard, and then it will be soft," one child said as he grasped the meaning of the sponge image. Letting go of habits of muscular holding, he allowed his thorax to relax.

Barbara devised many other games and stories for the purpose of establishing the child's awareness of the location of his bones and joints and their properly aligned relationships to one another. In order to improve posture and movement, the child needed enhanced awareness of the critical areas of bony support. For most children, these anatomical concepts were completely new. The usual body nomenclature and concepts passed on from adults to young children, imparted little understanding of how we are designed for movement. Many of the body part names, such as the terms waist, backbone or hips, had little functional significance. Other areas of the body with tremendous importance for posture and movement, such as the thigh joints, were virtually ignored. In order to enlarge their kinesthetic reference systems, Barbara introduced her tiny students to the spine, collar bones, sternum and ischia, and the workings of the joints of the arms, legs, feet and ribs. She intended to start children's kinesthetic education with a more accurate conceptual framework of the sort she had learned from Miss Todd.

To Barbara, the general lack of awareness of the major bones and joints among adults and older children was one of the great travesties of modern physical education. "How can a person become physically educated," she would complain, "unless they know where their bones are?" Realizing young nursery school students were not yet capable of absorbing the vocabulary of functional anatomy and kinesiology she learned from Miss Todd, Barbara searched for simple, playful ways of teaching the same information.

Awareness of the ischial tuberosities was derived from an exercise called "sitting on the spots." This involved sitting on a small stool painted with two round spots which marked the points of contact for the ischial tuberosities in a properly balanced sitting position. The memory of the "sitting bones" could then be recalled in a table lesson or in other movement practice. The children were also encouraged to feel their superficial bones and bony prominences. As the children touched their clavicles the image of "candy sticks" was suggested. The children could then imagine the candy sticks moving in exercises designed to free the shoulder girdle from the ribs. Greater awareness of the heels was developed by massaging them and then imagining they were large pieces of chalk which could scribble on the ceiling. The shape of the foot arches was absorbed as Barbara likened them to tents and bridges under which imaginary characters could hide, or as shovels that could scoop sand into piles.

To prepare for one of the table lessons, Barbara told the story of a mouse crawling down the steps of a tower. Then, as the child lay on his side, Barbara repeated the story with her tactile accompaniment. Supporting the child's abdomen and sternum with one hand, she used the other to indicate the location of each spinous process. These were construed as the steps of the imaginary tower the mouse climbed down in the direction of the pelvis. The goal of this table lesson was to build awareness of the location and length of the spine. In subsequent sessions, Barbara repeated the story as she massaged the muscles on either side of the thoracic spine. This additional tactile procedure was designed to encourage the release of tension in the extensor muscles and promote deeper breathing.

Another game called "sewing shoes and stockings," accompanied tactile techniques which stimulated the tibialis anterior and posterior into stronger action to support the medial arch of the foot. Each toe was related to the center of the foot through games such as "autos driving into the garage" or "birds flying into the birdhouse." A "playground slide" was imagined as the child rested on his back with knees bent toward the ceiling, to build better awareness of the aligned relationship between the second toe, knee joint and thigh socket. As Barbara's fingers traced up from the ankle to knee and then down from the knee to the thigh crease, the child imagined his favorite toy climbing the slide and then sliding downward. Other games were created for the upper body. To center the shoulders and arms, Barbara told of the travels of Peter and Molly Bunny. As she described their adventures, Barbara drew a line from the third finger, through the center of the arm, toward the inner end of the collar bone at the sternoclavicular joint.

Although Barbara worked to center all aspects of the child's body in a table lesson, she placed her greatest emphasis upon the importance of the spine. Barbara knew the relaxation of the spinal extensor muscles was a critical kinesthetic achievement for healthful functioning. Through the imagery of animal tails she encouraged the children to become aware of their vertebral columns and relax the surrounding muscles.

> The sensory awareness of the spine should continue throughout the body. The animal does this through the continuation of its spine as a tail. The child can do this too, through imagery. The child can stroke down the back of a puppet through the length of its tail. Then the teacher can stroke down the child's back and have him imagine his own tail uncurling down toward the floor.

To enhance understanding of the importance of balancing the body evenly around the spine, Barbara introduced the image of the "center line." A plumb line through a toy top was shown to introduce this image. Touching the center of the top of the head, she invited each child to imagine such a line through his own body. The children used their fingertips to trace up the front of the center line on the front of the body, as Barbara traced down the back of the line on their backs. This image was reinforced in all the children's movement activities, and special games for rolling, crawling and walking with the center line were also devised.

> The top has a center line just like our bodies. It turns around this line. Turn to the left around your center line and then turn to the right. Walk, taking your center line along with you.

With kinesthetic understanding of the balance and action centers of the body underway, Barbara worked to stimulate stronger use of the "crouch muscles" at the center of the body. These muscles, which she also sometimes referred to as the "pelvic muscles," were the psoas major along with the iliacus, the abdominal muscles and the adductors. There were games on the table for stimulating rectus abdominis and iliopsoas action, like "kissing" or "smelling" the knees while lying on the back. Another story called "knocking on doors" was told as the child brought opposite knees and elbows together, stimulating oblique abdominal action and reinforcing cross patterned coordination. When the children were strong enough, a slight variation of the traditional rhyme "Humpty Dumpty," [12] was used to accompany the action of a modified sit-up. Apart from these exercises which were done in individual lessons, Barbara devised strategies to encourage the use of strength-building developmental movement patterns for the group as a whole. For some children the opportunity to roll and crawl on the floor was not very appealing. Most children, however, did not need much encouragement and Barbara's ideas won them over easily.

Controversy about Barbara's teaching sometimes arose among the parents or from an occasional school administrator. Many adults thought physical education should be taught in light of the future use of the body in sports or dancing. Some nursery schools responded to this point of view by offering balls and bats to the boys and teaching dance-like responses to music to the girls. Although Barbara thought these activities were excellent for older children, she felt most nursery school children, "were not ready for it." It seemed to Barbara that younger children needed more experience in learning to relate the body parts to each other in the most basic movements. There was no point to introducing movement skills for which their bodies were not yet prepared. In a speech for the parents of students at Ruggles Street Nursery School, she tried to explain:

> The work the teachers and I have been doing with the children has been in the form of play that encouraged some form of the rolling, crawling, and squatting activities. These activities have been associated with the child of

under two years and therefore games have not been built around them. Children's games have been based largely on adult folk games and thus positions that involved the upright posture have predominated. Rolling, crawling and squatting favor the development of the deeper muscles of the body, the ones closest to the bones. Examples are the spinal muscles surrounding the spinal column, the pelvic muscles, those close to the leg and arm bones, and those in the center of the foot. To sit, stand, or walk well involves good development of these deeper muscles. To sit, stand, or walk less well is a result of depending too much on the muscles near the surface of the body.

It has been my experience that the young child who rolled, crawled, and squatted well continues to use these positions as he grows older, whenever he can make an opportunity. The child who never did them with great ease discards them the soonest. Adults like to see the child march—run—dance. But the child likes to wrestle, to lie on the floor and to tumble around. This, to the adult mind, seems silly and purposeless, but the child is doing what he needs to do to achieve strength and balance. Often, after a space of years, the rolling, crawling and squatting movements come back to the children in some of the sports—football, swimming, tennis, etc. What the world really does is to rush a child through these activities in a few months, discourage the continuance of them for several years and then expect good performance of them all at once.

Part of getting the children back into movement on the floor was to furnish play spaces with equipment which would interest them in doing so. Barbara modified many of the existing pieces of nursery equipment to be more in line with the size and proportions of a small child. Sandboxes were lowered into the ground to favor the use of the squatting position. Rugs and blankets were placed on the floor to soften and warm the surface so the children would be comfortable playing there. Large blocks were added to the sets of smaller ones to encourage the use of the larger muscles of the body in lifting and pushing. Padded boxes and cushions were placed around the floor to encourage the children to avoid postural strain by resting occasionally. Barbara said this would, "save the child's back from getting tired" and "teach good judgment in the use of the body."

Barbara disapproved of the use of the traditional slide in nursery schools. Sliding downward encouraged the child to pull "up the back" through his extensor muscles, which reinforced muscular holding patterns in a poorly integrated child. In contrast, sliding down a stair bannister gave the tactile experience of coming "up the front" of the abdomen and chest, a desirable sensation for the improvement of posture. As an alternative to the traditional slide, Barbara designed a "bannister slide," consisting of a short set of stairs beside a corresponding length of bannister just wide enough to center the child's thighs in his sockets. The children loved the bannister slide and Barbara considered applying for a patent to produce it commercially.

Although cost considerations forced Barbara to abandon the idea of the bannister slide, another of her designs for play equipment, the Tunnel Toy, was patented in 1933. Observing that children were more likely to get down on their hands and knees to crawl when there was something for them to move under or through, she invented the Tunnel Toy to encourage greater use of the crawling pattern. Her patent description explained the rationale:

> Modern research points to the fact that the exercise of crawling has great value in the development of children. Those children who have been most proficient in this exercise appear to be stronger and better developed. The pelvic muscles especially, are better developed by the use of four supports as in crawling, than by the use of two supports as in walking.
>
> It is an object of my invention to provide a toy which will be attractive to children so that they will use it extensively . . . in an instinctive and natural manner. . . . The exact dimensions of the tunnel will vary somewhat depending upon the age and size of the children for whose use it is primarily intended. A convenient size is twenty inches in length, twelve inches in height at the center of the opening measured from the top of the base and twelve inches in width. These dimensions . . . may be increased or diminished to adapt the tunnel toy to the most convenient and suitable use by an average child of predetermined age.
>
> It is desirable to provide the tunnel with inclined approaches (10). Crawling up and down inclined surfaces and changing from one level to another is beneficial to a child's development. In this case therefore the base of the tunnel is elevated four to six inches. Perforations (14) may be provided in the sides of the base (4) through which axles may be carried and the tunnel may thus be made convertible into a cart.
>
> Actual use of my tunnel toy has demonstrated that it has a great appeal to children who use it in a variety of ways for which its structure peculiarly adapts. Crawling into a hole is an instinctive behaviorism in which a child will indulge and one which should be encouraged by the provision of attractive facilities, because of its value. The rounded top of my tunnel is much more suitable and desirable for children to climb and sit upon than, for example the sharp surface of a horizontal bar. Children will sit astride upon the tunnel, walk the length thereof, climb on and jump off—all of which . . . are beneficial to the child's development. [13]

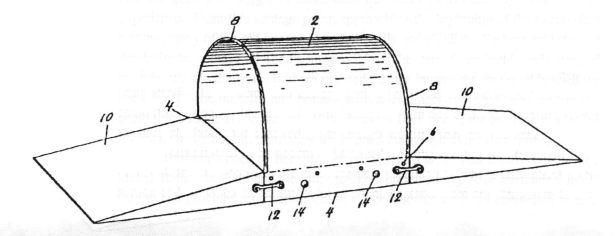

The Tunnel Toy went into production in late 1933. Initially, Barbara sold most of them in Boston. Invitations to lecture on her ideas and occasional local newspaper articles on the merits of her invention, followed. As nursery teachers trained in the Boston area moved elsewhere, Barbara received orders from schools and churches throughout the United States. Barbara modestly delighted in the attention that came with these developments and each new order buoyed her confidence in the growing public acceptance of her work.

Barbara organized some of her teaching ideas developed during this period into a guide for teachers and parents of three, four and five-year-olds called the *Posture Plays* (see *Part II*). Her curriculum focused on practice of the essential developmental movements. The proper performance of each movement pattern was delineated in detail enabling the adult to demonstrate or take part in the activity. Then, imaginative "plays" were described as a means for making practice of the movement more interesting for the children.

Barbara also began several storybooks during this period which were to be read to the children themselves. Most of these presented characters Barbara used in the table lessons and preserved the rhymes and stories the children knew from movement practice. However, one of the manuscripts, *The Children's Book*, was intended to stand on its own as a primer of kinesthetic education.

In *The Children's Book* (see *Part III*) simple awareness exercises, along with drawings which would appeal to children, were presented to foster the development of kinesthetic awareness. The simplified drawings of the human figure guided the child's discovery of bony landmarks essential to the balance of body weight and critical joints as action centers. Imagery of the movement behavior of cats was intended to acquaint children with the facile strength which comes through the release of spinal extensor tension and the coordination of movement and breath.

The Children's Book was Barbara's first formal attempt to develop a language of kinesthesia for her readers. The interactive style of the lessons foreshadow the approach she would eventually take in writing "the manuals" for which she is best known. Although the concepts used in *The Children's Book* were simple enough to appeal to the child, her ultimate goal was astoundingly profound—to restructure and refine the culturally transmitted awareness of the body. She sought for children, and ultimately for everyone, a renewal of our connection to "the natural," and the right to understand and preserve our kinesthetic legacy.

Drawing, Dance and New York

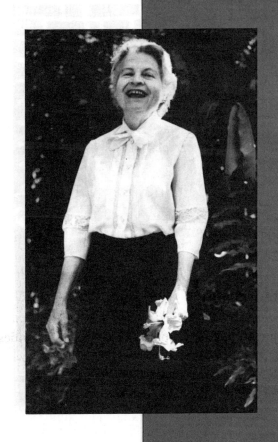

SOON AFTER THE SUCCESS OF THE TUNNEL TOY, Barbara's career was interrupted when the wife of one of her brothers died in childbirth. Realizing marriage and having her own family were no longer probable, Barbara took the children in. With financial help from her mother, she settled her new family into a tiny bungalow in Wellesley, Massachusetts and retreated from her career into a domestic life.

If this professional hiatus had to happen, it seemed to Barbara that it was at an ideal time. Miss Todd's influence was growing rapidly and, in Barbara's estimation, greater understanding of the work was beginning to take hold. Todd's teaching at Columbia University had been very successful, and in 1931, she was offered another university teaching position at the New School for Social Research. In association with her work at Columbia, Todd published *The Balancing of Forces in the Human Being: Its Application to Postural Patterns* in 1929. In 1934, following a radio broadcast about her work, Todd published a simple educational pamphlet called *First Principles of Body Balance*. By the mid 1930s, she was hard at work writing a more complete exposition of her ideas which was eagerly anticipated by Barbara and all Todd's studio teachers.

When *The Thinking Body* was published in 1937, Barbara was greatly relieved. Although she was confident about her skills as a "teacher of body movement," she was uncomfortable analyzing the work on an intellectual level. Barbara enjoyed reaching people through imagery and kinesthetic awareness. Explaining the process reminded her of Oberlin, where scholarly preoccupations drained her energy and tried her patience. Convinced the analysis of the work had been accomplished through *The Thinking Body*, Barbara felt as if a load had been taken from her own shoulders. She celebrated the accomplishment of Todd's classic work and became eager to return to the teaching.

In the mid-1940s, just when the children were old enough to need less of her supervision, Barbara's attention again was drawn homeward by the needs of her elderly mother. As the maiden sister and a nurse, Barbara was expected to handle the next major family crisis. Barbara tried to combine teaching with the care of her mother, but it became increasingly difficult. Her brothers and sisters were unable to understand Barbara's need to remain involved with her career and mocked her tendency to overdo as a "teacher of relaxation." For a time Barbara attempted to keep everything going. Gradually, it became obvious that her mother would require more care than she felt able to provide. With sadness, guilt and the disapproval of most of the family, Barbara placed her mother in a nursing home. As her own sixtieth birthday drew near, Barbara resolved to leave Massachusetts and rebuild her professional life.

Barbara yearned to get back into the teaching. She also realized she lacked the energy for working with nursery school children as she had in the past. Searching for a new direction, she found the desire to study drawing was also uppermost in her mind. Barbara had experimented with simple drawings as teaching aids while working in the nursery schools. She was a master of employing all the senses of a child in the process of kinesthetic learning. As Barbara explored various ways of presenting the imagery, she found that most concepts could be conveyed by touching the child as she told her playful stories in the table lessons. However, when working with groups of children rather than individuals, the use of tactile procedures was somewhat limited. In her work with groups, Barbara was pleased to see how much kinesthetic information could be conveyed to the children through the simple pictures she devised.

Visual imagery had been shown in Todd's studio to help pupils formulate the concepts which were the focus of the table teaching. Usually the pictures came from scientific textbooks and depicted some aspect of mechanics or human anatomy. Such illustrations, intended for technical study by students and professionals in those fields, contained much more information than Barbara needed or desired, and were, in fact, quite confusing. Rather than struggling to decipher the intended application to body alignment, Barbara often ignored the pictures and relied instead upon the teacher's touch and description of the imagery. Todd and the Boston studio teachers also used fanciful imagery which was equally troublesome. About this, Barbara wrote:

> Todd studied the science of movement so much that the image of the body in mechanical terms was very real to her. Such imagery was unreal and too complex for many. In the effort to simplify the imagery for the uninitiated, she and the other teachers made the imagery childish, almost laughable. I saw the good in the approach but wanted to remake all the imagery. You can't get rhythm into the lesson if it is too conscious. Miss Todd's lessons were too conscious, but that was the only way she knew how to do it.

By characterizing Todd's imagery as "too conscious," Barbara meant that a well-designed image should speak to kinesthesia on its own, with very little explanation or tactile interpretation. As Barbara ruminated over a new direction for herself in the teaching, she felt she should develop the imagery in this direction. Without knowing exactly how she would accomplish it, the desire to learn to draw motivated Barbara to pick herself up and move on.

In 1949, Barbara sold her bungalow for $3,000 and moved to New York City to study drawing with Mr. Robert Beverly Hale at the Art Student's League. Barbara felt completely at home in her studies and made friends with other students working there. She loved her art classes and immediately recognized parallels between Todd's work and Mr. Hale's "sensory approach" to anatomical drawing.

> Miss Todd used her hands in her therapy work to give direction in the student's body and she tried to teach her teachers to do the same. Mr. Hale taught a student to use his own hands in finding the location of parts of his structure. Mr. Hale demonstrated how to feel the size of a part, such as an elbow in the palm of your hand. He would trace the rim on the top of the pelvis of his body first on one side and then the other with the thumb and fingers of his hand.

Barbara also studied a wooden model of the pelvis, a small collection of bones, as well as pictures from various anatomy books to refine her understanding. Then, abstracting the musculoskeletal system into its simplest elements, she honed the forms of the muscles, joints and bones into simple visual images. Absorbing human anatomy through drawing became a new means of kinesthetic discovery for Barbara. Excited by this process, she began to share some of her experimentation with Miss Todd.

> Miss Todd liked to have me stop by and let her see what I had done and she was very encouraging in the way that it appealed to her. I could not do much but I have grown to see that it is the character of the little that counts. Does it have balance, rhythm, movement? People can only take in a little at a time.

Although supportive in their visits, Todd, by then well into her seventies, was too preoccupied to be of much help to Barbara. Todd was grappling with the development of her next book, *The Hidden You*. Failing health and her professional concerns necessitated much travel and time away from her home in New York. In the colder months, Todd visited the western states where she could relax and write in a milder climate. Staying with friends in California, she did some teaching, seeing the potential for building a clientele in Hollywood's film industry. Back in Boston and New York, many of the studio teachers had retired or were working less. Although they expressed some interest in Barbara's discoveries, they were rather resistent to anything new. Without much support from colleagues, Barbara's intuitions about developing her drawings as new imagery for the teaching were rather tentative at first.

Barbara did form an odd but ultimately productive intellectual alliance with Dr. Lulu Sweigard. Sweigard had been a student of Todd's during the Columbia years. Intrigued with the success Todd had achieved through her techniques and principles, Sweigard focused upon the scientific analysis of the work, hoping to document its validity through experimental studies. Between 1929 and 1931, Sweigard conducted a study of 200 individuals, "who had the posture teaching." [14] In 1939, she embarked upon a three-year study for her doctorate, which documented the patterns of bilateral skeletal alignment in 497 subjects. Based upon her findings, particularly from the first of these efforts, Sweigard concluded that the locations and directions of improved alignment for most of the students were largely the same. Change occurred in at least twelve consistent patterns, which were noted as she compared skeletal measurements before and after a semester of teaching. These findings provided the information Sweigard needed to systematize Todd's approach. Based upon her research she classified the imagery according to its application to, "Nine areas of the skeleton . . . whose location and alignment had the greatest influence upon the alignment of the structure as a whole." [15] With this new approach to the organization of the teaching, Sweigard began to develop her own unique role in the field of physical education, apart from Mabel Todd.

Having been a student of Miss Todd it is often assumed that I continue her method of teaching. This is true only in part. I accept her basic philosophy, but my teaching has its basis in the findings of two of my research studies and, therefore differs in approach quite markedly in many ways from that of Miss Todd or any of her pupils. [16]

Once they were acquainted, Barbara was invited to sit in on the classes Sweigard was teaching at New York University. Barbara was interested in Lulu's activities, not so much for their scientific slant, but because she was broadening the educational foundations of the teaching. Sweigard taught groups of people as well as individuals at the university. Within the class context, Barbara observed that even with much less reliance upon the teacher's exclusive attention and touch, students were learning kinesthetically and changing their movement habits.

The positioning of the students in Sweigard's approach was different from what Barbara had learned to use in giving private lessons. Todd's teachers usually positioned students on their sides so the teacher could touch both the front and the back of the body. Although Sweigard still conducted Todd's table work in the traditional manner in private lessons, she made greater use of the **constructive rest position** in her posture laboratories. In constructive rest, the students reclined on their backs with their knees bent and oriented to ceiling and their arms resting comfortably across the chest. In the absence of a teacher's tactile direction, the students had to think through the imagery on their own. The feeling of the weight of the body in the gravitational field or the touch of the surface of the body on the supporting surface provided the feedback.

Barbara briefly became Lulu's assistant, helping her not only with the tactile instruction of the students but also with the development of visual images for the class presentations. Barbara was pleased that Dr. Sweigard liked her drawings and spoke of the possibility of using them in a book she was planning. Although Barbara was reluctant to give over her drawing ideas to Sweigard wholesale, the support buoyed her confidence in charting new directions for the imagery.

In the early 1950s, the popularity of Sweigard's work was growing rapidly through the world of dance. Barbara was very interested in the dancers in the classes. Having taught for a few summers at a Girl Scout camp where the English Folk Dance Society also gathered, Barbara had tried some folk dancing. She liked the rhythmic repetition of movement which occurred in dancing and the way it enhanced kinesthetic awareness. The dancers she met in New York shared Barbara's keen interest in the body and she felt a strong kinship with them. When Sweigard found herself with many more requests for private lessons from dancers than she could possibly accommodate, Barbara opened her own studio in rooms rented near the Garment District to take on the overload.

Barbara realized that dancers, already being quite kinesthetically aware, could readily utilize what she was developing to enhance dance performance and avoid injuries. With some of the students, if special sensitivity to the work was evident, Barbara went beyond the usual table lesson procedure to share her latest drawings and ideas for new imagery. To her surprise, some of the dancers became very enthusiastic about her ideas and expressed their preference for Barbara's unique approach to the teaching.

Barbara's approach was certainly simpler and more casual than Dr. Sweigard's. Naturally, with all of her scientific background, the theoretical underpinnings of the teaching were uppermost in Dr. Sweigard's thinking. Working in an academic environment, it was important to supply the students with the logic and references they would need to understand the material intellectually. Barbara was more comfortable with building the student's confidence in the approach by relating her own story, or the development of former students, through the power of the principles. Barbara avoided intellectualizing the work, feeling that too much attention to the rationale ultimately detracted from the student's creative exploration of the imagery. It was more comfortable for Barbara to set the theoretical aspects aside or refer interested students to *The Thinking Body*. Barbara preferred to "keep it simple," insisting that making the changes the work implied was just "good common sense." A letter written to Barbara by Dr. Sweigard at the time, provides a glimpse of the differences of philosophy emerging between the two teachers.

January 23, 1957

You know the one marked feeling I have had about all those who try to carry on in some manner the work Miss Todd started—a lack of scientific background and hence inability to stand up to anyone in supporting the manner of the work. One wins by changing the person, but there is no winning by writing and by talking unless one can do it with readiness to cite facts and principles. Miss Todd had them in part, but still not enough; she lacked true research backing and was unable to think in those terms even after such research had been done. She truly abhorred the scientific attack as she let me know when we were working together. [17]

An entry from Barbara's diary seems to respond:

I was the only Boston studio teacher who kept records of pupils' work and what was taught them. I had the feeling that it was all research and records should be kept of it. Later when I came to New York and worked with Dr. Sweigard, she told me that what I had done would not be considered research, as it was conditioned by a personal evaluation.

My body is my lab and I don't have to walk to it or pay rent. Of course I know that some groups would say that this is not scientific and therefore cannot be depended upon. However time has proven that others who have used the same principles with their personal laboratories have come up with very similar experiences.

There is a difference between the way the mind accepts an idea, knowing it as
a theory or as an action. One is rigid and the other elastic and supple. The
object of the work is to teach kinesthetic awareness; everything else must be
subordinated to that. Kinesthetic awareness is our guide in the use of the
body—the pleasurable experience that makes joy out of movement and
makes movement into an art. We should not allow the subject matter to
eclipse the above purpose. The science of movement is mechanical, and does
not necessarily include kinesthetic awareness. Scholarship in the science of
movement can do much, but imagination and perception can do more.

Perhaps it was this dissimilarity in philosophy which was responsible for
the contrasting approaches of the two teachers toward the use of imagery. With the
imagery categorized to support the achievement of nine "lines of movement,"[18]
Sweigard focused specifically upon those goals. Drawing upon all of her previous
experiences, Barbara relied upon her intuitive sense of which image or principle
might open the door to awareness for each individual student. By adopting a casual,
conversational approach, Barbara could react to their unique needs and interests.
Finally, Barbara simply offered companionship in the wonder in kinesthetic discovery, sharing her latest inventions of imagery and listening enthusiastically to the students' description of their own. In comparing Clark and Sweigard, one student said:

I had ten lessons with Dr. Sweigard. Miss Clark had just come out and
was only charging about half Dr. Sweigard's fee and so I decided to work
with her. Dr. Sweigard was alright, I liked her. She was the type of character I could appreciate . . . but she had certain imagery that you had to
follow . . . I mean you **had** to follow her imagery. Miss Clark was so
much more laid back, and so much more into wanting you to create your
own imagery, and also into changing the imagery. You know images wear
out very quickly." [19]

It may have been the process of learning to draw, and hence, learning to see,
that released Barbara into this sort of improvisational approach to teaching. Mr.
Hale's classes exposed Barbara to artistic renditions of the human body which were
expressive of all her ideals of balance, centered strength and "the natural" in movement. Studying the bones and muscles revealed designs for action and relaxation
which awakened a new appreciation of what Todd had been after. Seeing sources of
visual imagery almost everywhere, Barbara was probably overstimulated by all the
possibilities. Her students were her confidants and their lessons were Barbara's
means of expression. That her students might not completely understand all aspects
of her discoveries was not a concern. She was certain that if they were motivated,
her students would continue to grow in the work as she had. What was obvious to
her would eventually become understandable to them, if they continued to explore
the approach creatively.

During this period, Barbara's copy of the Spalteholz-Spanner *Atlas of
Human Anatomy* was always open to the musculoskeletal system and she pored over

the pictures constantly. Introduced to the book by Miss Todd, Barbara considered it the best anatomy she had ever seen. Usually, several drawings for each area of the body were provided showing the layers of musculature, superficial to deep. The illustrations were ample in size, very detailed and subtly colored to delineate the bones from the ligaments, tendons and articular surfaces. Barbara found several illustrations which captured the alignment concepts in a strikingly beautiful way. She copied those drawings repeatedly, endeavoring to simplify the forms and extract their kinesthetic meaning.

> I studied the anatomy pictures—where the muscles attached and how bones met in the joints. I looked at these over and over, consistently—not just once in a while, but frequently, almost every day. With study, the anatomy picture opens up and becomes an active representation helping you to know the body better. This is what happens in the body as you focus upon an image and relate the parts to the whole.

As Barbara's confidence in her own approach strengthened, she left her position as Dr. Sweigard's assistant and enlarged her own private teaching. [20] Many young dancers, pursuing a professional future in New York, frequented Barbara's studio in the early 1950s. Some of them simply used Barbara's services to relieve the discomfort of injuries or as a means of recovery from a long season of performances. Others became committed to her approach.

One of the first professional modern dancers to work consistently with Barbara was Erick Hawkins. While recovering from back and knee injuries, Hawkins began to reexamine dance technique. Recalling that period, he wrote:

> Surely there must be a way for a dancer to train so that he would know how to protect his body from major injuries that might end his career, and minimize the minor ones that are such a frustrating interference with a dancer's life. [21]

In his break with the Martha Graham company, Hawkins began searching for possible alternatives to traditional training, which lead him to Dr. Sweigard, then to Miss Clark and an exhaustive study of Todd's writings. As Hawkins experimented with the application of their ideas to dance technique, he spread the word about Barbara.

There were other associations with dancers which enlarged the network of students for Barbara. Pauline Lawrence brought students from José Limon's company and studio. Katherine Litz, a soloist and comedic choreographer who suffered from a recurrent shoulder problem, also came for lessons. Sensing the importance of the work as an educational adjunct to the study of dance, Litz recommended Barbara to many of her students and associates.

Early on, it seemed that Barbara's approach might also make inroads into the domain of university physical education. Barbara's link to physical education was through the Forbes Hawkes family, who were themselves quite familiar with

Todd's teaching. Dr. Forbes Hawkes had been a prominent surgeon practicing in New York in Todd's day. His wife, Alice, took several lessons with Todd, as did their son John. John became interested in the teaching and tried to pursue further education in the field through a degree program at Columbia University. By then however, the curriculum was oriented toward the problems of rehabilitating disabled veterans of World War II. Since this was not the career he had in mind, John left the program to explore business pursuits.

In 1950, John's young wife, Winnie, contracted polio while pregnant in Paris. Winnie had been very active in sports and studied modern dance in Vermont at Bennington College; the paralysis was devastating to her. Using the family's considerable resources John and Winnie explored every known therapy for polio available at the time. Then, remembering Todd's work, Mrs. Alice Hawkes contacted Todd's New York studio and learned about Barbara. Barbara met with the family in New York and then traveled by train to John's Florida home to give table lessons to Winnie.

Winnie's improvement, through table work sessions and the movement practice Barbara suggested, was dramatically obvious to everyone. The family's interest in the teaching was rekindled and their enthusiasm for Barbara's work was made known to many of their associates. Among them was Dr. Gertrude Mooney, a professor of Physical Education teaching dance at the University of Florida. At the insistence of the Hawkes, Barbara and Mooney met to discuss the work on several occasions. Mooney liked Barbara and although she considered her approach a bit esoteric, she recommended her to Dr. Josephine Rathbone, a physical education professor at Teacher's College, Columbia University, New York. [22]

Nothing of substance ever came of Mooney's recommendation to Dr. Rathbone and Barbara dismissed the possibility of gaining academic acceptance for her work. The young students that surrounded her in New York held much more promise than any hopes of convincing those in "old physical education" of the value of the teaching. Drawing her students into her world of imagery, she was assured that they would be the ones who would "get the work over to people" in the future.

The first student Barbara really cultivated as a teacher was Joanne Emmons. Joanne had been studying dance in New York since 1946 and by 1948, she was performing some of Doris Humphrey's pieces and working with the Dance Notation Bureau on the process of notating them. Joanne was also studying with José Limon. As she progressed into Limon's advanced classes, her body began to rebel. A light case of polio in childhood had caused some muscle weakness and the strenuous dance movement, "was not making me better, it was making me worse." [23] The leg that was affected by the polio began to collapse mysteriously in leaps across the floor and her back pain was constant and often excruciating. Out of concern for a promising student, Limon's wife, Pauline Lawrence took Joanne to Sweigard and then to Barbara.

Although the back pain began to subside, it was clear to Barbara that Joanne's problems would take more than a few sessions on the table to work through. Having developed so many compensations in her body due to the polio, Barbara realized Joanne needed extensive work and a mentor to help her understand the teaching from many perspectives. Almost immediately Joanne became Barbara's creative confidant.

> At first, we would meet at a room in New York where she taught and lived; her table was there in a big sun parlor type situation. And we would meet each other and I would say, 'Oh, I have this wonderful new image about this,' and she might do the same to me. Miss Todd had always told Miss Clark that she was her favorite teacher and I could believe it. I loved it and right away my dancing began to change and my teachers noticed it. I would think, 'Oh, that is how it is supposed to feel,' and instead of pain it was gratifying to move. Before Miss Clark I had reached the point where I was ready to chuck the whole thing; I was so disillusioned. [24]

Their lessons evolved into a fast friendship in which Barbara nurtured Joanne's interest in applying the material to dance. Joanne began to consider developing a "pre-dance" technique. She reasoned that practice of the alignment principles in the most basic dance movements would prepare the student to withstand the rigors of more advanced training. To Barbara, it made perfect sense.

> Exercise in depth! What is necessary? Time and thought. People need activity to go along with alignment. Then they enjoy the action much more, having acquired sensory pleasure in better alignment and distribution of weight. This makes it possible to move more easily in and out or to and fro on their bony levers as the impulse for movement comes or the occasion requires. Animals return to center on all levers for rest and relaxation. People need to do the same. The rhythm of slow movement releases muscles to make new patterns.

The next student Barbara took in to groom as a teacher was a young actor with a magnificent speaking voice. André Bernard, like many in theater at the time, was working in dance to improve his basic movement patterns and physical presence on the stage. He described his first lesson with Miss Clark:

> After several lessons with Erick Hawkins I began to see that there was something in the movement that his people did that I thought was wonderful. But I didn't know how to get it into my own movement. Erick had an immense library of wonderful books and he would talk about them and suggest certain readings. In one of those discussions, I told him there was something that he was doing in movement and his good students were doing that eluded me—I didn't know how to get it. I asked him if there was anything that I could do to learn that. Then he mentioned Barbara Clark, saying 'you must go to her and she will show you what you need to know.'

So I did just that. I called her and made an appointment. I had my first
lesson which was a table lesson and a little bit of either sitting or standing
or something. When I came out to catch the bus that would take me home,
and stood in front of Carnegie Hall waiting for the bus, I can remember
thinking that it was very strange work. You see, I had been a chemical
engineering student, majoring in chemistry with a minor in mathematics,
studying what is obvious . . . for me, it was such a strange way to think.

I don't think I would have gone back had it not been for Erick. I thought
to myself, 'Erick is advising me to go and he is a very fine dancer and a
very intelligent person and he must know something that I don't know.'
So I decided to keep on going until I found out what that was, and that is
why I hung on. As I had more lessons, I began to get a reaction from the
images that I could perceive and then of course I really began to like it
more and more. [25]

André's sensitivity to the images and his grasp of Todd's principles were
strong indicators of his potential for the teaching. Along with his lessons, Barbara
began to encourage André to give aspects of the table teaching to her. Then, she
commented upon his conduct of the technique and offered direction. She liked the
quality of his touch and his steady, professional manner. His academic background
gave Barbara confidence he would be able to withstand scientific scrutiny.
Gradually, Barbara entrusted André with the traditions of Todd's table teaching.

André and Barbara also discussed her ideas for bringing the work more
solidly into the realm of "the educational." Barbara realized from working in the
nursery schools and observing Sweigard that the work need not be limited to therapeutic applications. Educationally, the material could be used to ameliorate simple
problems and provide understanding which could prevent further difficulties.

Early posture programs had a 'corrective character', but more recently, the
educational aspects of the procedure have been stressed. In particular,
those teachers who subscribe to the use of mental imagery as the dominant
factor in changing habits, emphasize the educational viewpoint.

As Barbara prepared to launch Joanne and André into their own teaching
careers, she went to John Hawkes for support in his knowledge of business and
other practical matters. Welcoming John's interest in the content of the work as
well, she hoped that he might eventually become involved in the teaching. In 1952,
the "Technique for Movement Association" was officially established. Joanne
Emmons described the beginning of the venture:

We had a meeting with John, André, Barbara and myself. Miss Clark said
that she wanted the work to grow, and she felt that a group was the way to
make that happen and that we were the key people and that we should all
get to know each other and have this organization. I was in favor of it
because I had seen how it worked with the Dance Notation Bureau. We
were to have a president, a treasurer and secretary. [26]

The group found an old handbag factory on 37th Street, off of Seventh Avenue in the Garment District, to serve as their studio. The owner was going into retirement and diminishing his level of business. There was large space with a good floor for dance, which was perfect for Joanne's classes. There was also a bath, dressing rooms and an alcove just large enough for Barbara and André to use in private lessons. John helped with the printing of the business cards and the flyers which advertised Joanne's classes. Barbara, the "honorary chairperson," quietly pulled strings and influenced decisions to insure that all would move forward successfully for the group. Focused on promoting the efforts of her students, Barbara insisted she was not in charge of Technique for Movement. However, there was another element in this decision her young colleagues, at first, knew little about.

In the early 1950s a lawsuit was brought against Mabel Todd by a New York medical association accusing her of practicing medicine without a license. Although the suit was not brought to trial, Barbara learned Miss Todd agreed to terminate her work in the state of New York as part of an out-of-court settlement. Todd closed her studio in the Roosevelt Hotel and dismissed Ruth Mitchell, at the time her only assistant. Although Todd's work on *The Hidden You* and her failing health had already reduced her influence in the teaching, the news of the scandal was a tremendous setback for Barbara. Clearly, it was best to advance the work through the efforts of the younger teachers and diminish attention upon herself and any association with Miss Todd.

Although officially in the background, Barbara was still somewhat authoritarian about how the work should be presented. With concern that Technique for Movement might attract the same sort of disfavor that had finished Miss Todd, she met with the two young teachers at length in preparation for their teaching. Guarding her brood with conservatism, Barbara planned ways of directing the work away from its therapeutic origins toward a new educational focus.

With Joanne, Barbara's attention focused on transposing the kinesthetic awareness learned in the alignment lessons, into the performance of basic dance techniques. Joanne was given some leeway to select the dance movement which was practiced, as long as Barbara could see the relationship to the alignment principles. For Joanne, the relationships were obvious.

> Pliés to me are basically thigh socket awareness. Leg swings are the same. Arm movements to me are basically rib socket awareness, although I first teach from the arm socket, as that is the easiest to follow. Sternal awareness is taught from the beginning—it leads in walks—runs—leaps. Balance is atlanto-occipital awareness, the focus of any emotional or intentional impulse. Spinal awareness must be also be taught from the beginning—the difference between a rounded back and a straight back. I try to give the awareness of the spring action of the lower spine and the building up of the spine vertebra by vertebra—head balanced on the top. All of this must be done with a lot of relaxation to allow the students to feel through the movement. [27]

Joanne's early pre-dance classes were simple applications of Barbara's image vocabulary to basic movement. The lessons typically began with the students lying down on the floor with the lower legs supported on a chair seat. In that position, they imagined the weight of the thighs dropping into the thigh sockets or the lengthening of the spine. Simple rolling actions were also incorporated into the work on the floor. Image exercises relating to the awareness of the ischia were practiced while sitting. The lever action of the legs was explored as students practiced moving from the sitting position to standing and then back to sitting again. In standing, thoughts would turn to the image of the pelvis resting on the tops of the thigh heads. This awareness was cultivated further as the students practiced the demi plié or performed a "slow, free walk to music." [28]

As the classes progressed, more of the images and anatomical concepts were presented for practice in the simple movement sequences described above. The movement repertoire also enlarged somewhat to include leg swings and arm movements. Eventually jumps and turns were added to the movement sequences. The improvisation experiences at the end of each class were an element of creativity which the students relished. Tied to the new lesson material of the day or reminding the students of a principle learned previously, the students were to explore their own interpretation of the imagery. Although the following list of improvisations does not represent a specific order of presentation, it does provide a glimpse of the wide range of kinesthetic experiences which were explored.

> Have a feeling of inner space; give your skeleton room to move.
> Picture lengthening the spine before each movement, take time to do it.
> Center your feet as you move.
> Dance with large festoons from ischia to fibula.
> Let the fingers of the serratus anterior lengthen as you move.
> Go from a feeling of space within to space without.
> Picture the large toe coming back to the heel as you move.
> Do a dance for only your legs.
> Relate the center of the foot to the femoral socket as you move.
> Centering your head at the top of the spine—do a head dance.
> Center your arms in their sockets as you move.
> Picture the iliacus as you move—let it move with you.
> Let your trapezius lengthen as you move.
> Let the impulse for your arms come from the base of your spine.
> Relate the thigh socket to the opposite arm socket as you move.
> Lengthen the angles of the trapezius as you move.
> Centering your feet at the talus—do a foot and ankle dance.
> Center the head on its level between the ischia as you move.
> Picture the whole spine as you move smoothly through all levels.
> Deep muscles of the pelvis dissolving into a swirling core of energy—
> dissolve into it and let your movement come out of this energy. [29]

Barbara was enthusiastic about the application of her work to the dance classes and watched them whenever she could. As the work with the dancers developed however, Joanne began to feel a bit inhibited by Barbara's watchful eye. As the classes progressed, Barbara said some of the students were "not ready" for the more challenging dance movements. She felt students should not be allowed to progress to more difficult material until they could maintain their alignment in basic movement. Agreeing in principle with Clark's concerns, Joanne was also sympathetic to the students' expectation that a pre-dance class should include some dancing. For Joanne, achieving balance between these concerns continued to be a challenge and sometimes a dilemma. For Barbara, there was no doubt.

> In beautiful movement, distortion must be avoided. The body must learn how to move with ease in proportion to the existing condition of strength. When a student is disturbed by the mechanics of movement it becomes difficult, if not impossible, for him to center his structure. Failing in this, the movement is done poorly and the student has a sense of defeat.

> The pattern of returning to center, to an awareness of balance or rest is the least understood and generally least practiced of all the components of dance. Of course, all movement involving effort deepens breathing action and increases circulation of the blood. This is exhilarating and makes you feel good. But if good weight support at the center of the structure has not been kept, although you may not notice any bad effect at the time, it will crop up later in a weakened structure.

André taught most of the table work lessons at the Technique for Movement studio. He worked with all the actors who came for sessions and most of the men. Barbara confined her efforts to teaching her longstanding students, helping André to plan his lessons and observing his work. She offered suggestions and also encouraged him to develop his intuitive understanding of the needs of each of his students.

> André's touch always helped me, and others liked his touch very much, too. It was nearer like my own. I suppose he imitated me to some degree. André caught on to the fact that it was the line of direction that helped people to grasp the image as well as the exactness. Touch is a sense approach. It can be exploited toward others if used unwisely. It needs to be kept impersonal.

André had difficulty with some of the table procedures and began to experiment with using only one hand to direct the visualization of the images. Barbara also found this was easier and helped the students to become more self-reliant. In some of the exercises, André and Barbara also instructed the students to touch their own bodies as they described the imagery. Doing less for the student through touch was a way to make the work more educational. Barbara hoped with the development of clearer, more sensitive imagery, the table teaching might become unnecessary.

Of course, the teacher can do a great deal to convey the concept of continuity in movement to his pupil through the sense of touch. But the use of a student's own touch has a future in its development too, I think. It depends on the clarity of the image and whether it lies within the range of a person's own experience. The teacher's touch can be conveyed to a group of students through the pointer directing attention to the details of a drawing. If one can get the imagery of a continuous stream or line flowing through the head of the pointer and keep the line flowing evenly and easily, with occasional pauses for accent, the dramatic effect can be terrific. I sense we can go far in this direction, but how far I do not know.

The *Technique for Movement Lessons* (see *Part II*), was a two-year curriculum of private lessons which Barbara prepared for André and other students who would later learn to teach the work. Although some lessons are missing or incomplete, what remains demonstrates Barbara's thinking about the necessities of the teaching and the appropriate order of presentation. The emphasis in these lessons was still upon the table work. In each lesson, new tactile procedures and movements were presented and described in detail. In subsequent lessons, the review of old exercises was indicated by references to their titles. Much repetition of material from previous lessons was suggested in the original manuscript. Probably more of this was described than was actually done. In practice, the teacher was free to decide which of the past learning experiences would be the most appropriate for individual students to review.

Barbara was also grappling with issues which were more educationally oriented in the lessons. Teaching materials, such as the skeleton, separate bones or pictures from the Spalteholz-Spanner *Atlas of Human Anatomy* were specified to accompany the "demonstrations" of anatomical concepts. Other aids, such as cloth patterns for the muscles or balls and cardboard tubes as models for bones and sockets, were shown to simplify the principles. Barbara's visual images, referred to as "designs," were shown to help students internalize the material.

The collaboration of the Technique for Movement group provided the new direction Barbara sought in moving to New York. By learning to draw, she found that graphic simplification of anatomical design could give powerful direction to the exploration of kinesthetic awareness. Her search for movement experiences which enhanced the meaning of her visual images, was deeply inspired by dance. As she watched her young colleagues creatively experimenting with the work among their own students, Barbara was aware of the continuance of Todd's legacy—she was convinced of its potential to develop in many new, important ways.

Writing
in
Pictures

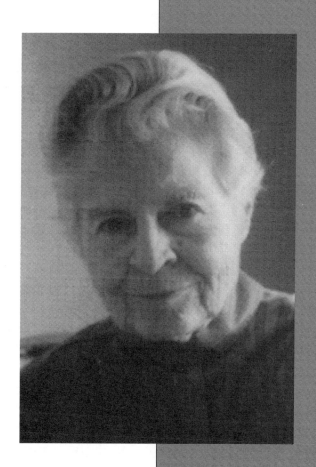

JUST AS BARBARA PREDICTED, there were many other students who became interested in the teaching by way of the Technique for Movement group. Among them was Anthony Mannino, an actor who taught at Herbert Berghoff's studio. About the time Barbara arrived in New York, Tony was in the process of starting his own acting school and exploring various movement techniques for his students. Tony had studied dance and fencing; however, his own problem with a back condition, which he felt "bordered on being hunchback," [30] motivated him to explore other alternatives. Through André, Tony learned about Barbara. In his first lesson, he experienced a vital connection to her work.

> In five minutes I knew that this was the right thing—so simple, so beautiful—I knew this was it! Through the imagery and knowing where the centers are, I was able to relax over-tense muscles and use those that were over-relaxed, getting better proportions and posture. Barbara was unassuming, dedicated and I bless her. The ease with which I am able to move around and rest, that I learned from her, has extended my life. [31]

Tony was one of the acting teachers, spun off from the Group Theatre, who had been influenced by the Stanislavski Method. Tony defined acting as simply, "doing something truthfully for a purpose." [32] It was to be a creative rather than imitative process. For Tony, the self-awareness and discipline gained through Barbara's approach to alignment was a tremendous enhancement to his own goals in teaching acting. Tony's students flocked to the Technique for Movement studio. They all studied Joanne's pre-dance technique and many had private table work sessions with André. Seeing the results of this combination of experiences, Tony felt he had found the rudiments of an ideal approach to movement. Hoping to incorporate the material into his school, Tony urged Barbara to structure her ideas into a basic movement curriculum for actors.

By 1956, Barbara had shaped the content of many new lessons for André and Joanne to teach at Tony's school. Yet, that year was the beginning of the end of the Technique for Movement Association. Joanne had married and was planning a family. André, weary from an exhausting schedule of performing and table lessons, decided to go south for a few months of rest. Closing the studio was disappointing for Barbara, but she was completely supportive of her two young friends and their needs as individuals. She knew André would eventually return to New York to continue the teaching. Joanne reassured Barbara she would also teach dance again, a few months after the birth of her baby. Shifting gears, Barbara graciously accepted the change and proceeded to cultivate Ethel Brodsky, a relatively inexperienced teacher, for the work at Tony's school.

The winter of 1956 also marked the conclusion of Barbara's relationship with Miss Todd. She learned of Todd's death from Mary E. Waddell, Todd's companion.

February 2, 1957

Our dear Mabel passed December 14th, 1956. An autopsy was performed. Mabel's case record will go down in the history of medicine as a rare one. Physicians of long experience marveled how she had lived into adult life. Also how she had lived since her heart attack. Mabel's great illness at the age of three years left her with unnatural kidneys. All of her internal organs were small, her blood stream was impaired and over a period of twenty-five years she gave herself iron shots.

She was in and out of the various hospitals but we always made it possible for her to come back home. . . . Over the period of two and one-half years that we lived together, she refused to take opiates, because she felt they were only to be used at the time of heart attacks. She was conscious and smiling twenty-five minutes before passing. She did not go into a coma, but found it hard to breathe. The doctor was here at 6:30 p.m. and told us 'she cannot live until morning.' At 7:30 p.m. she had passed.

We had a memorial service on December 19th. Her remains were cremated and sent on to Syracuse, New York for interment. The bulk of her estate goes to her cousins in New York State and she has remembered her friends with small gifts. Mabel was a true example of overcoming, as she demonstrated fourth dimensional thinking, lifting herself into a realm where pain could not remain. [33]

The sense of loss must have been profound for Barbara. Miss Todd had been at the center of her life for almost forty years. "It is difficult to think of so vibrant a personality coming to a close. I must think of her as going on." Some months later, Barbara learned the copyrights to Todd's books had been left to Dr. Sweigard. Although she rationalized that Sweigard's academic connections would make her the logical one to continue the publications, Barbara was slighted and shaken by the news. Like a child shunned momentarily by a disapproving parent, Barbara wrestled with worries that the decision was an indication Todd preferred Sweigard's approach to the teaching. Then, as if to soothe her own doubts, she rekindled all the support and approval she felt from Todd in their last meeting.

'I think you have been my favorite teacher.' Miss Todd said this to me the last time I was with her. The words came slowly and introspectively. Her eyes at first took on a backward glance as if she was thinking over the years, and then she focused them on me as she spoke.

Finally, to set the situation straight in her own mind Barbara wrote:

I know that other teachers had more in common with Miss Todd as friends and associates in some phases of the teaching. I was immature in some respects, which helped in relating to children, and Miss Todd was quite sophisticated. But when it came to creative, imaginative ideas in relation to the human body, I know she liked my clear cut and simplified thinking.

Barbara worked through this disappointment and her grief in losing Miss Todd. Approaching her seventieth birthday, she gathered the eager young Ethel Brodsky under her wing and prepared to move the teaching forward again at Tony Mannino's studio, Drama Tree. Initially, Barbara was very involved in the work there, preparing Ethel for each session. However, within a few months, Ethel left the teaching to be married. By then, André had returned from his respite in the south and was ready to begin working again. André took over the work at Tony's studio along with a new job in radio broadcasting. Because of his limited availability for private lessons, he restructured Barbara's material into classes which could be given to groups of students. Aspects of anatomy and the principles of posture were introduced in short lectures preceding the visualization and movement practice. In the lectures, Barbara's designs were presented on large charts to illustrate the imagery. While picturing the images, students practiced simple dance, pedestrian and developmental movements as well as concentrating quietly in constructive rest. To introduce new elements of awareness, the table procedures were simplified so students could perform them on each other, alternately giving and receiving what André called "tactile aid." Approving the direction he was taking with the classes, Barbara concluded "André was so efficient that I was able to stop observing and advising."

In visits with Joanne in New Jersey, Barbara could see the work in dance was also taking on a new dimension. After the birth of her child, Joanne began to study again. She had classes in Mary Wigman/Hanya Holm technique and studied with Merce Cunningham. Her teachers criticized her dancing for being overly relaxed. As Cunningham put it, her technique "didn't have any starch." [34] Although she refused to return to her old approach to dancing, which was riddled with tension and misplaced effort, Joanne realized she had further to go with her new ideas. Now, it was time to take what she had learned from Barbara and make it work in the performance of strenuous dance movement. For a while she assumed the role of the worst in class so she could concentrate on applying the imagery in new ways. The problem was to strengthen her body sensibly, using the imagery to stave off tension and insure that the movements were coordinated efficiently. Joanne progressed quickly and developed strategies for teaching her discoveries to others.

Joanne began to teach again at the Dance Notation Bureau, working primarily with students from Julliard and the High School of the Performing Arts. She expanded her pre-dance technique, applying the imagery and anatomical information to movement which was more challenging, technically and expressively. Convinced the alignment work need no longer be confined to beginning level or pre-dance applications, Joanne began to call her approach, "dance in depth." [35]

Barbara was awed by Joanne's progress and terribly proud of her. However, ever cautious about movements which might be harmful to the body, she watched Joanne's classes very critically. When she felt the movement was taking the students too far "off-center," she assailed her former student with criticism. In more than one instance, her protests actually stopped the class. Joanne tried to help Barbara understand what she was after. Asserting that some of Barbara's physical limitations might be due to the effort to "stay so carefully on-center," [36] Joanne encouraged her to be less conservative. Despite her age and lack of experience, Barbara did give some of the dance movements a try. But, whenever she went much beyond the pliés, she felt she suffered from it and complained to Joanne, "It took a day in bed to recover." [37]

Although the dissension between them was uncomfortable, Barbara understood that Joanne had really begun to "own the material." This was something Barbara knew should happen for all her students, as it had for herself with Miss Todd. Barbara and Joanne continued working together for several years. They met regularly to give table lessons to Joanne's children, to make costumes for her choreography and compare ideas concerning the development of the work. Whenever a young dancer asked Barbara to recommend a teacher, she would emphatically respond, "Joanne Emmons is the best that I have ever seen."

When Barbara visited Joanne's and André's classes, she was introduced as their teacher and the originator of the material the students were exploring. Making herself available for discussions with the students after class, Barbara learned from their reactions to the teaching. Many of their discoveries took place outside of class as they moved through their patterns of daily life. Thinking of one of the images, old tensions were discarded as the truth of skeletal balance was kinesthetically understood. Barbara marveled over how such basic concepts could have such a profound effect on the students. She identified with their independence and yearned to contribute further to their learning with the fruits of her long experience in the work. In considering this prospect, Barbara envisioned a series of books as a new means for sharing her drawings and lesson ideas. Her closest colleagues, André, Joanne, John, Tony and Katherine Litz, agreed that written material for individual practice would be a welcome addition to the study of alignment in classes. Barbara also pondered the possibility that her writing might become a new form of physical education for the public at large.

In the early 1960s, as Barbara considered the potential for writing as the next step in her career, she felt fairly confident. It would be a natural outgrowth of the writing she had done for the nursery schools and the Technique for Movement group. Sifting through the lesson material she had already developed, she could see there would be plenty of ideas to use. Having organized the material for her students to teach, she had a strong sense of its structure. Yet, it was still so difficult to begin.

> I think I talked to John Hawkes the most about this and he was very interested in helping me to write. I have to laugh whenever I think of how he was going to begin his part in it. He was used to typing so he rented a place for me in Miami, Florida and called it an office although I had apartment space in it. When it was fairly well set up, he sat down in front of the typewriter and looked at me as if expecting me to dictate to him what should be said.

> And I laughed and said, 'Why John, I am not so well organized as to have it
> all planned out in my mind and ready to go on paper.' He looked so sur-
> prised. Without a student before me, my mind seemed to be a blank. My
> conscious mind did not have the ability that was in my unconscious and I
> had not learned then how to release the latter. This too has to develop.

Barbara explored various approaches to writing, looking for something to
model her own work after. She felt the anatomy and kinesiology textbooks she
studied were too long-winded, distracting the reader from really learning anything.
Later, in a magazine article, she was pleased to see that experts agreed the typical
textbook was "filled with trivia and useless information," and was likely to "stunt
the inquiring mind." [38] Barbara also looked through Todd's books and articles for
ideas. However, she concluded that all but *First Principles of Body Balance*, were
too difficult for most readers to understand. Perhaps, it was Barbara's laconic
Vermont upbringing which shaped her preference for the writing found in several
public affairs pamphlets she collected. These handbooks, with titles like *Live Long
and Like It* or *Know Your Heart*, were published by a non-profit educational organization in New York and distributed for not much more than the cost of postage.
Barbara liked the simplicity and practicality of these manuals and felt they were
more in line with what she could do with the alignment ideas.

   With the format selected, the mechanics of how to get the ideas down on
paper still eluded Barbara. She felt ill prepared for the task. As she put it, "I was
taught to think, but not in the use of words in expressing my thoughts." She attend-
ed a series of lectures about newspaper reporting. However, comparing her goals
with those of journalism made her realize that describing the work was not enough.
Barbara wanted her words and pictures to fundamentally change the way her readers
regarded their bodies and approached movement. To do this, they would have to
become involved with the material on a sensory level. Finally, a discussion with a
lawyer provided the solution. "Why don't you try the question and answer method?"
he suggested. Barbara had used this approach in her work with young children; it
was the logical way to begin.

   In preparing to write the "manuals," Barbara also faced the problem of
reformulating the information ordinarily conveyed through the table procedures,
into clear directions the students could follow on their own. She approached this
problem with more assurance. Mr. Hale's sensory approach to drawing, as well as
André's success with simple tactile aids, proved that students could locate anatomical landmarks and trace the direction of the imagined actions independently.
Joanne's experience with "dance in depth" demonstrated that moving while visualizing provided sensory feedback which could be used for self-correction. Barbara
confidently concluded that these elements of self-instruction could readily promote
kinesthetic learning through the manuals, if the imagery was clear enough and the
reader was sufficiently motivated to improve.

All Barbara's more experienced students, Joanne, André, Tony, John and Katherine, had a hand in the development of the manual. As Barbara explored many different approaches in creating the lessons, the reactions of her students were carefully considered. Having so much advice, however, complicated matters. Not only did the students have preferences for certain imagery as individuals, but their backgrounds as dancers, actors or teachers also biased their views. Barbara put drawings, exercises or whole lessons in or out of the manual to the satisfaction of one person, only to find another disappointed. She simply could not please every-one. Gradually, Barbara realized that because of the circuitous nature of the materi-al there were many equally satisfying ways to begin. She later cited Alice Hawkes, backer of the project, as the co-author for helping her to finalize the decisions and keeping the project within their financial constraints.

Let's Enjoy Sitting–Standing–Walking (see *Part III*) was published in 1963. Focusing primarily on the pelvis and the axial skeleton, awareness of the tuberosi-ties of the ischia or "sitting bones" in the sitting position was logically followed by locating the thigh heads as the focus of balance in the standing position. The center of the ankle joint was explored in a simple exercise of ankle flexion to help the reader learn to support the pelvis through the "middle lines of the legs." Centering the joints of the legs then led into the image of an axis for the torso which was called the "center line."

In contrast to the emphasis upon the musculature seen in the *Technique for Movement Lessons*, Barbara curtailed discussion of the muscles as too difficult for the beginning student. However, imagery for relaxing the tension of the extensor muscles of the back was given and the diaphragm was also introduced. The image of the psoas major muscles as a "bridge," conveying traffic from the legs to the spine, was pictured in several movements suggested for practice.

Basic images for sitting, standing, and walking were the focus of most of the lessons. Two developmental movements, rolling and squatting, were explained and, "to keep the men involved," Barbara developed an image exercise related to the activity of tying one's shoes. Although she considered using more dance movement in *Let's Enjoy Sitting–Standing–Walking*, only the dance plié was introduced. Over the protest of her dance colleagues, Barbara decided that improved "sensory aware-ness" should be established in movements which were familiar, before venturing into anything more difficult.

> We absorb knowledge with the entire body as well as through the use of the mind alone. The animal uses all of the senses to help him keep his body weight properly distributed and to coordinate his body parts in plea-surable, comfortable, enjoyable movement. Sensory awareness lowers neuromuscular tension, allows better weight distribution and gives more endurance. Somewhat like the animals, when we as human beings say that we have to feel a thing out before expressing an opinion, we mean that we have to use a stronger sensory approach than we command at the moment.

> We have to correlate more of the senses to give us the clearest image of the idea we wish to have and express as our opinion. We discover the truth in simple things. We sense it in one way or another—seeing it, hearing it, feeling it. I am trying to make my written words have a sufficiently sensory approach to the subject so that they will produce some pattern of kinesthetic awareness in the body of the reader.

Former students and colleagues learned of *Let's Enjoy Sitting–Standing–Walking*, and soon the orders began to pour in. Many of the students wrote back to Barbara of the value of her book as an adjunct to the teaching. A few colleagues patiently corrected her grammatical flaws and urged her to reorganize aspects of the writing. Cora Belle Hunter, one of the last teachers to work in Todd's studio, was somewhat skeptical about the manual concept.

> I've been so involved in other activities I, as yet, haven't carefully gone through the book—the sketches are good; however, I must confess Barbara that when we put exercises in print and expect people to carry them out against their fixity of tensions which misguide the movement we are really doing something Mabel never did. Private lessons and the feel of the body vs. relaxation is so necessary in most cases. You've attempted a big thing. My pupils used to want me to write a book of exercises, my reply always was—the very best exercise can be carried through in the wrong way. So blessings on you and what you do! Mabel E. needs to be kept alive—her principles are breaking through in all fields and are what the educational world needs most. You deserve much for your interest and what you've done.[39]

All the reaction to the manual intensified Barbara's determination to continue with her plans for writing. It also clarified important differences between Todd's point of view and her own.

> [Todd] was intensely interested in **her** research into the subject. She analyzed the pupil from her own point of view. In her therapy work Todd's fingers quickly found the tense areas . . . and her mind was directed toward how [to] change what the pupil had done to himself. But also included is how to stop [the pupil] continuing in that destructive course. . . . In my teaching, I changed from the first attitude to the second and became involved in writing and drawing to illustrate.

One of the most avid supporters of Barbara's early writing efforts was Marilyn Monroe. Marilyn learned of Mabel Todd's work as early as 1953 through her study with Michael Chekhov.

> Chekhov has actors work on imagery associated with their characters and with 'images of fantasy' in order to develop imaginative flexibility. He explores in considerable depth the process of perfecting a character's dominant psychological gesture, and he combines his initial physical exercises with certain psychological themes the exercises explore. He then pro-

gresses to the principles underlying the composition of a good performance and the structures of plays. At every step, his aim is to broaden the actor's sense of responsibility and insight.

> Chekhov stresses the organic relationship between life and art. His view is that the same laws of composition govern the universe, 'the life of earth and man,' and all of the arts. As a corroboration of this insight he recommended that Monroe study Mabel Elsworth Todd's *The Thinking Body*, which became, Monroe later told her friend Ralph Roberts, her Bible. She would take years to absorb *The Thinking Body*, and although she never claimed to understand all of its technical information, she practiced many of its exercises and was influenced by Todd's way of situating the body within the continuum of human psychology and physiology. [40]

> Her's [Todd's] was a holistic view of human activity Monroe could identify with and practice; a teaching that could turn her toward a therapeutic inspection of herself and away from Hollywood's mechanical magnification and distortion of what were supposed to be her better parts. [41]

Marilyn's friend Ralph Roberts was an actor making most of his living as a masseur. Roberts knew André, and it was this connection which lead Marilyn to Barbara. Barbara gave Marilyn her first table lesson when the actress was hospitalized in New York at Columbia Presbyterian. Barbara was sympathetic to Marilyn's obvious exhaustion and tried to help her through the teaching. André also gave Marilyn several lessons. As soon as she was well enough, Marilyn left the city again to film *The Misfits*. Barbara continued to hear from her during that troubled time in California. Although she felt she could do little to help Marilyn personally, the star's enthusiastic interest in the material motivated Barbara to continue to develop the writing.

> A letter from Marilyn Monroe during her last years in California asked me if I could help her by mail. This may have had something to do with getting me into action on the manual. Marilyn also knew a publisher and said she would speak to him when the manual was ready.

Perhaps because of the association with Monroe, Barbara began to consider film as another medium for the communication of her ideas. In the mid-1960s she met Sherman Price, a director who specialized in the development of short educational films. Although Price did not study extensively with Barbara, they had long discussions about the work. This dialogue led them to the conclusion that Todd's teaching might be more broadly accepted through the medium of film.

> I've enclosed a paper . . . which explains the importance right now of utilizing the unique facilities of the motion picture medium to enable people to discover, despite their static-atomistic cultural bias, the dynamic connections of content transformations occurring in process and the invariant relationships which become apparent when they direct their attention to

these transformations as dynamic experiences. The immediate content orientation is the wide concern about social and environmental relations of man. But the basic material is support for the personal discovery that we, as a part of nature, have the facilities to self-generate higher-order, more dependably lasting information about how to see, think and act in resonance with the potentials of ourselves and our environment. I feel that this material—also probably to be cast in the form of a book with some title such as 'The Dynamic Alternative'—will give people the conceptual readiness to appreciate concepts such as yours more deeply. [42]

In 1967, Sherman Price worked up a story board (see *Appendix D*) which presented some of Barbara's teaching ideas through film. However, due to the enormous production costs, the project never materialized. Although Price continued to seek financial support for the project into the early 1970s, gradually they lost contact. Yet, Price's story board, *Balanced Movement and Relaxation*, serves as another example of Barbara's commitment to building public acceptance of the work.

Barbara renewed her interest in teaching children in the 1960s through a project at the Starpoint School for Brain Injured Children just outside New York. Barbara met the director of the school, Marguerite Slater, through their common membership in the National Arts Club. Mrs. Slater was disconcerted by the number of handicapped children who failed to make meaningful progress in her school. She was impatient with accepted methods of working with brain injured children and was in search of alternatives.

Many of the children are difficult to handle because they need more than to be taught. They must first be reached. The teacher's job is to bypass the brain's functional failures and manage somehow to get the learning in. Mrs. Slater . . . says that she uses every contact, every specialist, every proven method in the books and has sought and cultivated the cooperation of experts in special fields everywhere in an effort to find the best ways to bring learning to her young charges. [43]

Barbara's experience with giving table lessons to infants and children with a variety of handicaps intrigued Mrs. Slater. As a result of their discussions, another student of Barbara's, Jimmie Elmer, was trained to work at Starpoint School. Jimmie instituted many facets of Barbara's nursery school curriculum and gave table lessons to individual children for about a year. Barbara also became somewhat involved in the work there, observing all aspects of the program. Through this relationship, she was delighted to learn of the work of Glenn Doman and Dr. Carl Delcato at the Institute for the Achievement of Human Potential in Philadelphia. Their research reinforced many of Barbara's convictions about the importance of movement in child development.

By studying hundreds of injured children and hundreds of normal youngsters, the institute's medical group developed new theories about how
uninjured brains develop and how this normal pattern could be imposed on
injured brains. 'We began to find,' Doman continued, 'that the simple and
long-known basic activities of well children such as crawling and creep-
ing, are of the greatest possible importance to the brain. We learned that if
such activities are denied well children, because of cultural, environmental
or social factors, their potential is severely limited. The potential of brain
injured children is even more affected.' [44]

Although apparently effective, Barbara was unsure of the methods which
supported this philosophy. Treatment involved a routine of repetitive manipulations
of the child through movement patterns which were absent from his early development. Remembering her success with the gentle table procedures, Doman-Delcato's
approach seemed overly forceful. However, the emphasis upon "cross patterning,"
or programmed experience in movement which crossed the midline was fascinating
to Barbara. The idea was so similar to Todd's early work in which forces were pictured moving in diagonal pathways, from one of the thigh sockets to the opposite
sternoclavicular or atlanto-occipital joints. Thus, as Barbara began to plan her next
manual, cross patterning was very much on her mind.

Barbara was also ready to bring aspects of the alignment of the shoulder girdle
into her writing. *Let's Enjoy Sitting–Standing–Walking* had emphasized balancing the
core of the structure through the spine, pelvis and legs. Barbara cultivated awareness of
the pull of gravity through those parts of the body and led the reader to the precise location of the mechanisms of bony support. This was done in deliberate contrast to popular
approaches to posture which focused upon improving the appearance of the body by
holding muscular tension through the abdomen, shoulders and chest. Barbara considered such efforts misplaced attempts to defy the force of gravity. Instead, she wanted
her readers to learn to cooperate with its influence.

'Sit **up**—stand **up**—hold **up** your head.' How many of these commands,
that have been in use for so long a time, have really helped those that need
it? The directions have been wrongly used making people tense in their
superficial muscles. And when they try to relax the tension, their whole
support structure falls apart.

Vegetation symbolizes a better image of the vertical. Plants grow upward
toward the light. But in its earliest stages, vegetation grows downward to
get the leverage to grow up. This refers to the root system. Man should
develop similarly. The spine lengthens downward (as does exhalation) in
the back of the axis to give strength to come up in the front of the axis.
Body balance requires this opposition of forces.

With the work of "grounding" the body begun in *Let's Enjoy Sitting–
Standing–Walking*, Barbara felt she could move on to establish imagery for the
"reaction to gravity" in her next book. In doing this, Barbara revived the classic

image of the bicycle chain, which Todd used in *The Thinking Body,* as a metaphor for balancing the compression and tensile forces in the body.

> The balancing power between the compression members in the back and the tensile members in the front is like the bicycle chain. Should something happen to make either portion of the chain relax or contract more than the other, it could not be moved forward, around back, and up over the little wheel, and forward again smoothly; and its power for multiplying the muscular force from your body would be lost. So with the body-strength. The weight comes down the back and the power gaining in force as the weight accumulates toward the pelvic arch, would unbalance the structure if it were not balanced and checked by the lifting strength at the front of the spine and of the front muscle-wall connecting the pelvis with the thorax, the neck and head. . . . So it is not a purely fantastic analogy that is suggested between the body and the bicycle. Power, in the form of compression force comes down the back and turns forward through the pelvis, and in the form of tensile force it travels upward again from the pelvis to the top of the chain, through sternum, hyoid, mandible, to the base of the skull and down the spine again. It keeps the whole machine steady, so that the drive of the muscle force added to the weight can be continued into the legs and provide the strength to swing them in walking or running . . . . [45]

Barbara condensed Todd's discussion of the tensile and compression forces into one concise drawing which she called the "cycle image." The cycle became the central image for *How to Live in Your Axis–Your Vertical Line* (see *Part III*), published in 1968. The process of balancing the force of gravity "down the back" with suspensory forces "up the front" was the concern of many of the lessons.

André was particularly instrumental in the development of *How to Live in Your Axis.* In 1965, he accepted a teaching position in the Dance Department of New York University's Tisch School of the Arts. Barbara hoped her manual could be used by the dance students in his courses. She felt the cycle pattern was a necessity for dancers and its simplicity would appeal to them. However, because of the perceived sophistication of her prospective college level readers, *How to Live in Your Axis* presented a more abstract and perhaps, impersonal approach to the alignment material than she had used before. She abandoned the question and answer method, and played down her practical, pedestrian emphasis. Instead, she dealt with abstract lines of movement representing forces acting on or generated by the body.

While developing the lessons for *How to Live in Your Axis,* Barbara was very concerned that her drawings be anatomically accurate and proportionately sized. The original drawings developed for the manual were among the best of her career. However, out of worry over the limited budgets of college students, Barbara agreed to several cost-saving measures which reduced the size of the drawings and crowded text and illustrations together within the boundaries of a smaller page. As a result, Barbara was somewhat disappointed with the manual in its final published form. [46]

Barbara left New York City soon after finishing her work on the manual. Letting go of her rented rooms and leaving her possessions with friends, she traveled to see relatives and former students in various parts of the country. Barbara loved traveling, as Joanne Emmons described:

> When I knew Miss Clark, she was very active. She was always traveling around a lot, managing to visit some relative or another. She would go visit cousins in Albion, Michigan or go to be with her brother and his wife. Then she would go to Chicago to stay with her other brother, Tracy or visit the nieces she raised and their children. She would spend a week or two whenever she would go and sometimes she would be gone most of the summer. She traveled very light and lots of times when she was going to make a trip she would give up her apartment. Sometimes she would store a few things with me or with André and then she would come back and get another room. She wasn't that nomadic when I first knew her but she got that way in her seventies and then into her eighties and she loved it. She loved to get on the train and go and talk to people. She was much more outgoing as she got older. [47]

Riding the trains was a big part of the enjoyment of travel for Barbara, as well as the fleeting friendship of the people she met along the way. The changing landscape or the latest political scandal might start conversation, but inevitably Barbara found herself introducing some aspect of the work to her companions and sharing the manuals if they really seemed to be interested. She was surprised by the openness of most people to her ideas. It bolstered her conviction that the material could be useful to almost everyone. Barbara also became aware that the receptivity of many people to her ideas was due to their admiration of her own unusual youthfulness and vitality. It amused her to realize, for the first time in her life, she was far better off than most of her peers. Of course, she attributed this to the fact that her body alignment was "the best it has ever been." This opened up new possibilities for Barbara to philosophize about aging.

> To have youth is to be in action. The elderly have little or no action. They don't know that we have a large influence in determining the length of our own lives. They tend to think that we don't, so that they can do as they please, and then they blame the outcome on a force outside themselves. Self-control has much to do with longevity. We can grow old or we can grow up, the choice is ours to make. It is all in our approach to life, the attitude we take.

Confidence in the results of the work also had an effect on Barbara's drawing and writing. Feeling much of her earlier difficulty in the manuals had been the result of poor alignment and related psychological tension, she wrote:

> My problem has always been over-consciousness. Tension of the muscles holds me in the conscious so that I cannot express my own thoughts freely on paper. I am now writing better because I have less mechanical strain.

> My shoulders are more relaxed. My body is better integrated, and there-
> fore I have more kinesthetic awareness. I relate more of my sensory appa-
> ratus to the task. A changed environment is helpful in this. It stimulates
> the sensory awareness to a new approach to any problem.

When Barbara returned to New York in 1969, she arranged her routine once
again for concentrated work on the next manual. This time, however, she was to be
without the assistance of Joanne Emmons, who had moved to New Mexico with her
family. Barbara knew the association with dance and dancers was vital to the teaching. In his position at New York University, André was working almost exclusively
with dancers. Sweigard had also built her career in the world of dance. Barbara
found she missed the affiliation with dance she found so stimulating in her association with Joanne. Feeling the need to "get back into movement," Barbara, at the age
of eighty, enrolled in a series of social dance lessons offered near her apartment.

> Returning to NYC after several months in the west, I wanted a fresh start
> for a third manual. Personally I needed more discipline in foot coordina-
> tion, so I enrolled in a Social Dance course where I could apply my ideas
> of mind-body integration along with the concepts of teaching dance.

Barbara carefully diagrammed the floor patterns of the foxtrot, rumba,
samba, cha-cha and disco in her notebook for the class. Terse directions were rather
impatiently inserted by her teacher about the proper execution of the steps. These
comments, along with Barbara's own reflections on her process of learning, indicate
she was probably not the best dancer in the class.

> My rhythm and posture are good but I need help in the timing of the steps.
> Dancing well depends on taking one's weight on one thigh head at a time.
> This is my weakest point. I especially like the class in the group teaching
> of men and women as well as the usual couple dance performance. I
> found that women have the best of the situation alignment-wise. In the
> woman's part of going backward, the toe-heel action comes to the fore.
> And also the hand support that a man gives a woman comes at the weakest
> part of the back where the thoracic curve passes into the lumbar curve.
> The spine is balanced and straightened by being held a little forward. This
> strengthens the psoas action where it begins to suspend the thighs and
> pelvis.

The challenge of coordinating the steps in social dance stimulated Barbara
to investigate the dynamics of foot balance. She had little previous experience to
build on; Todd and the other teachers had given only cursory attention to the foot.
Barbara studied her set of foot bones daily, fitting them together like the pieces of a
puzzle. Guided by the illustrations in the *Atlas of Human Anatomy*, she attempted
to locate each bone in her own body. Probing her feet from all angles, Barbara
investigated the significance of each articulation. Imagining their combined actions
in movement, Barbara discovered balance through the centers of her feet.

The wealth of knowledge about the foot, disclosed through methodical examination of its articulations, led to similar investigations of other joints. By bringing focus to the joints, Barbara asserted she was moving away from "old physical education" and its emphasis on the "muscle sense." With this distinction, she was pleased to be in accord with the latest scientific research. James J. Gibson's book, *The Senses Considered as Perceptual Systems* was her reference in this matter.

> Muscles and joints are quite different structures. The muscle pulls; the joint rotates. The muscle varies in length; the joint varies in angle. The muscles are attached to the bones by tendons so as to form levers; the bones are fitted neatly together at bearings. There are receptors in the muscles and tendons on the one hand, and in the ligaments and capsules of the joints on the other hand, but their function is surely different. The mechanics of an elastic muscle is not the same as the mechanics of a bearing or a hinge. The evidence strongly suggests that the muscle sensitivity is irrelevant for the perception of space and movement, whereas joint sensitivity is very important for it. In short, we detect the angles of our joints, not the lengths of our muscles. It is not often realized, even by anatomists, that it is the function of a joint not merely to permit mobility of the articulated bones but also to register the relative position and movement of the bones. In the old terminology, each joint is a 'sense organ.' [48]

This information confirmed what Barbara had already concluded was the most effective imagery for the teaching. In reflecting on this she wrote, "Structure does not seem to change much through muscle action. Bone angles seem to be more vivid to the imagination in shifting the balance which effects the muscles."

In developing lessons for the next manual, Barbara became convinced that the pattern of balance she had discovered for the foot could be applied to many other joints. With the "heel pattern" established as one of the cornerstones for the writing, Barbara began the search for visual elements to use as imagery. With continued exposure to lectures and workshops at the National Arts Club, she became increasingly responsive to the use of graphic design in city billboards, newspaper advertisements and poster art. Viewing these materials as a part of the urban terrain, she became aware of the simplicity of the most successful graphics, as well as their eye-catching appeal. As she collected and studied these materials, Barbara experimented with new ways of presenting her imagery. Playing with abstracting the designs of anatomical structures, she superimposed geometric shapes over key bones, joints and muscles. Slight distortion of anatomical reality became a new way to make a kinesthetic point. "Prodding needs to be dramatic to get people's attention, as well as being correct in principle," she wrote.

Since the process of manipulating the skeleton of the foot had been so helpful to Barbara, she explored various ways of making models of the bones for her readers. She placed drawings of the top, bottom, front, back, right and left sides of the ankle and heel bones on sheets of thin cardboard. These views were arranged in a pattern which could be folded to create boxes, roughly the size of the bones. With the boxes constructed, each view could be seen in its proper place and a sense of the mass of the bones was conveyed. She hoped students would follow her suggestion to put the two models together, to gain awareness of the subtalar joints. For Barbara, understanding the balance of the ankle bone, located below the tibia and fibula, behind the navicular and on top of the heel, was the essence of centering the foot.

Barbara explored further applications of the cube design by methodically visualizing the front, back, top and bottom views of other anatomical structures. To stimulate others to think the same way, Barbara constructed drawings depicting the body in boxes. In one drawing, the foot bones were shown as little cubes, stacked upon each other, with the knee, pelvis and head as proportionately larger cubes. In another drawing, she changed the cycle image into a rectangle with distinct corners. Other images combined the cubes and elements of the cycle pattern.

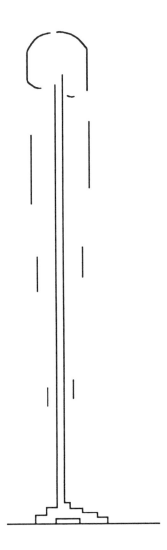

Although these drawings were more mechanical in feeling than any imagery she had drawn before, Barbara felt this served a useful purpose. Picturing the bones or the contours of the body as planes brought about a new dimension in kinesthetic experiencing. Attention could be drawn to the substantial importance of the "over the top" and "underneath" elements of the cycle. For Barbara, this represented an awakening, the birth of a new essential ingredient in the exploration of body alignment—the dimension of depth. Her discovery of this new emphasis became another major theme in the manual, as evidenced by the title she devised, *Body Proportion Needs Depth – Front to Back.*

> Let's enclose the center line or axis with four planes. Then we will know where the front of the body leaves off and the sides begin. The concept of depth is needed because we tend to stand, sit and walk at the front and sides of the body. We are not familiar with the central action or line up. The body has depth. You have a front and back and also a right and left. Box the body and go inside—then un-box it.

In teaching young dancers and other performing artists in New York in the early seventies, Barbara became aware of a resurgence of interest in Todd's work. The students also spoke of exploring Alexander technique, Feldenkrais work and other approaches, both old and new, which served to bridge the gap between mind and body. Barbara was pleased but not really surprised by the new acceptance of such ideas, reminding her students much of this had been foreseen by Miss Todd, in *The Hidden You.*

> The future holds for man the ever-increasing experience of consciousness, and the years add to his capacity for acceptance, qualification and control. Through knowledge, sensitive appreciation and self-expression, man continues to evolve. He forms a pattern of unity of forces, but it would be well if he were to increase his sensitiveness to the minute stimuli within, which influence his behavior, and to environmental stimuli. These together combine to affect his emotional thinking and responses. Man still lives dangerously and the habit of meeting emergencies is a part of his inheritance. The old mechanisms operate in the unconscious in their habitual way. Conscious control of conditions is only possible through recognition of the many forces involved. [49]

Barbara was encouraged by the new receptive climate for her ideas. At the same time, she realized the titles she had previously used for her work, such as "structural hygiene," "natural posture" or "body alignment," were dated, and might limit appreciation of the far-reaching implications of the teaching. "Letting go of the past," Barbara urged all her students and teachers to refer to the work as "mind-body integration." Perhaps thinking of *The Hidden You*, Barbara also began to imply the existence of a relationship between the process of integrating mind and body and the symptoms of national distress, which were so evident during that period. In assessing the world situation Barbara suggested, "Nixon won't know what to do until he can let go of those shoulders." Concerned over the future of the women's movement she concluded, "Women will never be liberated until they get out of high heeled shoes."

Barbara's practical perspective also spoke to the unrest in the world of modern dance. In the late sixties and early seventies, many of her students were of the "post-modern dance" or "new dance" persuasion. [50] They were disenchanted with the traditional approaches to technique which damaged bodies and accepted physical suffering as the way to improve. The social and political traditions of dance were also questioned by these young people. Traditional dance protocol placed choreographers and teachers in positions of unquestioned authority. Students, attempting to progress through this system, often experienced the loss of personal identity in the attempt to please their elders. Rejecting old imitative dance technique conventions and paternalistic hierarchies in companies and schools, students began to train exclusively through improvisation and to express their joy in dancing through loosely structured contact jams. [51]

Barbara gave many of these young explorers of post-modern dance a further sense of fascination with simple pedestrian movement. Working from the inside, with the play of imagery upon kinesthetic awareness, they endeavored to perform sitting, standing, walking, squatting, rolling and crawling, efficiently and without tension. Moving without any of the usual stylistic adornments, they were challenged by the complexity of moving simply. The strength and ease they discovered as they balanced through the centers of their joints surprised and empowered them take further physical risk, without fear of injury. That they were learning so much about movement from this tiny 80-year-old woman, so entirely disconnected from the usual trappings of the New York modern dance scene, must have delighted them and added to their sense of rebellion.

Barbara cared very little about her possible influence upon modern dance in this period of radical change. But the enthusiasm of the students did give her a sense of urgency about completing *Body Proportion Needs Depth* and organizing her ideas for another manual. Barbara left New York City before this transpired. After a period of travel and visits with former students and relatives, she settled in Illinois and published *Body Proportion Needs Depth – Front to Back* in 1973.

My dance colleagues and I at the University of Illinois were privileged to be a part of Barbara's process as she worked and reworked her ideas for the writing. We learned by observing what she valued, what she discarded and what she tenaciously achieved. Her creative interest in the material permeated everything she did. Even her daily discipline of "naps" was a way of working. She used these periods not only to recoup from the work of the day, but also to imaginatively explore the impact of her most imminent image or perplexing challenge. During these periods of rest, she utilized the full spectrum of consciousness to explore kinesthesia as her ultimate source of truth. They were times for synthesis of the functioning of the mind with the experience of the body. They were times of kinesthetic discovery. Often, coming out of a nap with a new idea, Barbara was aroused into a frenzy of drawing or writing.

> It starts as a feeling and becomes a thought. When the ideas come I can't get them down fast enough. Many of them leave me, but then they come back again.

As Barbara shared her latest ideas with us, she often spoke as if she really did not consider herself to be in charge of the discoveries. Instead, she said her "unconscious" mind was guiding her toward new awareness. Barbara often asserted that too much "conscious" activity on one's body alignment actually got in the way. She insisted that everyone could access the wisdom of the body, if only we had better understanding of the differences between these two aspects of mind.

> Too much thinking acts as a restriction. The thinking brain plans the meals. The unthinking brain eats. The thinking brain selects the clothes you wear. The unthinking brain puts them on and takes them off each day. The unthinking brain is the one you play with, the one you laugh with, the always comfortable one, the one with which you can really relax.

As she identified connections between her evolving ideas, Barbara crafted them into forms which would make what she called "suitable imagery." Visually, it was a matter of extracting a design from the musculo-skeletal anatomy and imbuing it with the subtle feeling of centered balance. Verbally, it was the process of finding the words and the rhythmic combinations of phrases which would guide the reader to this new source of integration or release. Barbara's ultimate choices of imagery to use in the writing were based on judgments of whether the imagery would "appeal to people," that is, be incorporated into their thinking easily.

> It takes imagination to use imagery. You have to have the power to think in a new form, a new way. But to make a change for the better in your alignment you also need a suitable image; one that affects the neuro-muscular organization in a way that will alter it. A way that will send the impulse over a new path, while at the same time blocking the old. Stylized images and unrealistic images should not be used.

Avoiding mechanical analogies or purely fanciful metaphors with little relationship to the human body, Barbara developed imagery which was masterfully sensitive, subtle and peaceful. Suggesting her latest image to her cadre of students, she would watch for the response, anticipating that a "suitable image" would lead them effortlessly into enhanced awareness.

> Awareness should be like the ripening of fruit. When it is ripe it falls off the tree. You don't have to reach for it.

Barbara continued work on the manuals well into her eighties, actively exploring movement to accompany her imagery. Although she recognized the value of working with the images at rest, she also felt there was no harm and much intrinsic value, in associating simple actions with the visualization process.

> People need activity to go along with alignment. They then enjoy the action much more, having acquired sensory pleasure in better alignment and distribution of weight. This makes it possible to move more easily in and out, or to and fro on their bony levers as the impulse for movement comes or occasion requires. The animal returns to center on all levers for rest and relaxation. People need to do the same.

Yet, Clark's movement accompaniments for the imagery were not exercises in the conventional sense.

> You need to use your mind as you exercise. If you don't your body loses out. You have to train for improvement in whatever you do—walk, sit, sleep. It is not so much what you do but what you think as you do it. We are teaching the **how** of movement and simplifying it to a knowledge of bones and muscles and their use to attain the best body alignment in movement or at rest. We teach in a way that one will sense this through a better feeling in the body as one moves in any daily activity or sports. This is encouraged through the mental pictures . . . rather than conscious direction of the specific bones or muscles, without their relation to the body as a whole.

> We should not try to create the image within the body from a muscular concept. You just hold the image in mind—you **see** it and in this way it comes to pass. You become what you are visualizing or thinking about. You defeat your purpose if you tense your muscles to bring it about. You cannot make it happen. It happens as a result of mind-body thought or integration.

As she structured the imagery and movement practice into lessons, Barbara deliberately avoided the tendency to dominate or overly organize the student's experience. In her opinion, a pedantic approach was ultimately quite destructive to kinesthetic learning. Instead she hoped the lessons would stimulate interest in the work and encourage the student to discover balance in his own unique way.

> Body movement in general is an inheritance directed by the unconscious. Body movement can be affected by conscious suggestion; but this needs to be kept in the suggestive field and not allowed to be overly directive. Ideas should move from one to the next briefly. The reader should be able to find himself in what is written or drawn. As the person gets the action, he will understand more and need less explanation.

> Use a familiar movement as 'the jump' to start interest. Then, gradually lead into simple analysis of what it does for the body, how it is done, feeling it happen, instead of forcing. This gives the opportunity to suggest an approach for creating action from the inside rather than trying to bring it about from the outside. This can be done with exercises for adults as well as games for children. Let the student participate in the discovery of movement.

Barbara sometimes laughingly speculated about the chances that she would "make it to 100." Although she was an amazing example of health and vitality in aging, life gradually became more difficult for her. As time passed, those of us helping her realized how essential our assistance had become. We were fairly unconcerned about some loss of hearing, but when she agreed to see an ophthalmologist, we were surprised to learn that glaucoma and cataracts had seriously impaired her vision. Perhaps, we should have suspected some of this because of the emphasis she placed on the senses as she developed lessons for her last manual, *The Body is Round—Use All the Radii*. It is probably accurate to say that Barbara's creative process always reflected what she needed to do most urgently for herself. She was completely assured even in her last years, that she could improve her functioning and restore her health by perfecting her alignment and self-awareness.

> In realigning the body, the individual needs to be willing to start disciplining his body. This means recalling an image and giving it thought. It means facing one's difficulty as it is and slowly changing it, a little at a time.

At the age eighty-six, Barbara had her first major setback. Hit by a child racing his bicycle down the sidewalk where she was walking, she fell and broke her leg. Barbara would want the world to know it was only a crack in her greater trochanter and the head of her femur remained strong and well aligned in the socket. The doctors operated anyway, pinning the bone back together and confining her to a walker for several months. The experience convinced Barbara that she needed the walker as a safety measure, and she used it the rest of her life. Not long after the fall, thinking that better vision might have helped her avoid the accident, Barbara agreed to have cataract surgery on both eyes. Without the immediate replacement of the lenses with implants, Barbara was quite disoriented by the procedure. The glasses she was given were heavy and uncomfortable and Barbara had trouble making the adjustment. Knowing I would be leaving the area soon for Arizona, I became concerned that it might be difficult for her to manage on her own.

I found a small nursing home for Barbara on the outskirts of town. When I nervously proposed the move there she accepted the idea easily, saying "Well, why didn't you think of it sooner?" As she settled into her room overlooking a cornfield, she said the scene reminded her of Vermont. She assured me that change was always good and the features of her room and its view made it the best possible place for her. Before we left the area, I found Barbara a small, well-balanced rocking chair which she planned to use for exercise. Our return visits would always find her there—rocking to center herself in her thigh sockets. On October 18, 1982, Barbara Clark died in her sleep of natural causes. She was ninety-three years old.

EPILOGUE

IN TALKING WITH HER STUDENTS AND COLLEAGUES about Barbara Clark's life and work, we often concluded our discussions with speculation about her most important and enduring contributions. Her special genius for crafting imagery so expressive of the kinesthetic realm, was uppermost for everyone.

As I pieced together the lessons for *The Body Is Round–Use All the Radii,* it occurred to me that Barbara's choice of instructional manuals as the mode for presenting her imagery was somewhat ironic. Of course, the choice was made because she believed all people could be helped by the material and had the right to be aware of it. The familiar "step by step" tone of a "manual" was adopted to engage the readers' attention and give them confidence about learning something new. To present the material as she created it, as the spinning of a magnificent web, would have separated Barbara from the people she was most interested in reaching and compromised her ultimate goal. Thus, she chose the most prosaic of expressive forms to extend her imagery to "the public," and the recognition of much of her genius was relinquished through her steadfast commitment to make sense in their terms. Of this André Bernard said:

> Clark was much more abstract than Todd or Sweigard. She was a master in the use and creation of imagery. But, it was very hard to understand Barbara unless you were in her world. In writing the manuals, Barbara thought that this was her opportunity to reach John Doe—Mr. Average and she really thought that if she made it simple enough that she could do that. She did not realize that her work is like poetry and to appreciate it one must have some kind of identification with the kinesthesia of the poet. Clark thought everyone would see what she saw, and that was the flaw in her teaching. [52]

Many of the individuals who served as sources for this book also remembered Barbara as a gifted teacher. As Joanne Emmons put it, "Miss Clark gave me the sense of my self." [53] Perhaps this sense of self is no more than knowledge of the primary reality—mind and body integrated as one. Barbara's teaching could be characterized as a process of mapping that reality, by awakening and refining the acuity of the kinesthetic sense. Her imagery of elements of skeletal design directed the discovery of key kinesthetic landmarks. Her portrayal of pathways of support and release guided exploration through the inner landscape in between. This process could be quite self-revelatory, particularly for those of us confined and confused by the unrealities of dance. Yet, the experience of self-nurturing engendered by Barbara's teaching was much richer than this notion implies.

A lesson with Barbara always began very casually. She would get a snack from her kitchen and there was talk of the events of the week. Inevitably the discussion led back to something she had learned from Todd or her country life in Vermont. This was not to dwell in the past, as older people sometimes made the mistake of doing, she insisted. Instead we were taking from the past those experiences which would help us understand the present and prepare us for the future.

As the afternoon went on, there were the pictures to study in the anatomy or from Barbara's own collection of drawings. For me, the most important pictures were of the shoulders and neck, the thorax and diaphragm. As we looked at them together, her words would complete the imagery—depth of the shoulder girdle, ease through the intercostal muscles, lengthening the breath. I know these pictures were selected with a sense of what I needed to learn in my body, but they were never presented in that way. Instead, they were offered as the objects of her own intense preoccupation and I was simply invited to share her pleasure in exploring them.

The times when she would insist that I lie down, because I was obviously too tired to take a lesson, were lessons in themselves. Overtly, she did little for me during those times. As she adjusted my cushions or drew the curtain so the light would be less bright, she said very little. Sitting nearby she would center herself and turn inward. Following her into that quiet, I connected to the wisdom in my bones.

When we took walks through the halls of her apartment building or climbed the fire escape stairs, watching her taught me to work actively with the imagery. As we moved together she would make sure that I did not try too hard. A running course of conversation diverted my attention, punctuated by her cutting sense of humor which kept it fun. She wanted me to take a light touch with the imagery and dispense with an overly conscientious nature which could only interfere.

Her permission to learn like this, in the manner of a child learning through effortless identification, set my own creative process into motion. She loved my stories of how thinking of an image got me through a difficult technique class or helped me make a controversial point without losing my composure. As I began to develop my own imagery, she was delighted. "That is very good," she would say as she digested my image through her own experience, and then she would talk about how I could use that idea with my own students someday.

In thinking back on this woman who fundamentally changed my life, I am reminded that our friendship took place in a era in which a bewildering array of gurus, healers and movements related to self-realization were beginning to emerge. With Barbara, the process of personal change was very practical and straightforward, offered to others with no strings attached. It was the sharing of a kinesthetic legacy, made accessible through a creed of simple truths:

"Remember the natural."
> Pay attention to the rhythms of the natural world and know that we are a part of it.

"Keep it in the positive."
> Let go of what cannot be changed and focus on what is possible.

"Find your body balance."
> It is a source of inner integrity which brings balance into our lives.

NOTES

Introduction

1. Marsha Paludan, a former faculty member in dance at the University of Illinois, arranged Clark's session at the conference and facilitated our acquaintance with her.
2. Barbara Clark commonly used the terms "the work" or "the teaching" to refer to the philosophy, techniques and principles which were begun by Mabel Todd.

The Early Years

3. Mabel Elsworth Todd, "Our Strains and Tensions," *Progressive Education* 8 (1931), 244.
4. Todd, "Our Strains and Tensions," 245.
5. Mabel Elsworth Todd, "Balancing of Forces in the Human Being; Its Application to Postural Patterns," 1929. Reprint. *Early Writings 1920 - 1934* (New York: Dance Horizons, 1977), 50.
6. Todd, "Balancing of Forces," 49-50.
7. Jesse Feiring Williams, *The Principles of Physical Education*, 8th ed. (Philadelphia: WB Saunders Company, 1964), 333.
8. *Announcement of the Teachers College, School of Education, School of Practical Arts, 1929-1930* (New York: Teachers College, Columbia University, 1929), 216.
9. Of the students who continued to study and write about Todd's ideas in the process of completing their own degrees, Lulu Sweigard is the best known. Although some sources speculated that Ida Rolf also studied with Todd at Columbia; such reports could not be confirmed.

The Children's Teaching

10. "Snugging" was a term Clark used to describe tactile gestures which moved inward toward the center of the body, from the distal to the proximal end of a bony segment or from an area of muscular holding to a location of bony support.
11. Joanne Emmons, letter to author, 3 September 1984.
12. The Humpty Dumpty rhyme and exercise are described under "Backward Roll - 1/4 Way" in *Part II, Posture Plays.*
13. Barbara Clark, US Patent No. 1917018, 4 July 1933, Clark Papers, Clark Manuals Trust, Tempe, Arizona.

Drawing and Dance in New York

14. Lulu E. Sweigard, *Human Movement Potential: Its Ideokinetic Facilitation,* (New York: Dodd, Mead and Company, 1974), 187.
15. Sweigard, *Human Movement Potential*, 193.
16. Lulu E. Sweigard, letter to author, 16 March 1972.
17. Lulu E. Sweigard, letter to Barbara Clark, 23 January 1957, Clark Papers.
18. Sweigard, *Human Movement Potential*, 192.
19. Joanne Emmons, telephone interview with author, 16 July 1988.
20. Although she continued to send Clark private students for several years, there was probably some sensitivity on Sweigard's part as she became aware that some students preferred the approach of her former assistant. Likewise, Clark bristled when she heard her ideas were dismissed by Sweigard as "unscientific." Although their correspondence revealed the two teachers extended a good measure of companionship to one another for many years, a rivalry did develop between them.
21. Beverly Brown, "Training to Dance with Erick Hawkins," *Erick Hawkins: Theory and*

Training, ed. Richard Lorber (New York: The American Dance Guild, Inc., 1979), 9.

22. Gertrude Mooney, carbon copy of a letter to Dr. Josephine Rathbone, 6 February 1953, Clark Papers.
23. Joanne Emmons, telephone interview with author, 16 July 1988.
24. Emmons, telephone interview, 16 July 1988.
25. André Bernard, telephone interview with author, 8 August 1988.
26. Emmons, telephone interview, 16 July 1988.
27. Joanne Emmons, Notes for PreDance I, n.d., Clark Papers.
28. Emmons, Notes for Predance I.
29. Emmons, Notes for Predance I.

Writing in Pictures

30. Anthony Mannino, telephone interview with author, August 1988.
31. Mannino, telephone interview, August 1988.
32. André Bernard, telephone interview with author, 8 August 1988.
33. Mary E. Waddell, letter to Barbara Clark, South Pasadena, California, 2 February 1957, Clark Papers.
34. Joanne Emmons, interview with author, Albuquerque, New Mexico, 7 August 1989.
35. Emmons, interview, 7 August 1989.
36. Emmons, interview, 7 August 1989.
37. Emmons, interview, 7 August 1989.
38. Joseph Margolis, *"The Trouble with Textbooks,"* Redbook Magazine, March 1965, 65.
39. Cora Belle Hunter, letter to Barbara Clark, n.d., Clark Papers.
40. Carl E. Rollyson Jr. *Marilyn Monroe: A Life of the Actress*, No. 39 *Studies in Cinema*, (Ann Arbor: U.M.I. Research Press, 1986), 45.
41. Rollyson, *Marilyn Monroe*, 60.
42. Sherman Price, letter to Barbara Clark, 9 August 1970, Clark Papers.
43. "Starpoint: Special Training Techniques," *Reporter Dispatch*, 30 January 1964.
44. Christina Kirk, "A New Road to Normalcy for the Retarded Child," *Sunday News*, 18 October 1964.
45. Mabel Elsworth Todd, *The Thinking Body*, 1937. Reprint. (New York: Dance Horizons Inc., 1972), 215.
46. For the edition of *How to Live in Your Axis - Your Vertical Line* presented in *Part III*, the illustrations have been redrawn based on those found in Clark's original manuscript.
47. Joanne Emmons, telephone interview with author, 16 July 1988.
48. James J. Gibson, *The Senses Considered as Perceptual Systems*, (Boston: Houghton Mifflin Company, 1966), 109.
49. Mabel Elsworth Todd, *The Hidden You*, 1953. Reprint. (New York: Dance Horizons Inc., n.d.), 92.
50. Mary Fulkerson, David Woodberry and Nancy Topf were among Clark's students in New York during this period.
51. For further discussion see Cynthia J. Novak, *Sharing the Dance: Contact Improvisation and American Culture*, (Madison: The University of Wisconsin Press, 1990).

Epilogue

52. André Bernard, telephone interview with author, 8 August 1988.
53. Joanne Emmons, interview with author, Albuquerque, New Mexico, 7 August 1989.

Part II

Each One— Teach One

Posture Plays

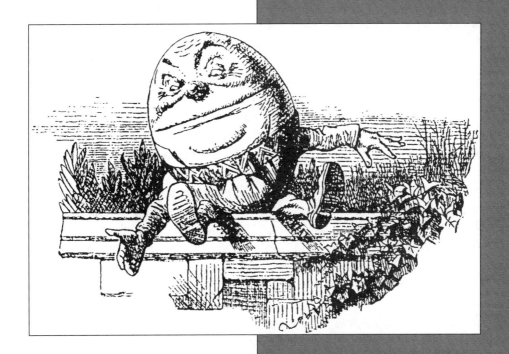

INTRODUCTION

To form good postural habits, children require activities which encourage them to develop good body support in movement. Generally, the preschool child of two to five years lacks the muscular endurance to maintain good balance and coordination in the upright positions of sitting and standing for long periods. If the child is in the vertical plane too much of the time, his body will strain to support itself. Therefore, nursery, kindergarten and primary school programs should include more scientific use of movement activities in the horizontal and semi-vertical planes. Particular attention should be given to rolling, crawling, squatting and other fundamental movements and positions used by nature in developing the child's body.

The *Posture Plays* are planned for the use of teachers with their groups and for mothers and nurses with children in the home. Explanations and descriptions of the correct coordination of movements used in the plays are given to aid the understanding of the adult. These instructions form a standard by which children's postural habits may be observed and will aid the adult in perfecting his own movement. However, specific directions for physical movement should not be given to the child. Instead, movement images are suggested in the plays to stimulate the joints and muscles to carry out improved movement patterns.

With attention centered on an idea for dramatic play, a story or verse, or an image of animal action, the child's interest will be aroused. With a background of enjoyable sensory experiences associated with the actions, the child can begin to develop his own rhythm. The movements should be slow, rhythmical and flowing. This will allow the most complete action through the muscle structure, since tense muscles will be relaxed and weaker ones stimulated into action. Repetition of the plays and observation of other children should be encouraged to improve form.

Because the interests of the mechanical age have taken away from awareness of our natural environment, much emphasis in the plays is given to nature. The movement of animals serves as excellent imagery for physical rhythm and coordination. The domesticated animals, like the cow, horse, sheep, pig, dog or cat, will best serve our purpose. Although these animals seem very ordinary to the average adult, they are fascinating to small children. Of the animals in a zoo, the elephant, buffalo, deer and polar bear are the better choices. Until a little child has developed a good sense of security with the idea of the domestic animals, it is not advisable to have them think of the fiercer ones. For our purposes, the tension associated with those animals could interfere with the best action of the muscles, especially the intercostals and diaphragm.

With each new suggestion, the child should be given the opportunity to place full attention on the new idea until it has made an impression. In line with this principle, only one major new image should be presented in each session of body movement practice. Use this new image long enough to satisfy the child's normal span of attention, but do not carry the idea to the point of boredom. Set a goal or dramatic climax for the end of the play. Lacking an "end" to build to, makes the action grow monotonous and dulls the senses.

The plays described on the following pages should serve to stimulate the use of other activities of this type. The plays can be adapted according to the interests of the children. It is their love of balance and motion (kinesthetic sense) that we are cultivating. In their undirected play, interest in activity itself needs very little external dress. The simpler the story, the more realistic the image, the greater the child's joy of expression and intelligence in action will be.

ROLLING

A child's body proportions are well adapted to rolling. The head is large, the legs are short, the body rounded and the muscle structure very pliable. The rolling action develops the deep muscles of the back, abdomen, thighs, and shoulders and thereby lessens lordosis (sway back), abdominal protuberance, uneven hips and shoulders, and poor head carriage. As the position of the body changes from the back, to the side, to the front, all the muscles of the trunk are being exercised. In this way the back muscles develop sufficient strength to maintain an erect spine and well-balanced head. The front muscles become strong enough to furnish good organic support and the straighter front line that is desired for good alignment.

Sideways Rolling

The aim of rolling sideways is to lengthen the axis. A baby is more relaxed as he begins to roll sideways than an older child or adult. The body proportions of the baby favor an easy tumbling sideways which helps him use the muscles along his axis. You will observe preschool children rolling sideways in various ways. The ones who have been allowed to roll freely during and since babyhood will be the most skillful in coordinating legs, arms and head, as the body slowly turns itself. Those less proficient will show more dislike of the floor and less enjoyment in their coordination. Many of the less proficient children tend to force the turn with tension of the surface muscles and their lower legs and arms. This can shorten the axis and make it rigid, which is the opposite of our aim. These children should learn to roll through practice with imagery and unconscious imitation of other children rather than by direction.

Directions for the Parent or Teacher

1. Lie on the back with the knees easily flexed so the feet rest flat on the floor. The arms should rest at the sides of the body.
2. Relax the shoulders, neck and buttocks until the body weight is centered in the lower middle area of the body between the hips. Keep attention on this throughout the exercise.
3. Relax one arm and bring it close to your side as you slowly roll the body onto that side. Let the other arm fall slowly upward and over the face as you progress.
4. Allow the legs to straighten slowly as the body continues to roll to the abdomen and on to the other side. As the rolling continues on to the back, allow the legs to slowly draw up to the position described in *Step One* and the arm to return to your side.
5. This completes one revolution or sideways roll of the body. Reverse the position of the arms in *Step Three* to roll in the other direction.
6. Imitating the action of a bag of sand being rolled will help the adult to move with ease. With the children, the play being dramatized will determine the number of rolls in one direction before rolling to the other side. One to six rolls is the usual number.

Plays for Sideways Rolling

1. Rolling a Barrel

   As broken chords are played on the piano very slowly and evenly, an adult rolls a small keg or barrel over the floor. If possible, each child in the group should be given the opportunity to roll the object. Keep the child's attention centered on the very slow movement of the barrel to the music. In this way, the child's nervous tension will become somewhat relaxed and he will be prepared to imitate the experience he has observed. Then, the children, singly or in a group, can dramatize the sensory experience of rolling kegs or barrels themselves. The children lie down on the floor and slowly turn their bodies from the back, to the side, to the front, to the other side and so on. See that the children are spaced over the floor so each child has plenty of room. Five or six revolutions is enough to do at one time. A smaller object such as a rolling pin may also be used. A ball is not good imagery because of its association with speed and excited motion.

2. Waves Rolling onto the Beach
   The children can discuss the ocean and trips to the beach. Then, the following ideas can be used for dramatic play:

   > Waves move so quietly you have to listen to hear them.
   > Waves are lying down and sleeping on the ocean floor.
   > Lying on the beach, feet like the feeling of warm sand.

3. Tail Image
   The "tail image" [described under *Breathing in the Rest Positions*] is also helpful in rolling. It serves as a challenge to use with children who respond well to the aims of rolling slowly and evenly.

Sideways Roll with Legs and Arms Extended

This variation of the sideways roll continues the aim of lengthening the spinal axis. This position allows relaxation of the muscles that may hold the lumbar spine in too great a curve. The action of gently attempting to "scratch" the back on a flat surface will stimulate the development of the opposing muscles. The adult's knees will be flexed somewhat in this exercise because of the length of the legs.

Directions for Parent or Teacher

1. Lie on the back on the floor with the knees flexed on the abdomen. The arms rest on the floor at the sides of the body.
2. Straighten the legs and arms toward the ceiling. Allow the weight of the arms and legs to fall back toward the body.
3. Gently "scratch" the lower back on the floor while you relax the muscles of the shoulders, rib carriage, buttocks and knees.
4. Keep the body weight centered in the lower body between the hips, as you fall to one side.
5. With knees flexed on the abdomen and arms relaxed at the sides of the body, return to the back lying position as easily as possible. Then, straighten both legs and arms toward the ceiling as in *Step Two*. Gently scratch the back and relax as in *Step Three*. Keep body weight centered and fall to the opposite side.

Plays for Sideways Rolling with Legs and Arms Extended

Ponies Scratch Their Backs
Use the image of ponies rolling in the grass and scratching their backs as they play.

Backward Roll - 1/4 Way

The complete backward roll is a more difficult form of rolling than the side roll. At first, only the easy portion of it should be used with young children. The action consists of slowly falling backward from a sitting position to lying on the back and then returning to the sitting position. This simple exercise is quite a feat to the child of two to three years of age. To roll backward and then come up again, without the aid of the arms, requires considerable development of the abdominal muscles. At first, the children will be obliged to touch their hands and elbows to the floor to keep from bumping their heads as they go down. They will use the same method to raise themselves up from the floor to return to the sitting position. This shows the weakness in the muscles of the average small child. To roll down and up rhythmically, with the body and legs coordinating well, will require considerable practice by the child as well as the teacher.

Directions for Parent or Teacher

1. Sit on the floor with the knees flexed. Grasp the thighs just below the knees. The feet should be flat on the floor.
2. Center the weight in the lower middle area of the body between the hips by relaxing the arms and legs.
3. Allow the hands to release their hold and slide down the back of the thighs as the body rolls backward to rest on the back. The legs will fold toward the abdomen like the blades of a jackknife.
4. With a little kick of the lower legs and the assistance of the hands on the backs of the thighs, roll forward to the sitting position.
5. The adult should strive for a slow rate of speed in both the rolling down and rolling up, to interest the child in going slowly. It will help the adult to control the rate of falling by centering the action in the deep abdominal muscles.

Plays for Backward Rolling – 1/4 Way

1. Humpty Dumpty
   This play will develop the spinal and abdominal muscles to give stronger more flexible backs and straighter abdominal lines. The play is based on a version of the Humpty Dumpty rhyme. Humpty Dumpty can be represented by drawing a face and body on a small sack of meal or a darning egg. The small sack of meal or sawdust would probably convey the best visual and tactile sense of the body weight in action. Only the face and body of Humpty Dumpty need be drawn on the puppet. Since we are interested in focusing the child's attention on the muscles of the back and pelvis, it is better not to include the legs or arms. Each child should be allowed to be the director of Humpty Dumpty's actions, which consist of allowing the puppet to fall down and sitting it up again as the verse is repeated.

   > Humpty Dumpty sat on a wall,
   > Humpty Dumpty had a great fall,
   > But Humpty Dumpty did not cry,
   > He said, "I can sit up again, if I try."

   When the rhyme and action are familiar, the children can play Humpty Dumpty. The children sit facing the same way on the "wall," which can be represented by a line on the floor. The verse begins and as the second line is expressed, the children roll backward on their backs. The children remain on their backs for the third line of the verse. This line can be hastened a little for greater interest. They roll up to the sitting position on the fourth line. Three or four repetitions of the verse are sufficient for one period of play.

2. For variety, Humpty Dumpty can also roll on the back from side to side in the folded position. Use this addition to the verse and roll three or four times each way:

> Now if you please, hold tight to both knees.
> First we'll roll and look at Polly.
> Then we'll roll and look at Molly.

3. The rolling backward action can also be practiced to this verse, sung to the tune of "Row, Row, Row Your Boat."

> Head to toes and toes to head,
> That's the way to go,
> Merrily, merrily, merrily, merrily,
> Rocking to and fro.

CRAWLING

The horizontal position taken in crawling gives the body a large base of support by means of four uprights. The spinal column is well supported in this way which gives it length. Crawling prepares for walking by using the psoas and iliacus muscles to swing the thighs forward. Crawling also exercises the shoulder girdle and promotes an even development between the shoulders and hips. The action of the arms and legs is an interplay of movement back and forth through the body which instills good habits of coordination. Most children are accustomed to crawling in undirected play. Usually, the motive is to cover the ground rapidly. To aid children in improving their coordination, slower crawling should be encouraged.

Directions for Parent or Teacher
1. Position the body on all fours—hands and knees. The knees should be three to four inches apart. Each hand should rest on the floor directly under its shoulder with the fingers pointing slightly inward. The thumb is relaxed and close to the palm of the hand. The elbows should be relaxed and slightly bent.
2. The thighs should take more of the body weight than the shoulders. Rocking backward slightly in the crawling position, will help move the body weight back to balance over the knees.
3. Think of the back as broad and flat like a table top, with the spine passing in a long, continuous line through its center. The eyes should be directed straight down at the floor. Keep a snug abdominal line as does an animal.

Plays for the Crawling Position

1. Images for Good Balance in the Crawling Position.
    Proper balance of the child's body in the crawling position can be encouraged with plays which stimulate the child to fold back into the thigh joints. Use the idea of the crouching bunny to move the weight off the arms and into the pelvis and legs. The exercise of picking up a spoon or other clean object with the mouth with the hands placed in the lap also may be used. Use imagery of the duck diving for worms or the robin picking up bugs with his beak.

2. The Cat
    On the hands and knees with the head hanging down, purr like a cat. Feel the sound vibrations come up against the small of the back. Then, arch the back at the waistline and hiss.

3. The Dog Stretch
    [Specific directions for movements to accompany this verse were not given.]

He stretches his two paws
To the tips of the claws,
The paws open very slowly
While he yawns.

Keep the waist up,
There's a good pup.

He stretches out full length
Just to test his strength,
He wakes up very slowly
As he yawns.

Keep the waist up,
There's a good pup.

Then, the hind legs to a point
Stretch the muscles of the joint,
While he feels all soft and rolly
And he yawns.

Keep the waist up,
There's a good pup.

Now he arches his back up
Like a strong and wiry pup,
He sits back on his heels so slowly
And he yawns.

Keep the waist up,
There's a good pup.

Crawling Forward on Hands and Knees

Directions For Parents and Teachers

1. Assume the crawling position.
2. Crawl forward in a straight line very slowly: draw up the left knee and put it down a few inches in advance, draw up the right hand and put it down a few inches in advance, draw up the right knee and put it down a few inches in advance, draw up the left hand and put it down a few inches in advance. Continue in this order.
3. Relax the ankles and feet to allow the movement of the thighs to come from deep within the body. The lower legs and toes will just clear the floor.

Plays for Crawling Forward on Hands and Knees

1. Horses Drawing a Heavy Load
    Think of the slow walk of a horse. In crawling, relax each wrist and let the hand hang down like a hoof. The tips of the fingers will drag over the floor. The horse pulls his load with the strength of his hind quarters The pull is actually a push of his hind legs against the ground which pushes his whole weight forward against the harness.

2. Little Bo Peep
    Imitating the butting head action of sheep will aid in keeping the head and back in alignment. The action also stimulates the use of the spinal and deep abdominal muscles. Sing the verse "Little Bo Peep," as the children try the action.

3. Crawl along a line on the floor or crawl between large blocks.

4. For alternating slow with faster rhythms in crawling, use the following verse:

    > Turtle, turtle on your way, why are you so slow?
    > No one else in all this world takes so long to go.
    > To the foot of yonder tree, run a race with me —
    > Who is then the better beast, we will surely see.

Crawling Backward on Hands and Knees

Crawling backward helps children develop slower, better coordinated action. It is less familiar and therefore, they are less likely to associate it with rapid motion. Crawling backward is often employed by the baby before the forward crawl. In moving backward, the heavier pelvic end of the body leads. This centers the weight in the pelvis, stimulating the action of the pelvic muscles. These muscles should be very well developed to support the spinal curves. The sitting and standing positions tend to pull the curves out of line.

Directions for Parents and Teachers

1. Assume the crawling position.
2. Slowly crawl backward in a straight line: draw up the right hand and put it down a few inches to the rear, draw up the left knee and put it back a few inches, draw up the left hand and put it down a few inches to the rear, draw up the right knee and put it back a few inches.

Plays for Crawling Backward

1. Crawling backward following a line on the floor.
2. Place a pillow against a wall as the goal or target. Crawling backward toward the pillow with the pelvis leading the way. The image of "Pretend Eyes" introduced in the *Plays for Walking Backward* can be used in this exercise.
3. Use the image of ponies backing out of stalls. Let the child decide what color pony to be.
4. Use the image of a train, engine at the sacrum and caboose at the head.
5. Take a bean bag or other soft, weighted toy "for a ride" on the back of the pelvis. This will slow the rhythm and encourage balance in backward and forward crawling.

Crawling on Hands and Feet

Crawling on hands and feet is a more difficult form of crawling for the average child. Most children move slowly in this pattern. A few children become proficient enough to move rapidly. This action is particularly good for the development of the pelvic muscles and those in the front of the thighs, lower legs and feet.

Directions for Parent or Teacher

1. The position of the adult's hands and feet will vary according to body proportions, muscle strength and flexibility of the joints. In the beginning, it may be easier to use the fingertips and ball of the foot rather than the whole foot or palm of the hand. The legs and pelvic muscles should take more of the weight than the shoulders and arms.
2. Think of progressing easily forward as if you were going to walk. Each foot steps toward the hand on the same side of the body. The arms are used to balance the action of the legs.
3. Crawl in a straight line forward: draw up the right foot and put it down a few inches in advance, draw up the right hand and put it down a few inches in advance, draw up the left foot and put it down a few inches in advance, draw up the left hand and put it down a few inches in advance.
4. As movement continues and the coordination becomes easier, there will be a slight sway of the body from side to side.

Plays for Crawling on Hands and Feet

[Images of a "Polar Bear" and an "Elephant" were suggested, but not described.]

SITTING

To maintain an erect spine in the sitting position, requires good development of the muscles close to the center of the body. To balance the weight of the shoulders and head well in the vertical plane, depends on the development of the pelvic, thigh and spinal muscles. Children should use sitting positions that stimulate the action of these muscles. Several sitting positions used by young children in play will be considered.

In sitting on the heels or between the heels, it is easy to keep the body erect. Although sometimes uncomfortable for the average adult, the position is excellent for children. Because their legs are short and their muscles pliable, they are able to maintain the position easily.

Sitting with the legs straight out in front is not advised if the muscles in the back of the pelvis and legs restrict leg action. Held for too long, the positioning may result in a rounded back, protruding abdomen, drooping shoulders, forward head, and a sunken chest. Sitting with legs in front of the body and the knees flexed is easier for most children.

Adults often take a cross-legged position when sitting on the floor. When there is good development of the pelvic, inner thigh and spinal muscles, the body can balance well in this position. If there is inadequate development of these muscles, the body will tire quickly of the effort. Sitting with one leg flexed and one leg crossed under may be easier. However, there should be frequent alternation of the legs to avoid uneven development of the right and left sides of the body.

The squatting position is often used by children beginning at about two years of age. They take the position frequently as it is well suited to their size and proportions. Moving in and out of the squatting position is excellent exercise for the child because it develops strength in the psoas, iliacus and adductor muscles. Maintaining the position also lengthens the muscles in the back of the pelvis and thighs. In undirected play, the child often uses the squatting position for comparatively long periods of time. The length of time the child maintains the squatting position can be left to his own physical inclination, since it is so well adapted to his developmental needs.

Children should not be expected to maintain any of the other sitting positions for many minutes at a time, however. In directed play periods or whenever the children are to refrain from moving, as in singing or listening to stories, they may grow tired of sitting. The teacher should suggest that the whole group change frequently from one sitting position to another.

Sitting on chairs should not be done unless the chairs are of proper size for young children. The seat height should be slightly less than the lower leg length and the seat depth less than the length of the thigh. The thigh muscle jacket, covering the buttocks and knees, should be loose enough to allow the thighs to flex fully in their sockets. The feet should rest fully on the floor in front of the chair. The body cannot balance well on the sitting bones (ischial tuberosities) unless the feet can rest comfortably. Support for the back is usually not necessary for the child. For the adult, back support is helpful at each end of the lumbar curve.

Sitting On or Between the Heels

Directions for Parents and Teachers

1. Kneel on the floor with the feet slightly turned inward. The body rests on the floor between the feet or may be partially supported by them.
2. Keep the spine properly erect by maintaining a long line through the center of the body from crown of the head to the area between the sitting bones.
3. Relax the muscles of the lower legs, giving special attention to the ankles and feet. For comfort in this position, the shoes should not bind or be stiff. It may be necessary to remove them.

Plays for Sitting On or Between the Heels

[The images of "Japanese Bowing" and "The Bedouin" were suggested but not described. These plays probably made use of a bowing motion while sitting on or between the heels. The images suggest movement from a vertical position toward the floor and then back to the upright.]

Sitting with Both Knees Flexed

Directions for Parents and Teachers

1. Sit on the floor with the legs in front of the body and parallel to each other. The knees will be flexed and the feet should rest on the floor. The hands may rest in the lap, on the knees or over the lower legs.
2. Support the body weight in the lower middle area of the body between the hips by relaxing any tension in the shoulders, buttocks and knees. Keep a snug line, up and down and across the abdomen, as does the animal.
3. The main thing in sitting is to keep the sit bones under the center of the body and the head balanced easily in between. Keep the body erect by thinking of supporting a weight on the head.

Plays for Sitting with Both Knees Flexed

1. Playing Boat

   Sing the poem, "Lightly Row," as the children sit on the floor with the knees flexed and the hands clasped around the knees. On the first verse the child sways gently forward and back as if rocking forward and back on the waves. On the second verse, the child sways side to side as if the boat were rocking sideways.

   > Lightly row, lightly row,
   > O'er the sparkling waves we go.
   > Smoothly glide, smoothly glide,
   > O'er the deep, blue tide.
   >
   > Let the winds and waters be,
   > Mingled in our Melody.
   > Smoothly glide, smoothly glide,
   > O'er the silent tide.

2. The image of a Merry-Go-Round can also be used this position. The feet step around in a circle, spinning the body around its axis.

The Squatting Position

Directions for Parents and Teachers

1. Sitting and squatting are alike in their action. Squatting is a good image to think of as you sit. Squatting is the sitting action carried to its completion.
2. With the feet in the usual standing position, squat down to the floor by folding the thighs close to the body. The hands may rest on the knees or clasp the front of them.
3. Keep the body balanced by using the deep pelvic muscles in the lower middle area of the body between the hips. Relax the knees, buttocks, shoulders and arms.
4. Often, adults will not be able to touch the heels to the floor in this position. As a substitute, one can remain on the balls of both feet, supporting the elevated heels with a board. It may be easier to separate the feet to balance over the whole foot on one side and over the ball of foot and toes of the other. In the latter case, alternate the feet frequently.

Plays for Squatting

1. The Chicken

   In this play, the children move about in the squatting position.

   > Be a little chicken
   > Hopping on a griddle.
   > How far can she hop?
   > That's just the riddle.

2. The Dog

In this play, the children wiggle the spine while maintaining balance in the squatting position.

> Bend your nice long legs
> Like a dog that begs,
> And sit on them.
>
> Be a dog with a flea
> Rub it off on a tree,
> Then walk, one - two - three.

3. The Butterfly

This play dramatizes moving from a squatting position into standing by slowly unfolding the legs and arms. Then, the children can "flutter" around the room.

> Be a fuzzy caterpillar, all nice and soft,
> Unfold your legs and wings to fly aloft.
> For now you are butterfly, handsome and gay,
> What more could you wish for, all in one day?

4. [Images of a "Duck Walk" and "Telescoping Together" were also suggested, but not described. The "Duck Walk" idea suggests walking while in the squatting position. The image of "Telescoping Together" may have been a way of thinking about folding into the squat from a standing position.]

STANDING

In standing, there is a long line of weight balanced on end, supported by only two uprights. For this reason, the standing position is more difficult for most little children. Too much standing increases the tendency to develop lordosis (sway back), abdominal protuberance, uneven hips and shoulders and poor head carriage. Most preschool children will be helped by practicing more diversified forms of vertical carriage such as walking backward or walking with a weight on the head. However, if the child's muscles are not strong, he should assume the positions described earlier, which are more favorable to body development.

In school activities, in which the children are in a circle and holding hands, adults and older children should take care not to pull the smaller child's hands and arms up too far. When the child's arms are pulled upward it is more difficult for him to maintain good body balance. When children are standing and also using their hands and arms in work or play, watch for signs of tension in their shoulders. When they are standing and also lifting, carrying or chopping with arms, encourage them to distribute arm action down through the whole back. When moving heavy loads, teach them to use the legs to push the weight rather than using the rib case and shoulders to pull it.

Plays for Standing

1. [This poem called the "Lobster's Tail" may have been used to build awareness of relaxation at the end of the spine in the standing position.]

> Be a Lobster good to eat,
> Tail curled down between your feet,
> As you stand.

2. [The "tail image," described under *Breathing in the Rest Positions* was also used in the standing position.]

Walking Backward

With attention centered so much of the time on moving in a forward direction, the abdomen and chin tend to be thrust forward. This increases the depth of the spinal curves at the waistline and neck, and shortens the spinal muscles. By reversing the direction of movement for a short distance, the opposite points will be emphasized; the lower back and the back of the head will tend to lead. In walking backward, as in crawling backward, the back muscles tend to lengthen naturally. Walking backward is also helpful in developing freer motion at the thigh and ankle joints.

Directions for Parent or Teacher

1. Stand easily erect. Relax the arms and let them hang perfectly free. Relax the thighs and let them move rhythmically from the center of the body.
2. Walk backward very slowly with short steps and a very deliberate and flexible toe to heel action in a straight a line.

Play for Walking Backward

Pretend Eyes

1. Place a small mask on the back of the child's head. The mask provides a reason for the child to imagine "pretend eyes" on the back of the head. All the children in the group should be allowed to try the mask on in this way. If it is possible, let them use a mirror to see how they look. Then suggest they try walking backward using their "pretend eyes."
2. Clear a space eight to twelve feet long and place a small chair at the end of it. The chair is the "goal" of walking backward. The space between the chair and the starting position or "home base" should be eight to ten feet long. The space should be wide enough to allow four feet of clear space on either side. There should no apprehension about hitting anything or distraction from other children who may be participating.
3. The child puts on the mask and stands on "home base." He should be directly in line with the front of his assigned chair, but with his back toward it. The child turns and looks at the chair with his "real eyes" and then begins to walk backward toward the chair sensing its position with his "pretend eyes." Ideally, the child walks toward the chair and sits down without turning his head to see where he is going. At first, most children will look to check on their progress several times. As they gain confidence in walking backward, they will take pleasure in moving smoothly and finding the middle of the chair with their "pretend eyes."

Walking Forward

Improved body balance in walking forward can be encouraged by having the child slow his rhythm, placing the feet carefully in each step.

Play for Walking Forward

Draw attention to the seesaw action of the foot at the ankle joint. Point out that the heel drops down below the ankle as the front of the foot swings up. The image of the seesaw can be used as the children walk down two parallel lines placed four or five inches apart on the floor. The middle of each heel and the second toe should contact the line on each step. The children can be reminded of the seesaw ankle action by singing the following verse:

> Seesaw, Margery Daw,
> Jacky shall have a new master;
> Jacky must have but a penny a day,
> Because he can't work any faster.

Walking with a Weight on the Head

Sitting, standing or walking with a weight on the head is excellent for strengthening the back muscles and improving the balance of the head and upper body. A soft substance which shapes to the top of the head is better than a hard, flat object. A very light weight should be used with small children to prevent strain or dislike for the action.

Directions for Parent or Teacher

1. Fold a light blanket or sweater into a square of about nine inches and place it on the top of the head.
2. Support the weight on the head from the base of the spinal column. Relax the arms and let them hang perfectly free.
3. Proceed forward slowly with short steps, letting the thighs swing directly forward from the center of the body.

Play for Walking with a Weight on the Head

A small light-weight bean bag can be used on a child's head. Strain in the neck indicates the weight is too heavy or the child is proceeding too rapidly. Walking down a line or crack on the floor while balancing the weight will slow the rhythm. A rhyme can also be sung while the child is walking.

> Seesaw sacerdown,
> This is the way to London Town,
> One foot up, the other down,
> Seesaw sacerdown.

Climbing the Stairs

It is difficult for young children to use most stairways because the steps are too large for their body proportions. For learning to climb stairs, the child should have steps that are broad and no more than two inches in height. On a such a small staircase, the child should be able to keep his balance without the use of hand support on the bannister. He should also be able to use each leg alternately and equally. On adult-sized stairs, the child should be allowed to climb up on hands and feet. On the way down, the child can sit on the stairs and lower himself one stair at a time.

Directions for Parent or Teacher

1. Balance the body weight in the pelvic area. Relax the shoulders and rib case and keep the spine long.
2. Fold the thigh at the hip joint and slide the whole foot onto the stair. When the body is balanced over that foot, place the other foot onto the second stair. When the body is balanced well over the foot on the second stair, leave the first stair behind and continue to the third stair.
3. Continue to move up the steps in this way, folding at the hip joints and taking the weight easily and rhythmically.

Play for Climbing the Stairs

The Pedaling Tricycle

The child can climb the stairs thinking of pushing away from each step just as he pushes down on the pedal of a tricycle. In other words, it is the pushing down that helps him to go up.

JUMPING

In jumping, the pelvic and thigh muscles must be employed, which directly stimulates their development. The thighs and hips have the heaviest bones, strongest muscles and the fewest articulations. Just as the lion and tiger leap through the strong muscles moving these basic bones, man should also center and move from this base of power.

Directions for Parent or Teacher

1. Stand with the arms relaxed and hanging free, without tension in the knees or lower legs. Let the chest relax and breath easily.
2. Prepare for the jump by letting go of the muscles of the chest, and centering attention on the pelvic muscles. Lower the weight into a semi-squat by folding the ankle, knee and hip joints.
3. The best coordination of the legs and pelvis will occur if the jump is directed slightly forward on a diagonal line rather than directly upward on a vertical line.

Plays for Jumping

1. Animals

    Have the children use imagery of animals, especially of the cat family. Think of the jump being like the spring of an animal. Emphasize the springiness of jump rather than the height of jump.

2. Jack Be Nimble

Use the rhyme "Jack Be Nimble" to give children experience in the preparation for jumping by folding in the thigh, knee and ankle joints. Have the children rhythmically bounce by flexing and extending softly in those joints as they say:

> Jack be nimble, Jack be quick,

The children should lower into a semi-squat position as you start the next line, and on "over," they jump forward and up.

> Jack jumps over the candlestick.

The last line is the recovery from the jump or the landing. Remind the children to land with easy action in the joints by encouraging them to land "quietly" or "softly."

3. Rocket Countdown

Use the imagery of a rocket's countdown as the children fold into the leg joints to prepare for jumping. With each individual child, the teacher can count down while touching various levels of the spine. The countdown begins at the neck level as you say "five." Continue the countdown touching lower levels of the spine with each count. You will end with "one" at the base of the spine or sacrum. With awareness at the base of the spine the child is ready for a big jump.

RESTING

For most children, nap time becomes a negative phase which is wrongly associated with confinement, illness, punishment or boredom. The average mother or nurse insists upon a rest period. Without one, the child will become fatigued toward the end of the day. He may be easily irritated and show less willingness to cooperate with companions or those who take care of him. At mealtime, his consumption of food may be below the usual. At night, even if he falls asleep immediately upon getting into bed, he is apt to be more restless than if he had not been so exhausted. Thus, the need for a rest period is not questioned by most parents and educators. How the rest period should be spent for the best advantage to the growing body and how to gain the child's cooperation in it should be uppermost in their thinking.

Rest should be treated casually. The animal rests frequently and so should the child. Provide places for casual resting in the play room, in a padded box or in the Tunnel Toy. Animals look comfortable when they rest. They are quite deliberate in the way in which they place themselves for a nap. They seem to enjoy the position and the sense of comfort it gives them.

There are three comfortable resting positions to consider in teaching body movement to young children: resting on the back, resting face downward and resting on the side. In these, the bony structure adapts itself readily to its support. These positions also help to maintain the body weight near the center of the body. Suggestions are also given for teaching relaxed breathing in any of the resting positions.

Resting on the Back

Tight pelvic and lower back muscles can increase the tendency to lordosis and abdominal protuberance. The position of lying on the back with the knees flexed and feet resting flat on the supporting surface is especially helpful for relaxing these muscles that might hold the lower back in too pronounced an inward curve. Gradually, the lumbar curve can relax into greater length in this position. However, it should never be forcefully flattened.

Directions Parent or Teacher

1. Lie on the back with the knees easily flexed so the feet rest on the floor. It is best to remove the shoes for resting. Some relaxation may be achieved with a medium height heel on the shoes. High heels should not be used because the height of the heel extends the foot at the ankle joint. This contracts the muscles in the back of the leg.
2. If it is hard to relax in this position, allow one leg to extend downward and rest full length on the floor. Change legs by drawing the extended one up to the flexed position, and straightening the other leg downward to rest full length on the floor. Alternate the legs in this way for a few moments and then flex both knees again.
3. In the beginning, a helpful variation of this position involves placing the lower legs and feet on a low chair seat. This position allows the weight of the thighs to rest in the pelvis at the thigh joints. This encourages the development of the pattern of control of the legs by the deep pelvic muscles. The use of imagery and action to increase toe and ankle action while in this position also stimulates development of these muscles.
4. The arms can relax full length at the sides of the body with the palms and arms turned up toward the ceiling. Or the lower arms can bend at right angles to the upper arms with the palms of the hands on the upper abdomen. The elbows should remain close to the sides of the body.
5. The arms can also lap over (encircling) the front of the body above the breasts. The elbows will point towards the ceiling. The lower arms will hang downward over the sides of the body with the palms toward the body. Occasionally alternate the position of the arms.

Resting Face Downward

This position helps to relax muscles that may hold the upper back in too pronounced a backward curve. It straightens and lengthens the entire spinal column. This position requires a very firm surface such as the floor. The springs and mattress of a child's bed should not sag in the middle. Poor support in this position increases the tendency to develop lordosis, abdominal protuberance and generally poor posture. A pillow should not be used under the head in this position. Placing the upper body on a higher level than the rest of the body could produce strain in the neck and shoulders.

Directions for Parent or Teacher

1. Lie face downward with the front of the thighs, abdomen, and chest resting on the floor or bed.
2. The arms should be close to the sides of the body with the backs of the hands resting on the floor and the palms upward.

3. The feet will be extended with the toes pointing slightly inward. If the legs are bowed or ankles pronated, let the toes hang over the edge of the mattress in this position, with the feet parallel.
4. Turn the head so either side of the face rests on the floor. Alternate the position of the head frequently.

Resting on the Side

Lying on the right or left side of the body with the thighs flexed, allows the rib carriage to lengthen downward. This strengthens the abdominal and lower back muscles. Balancing the structure on its side also keeps the body rounded and the hips narrowed.

Directions for Parent or Teacher

1. Lie on the floor with the middle of either side resting on the floor. Pay attention to positioning the exact middle side of the head, rib case, hips and thighs. The side seam of a cloth doll serves as a good image in doing this.
2. The adult will find that a folded blanket or pillow placed under the side of the head, is necessary for proper support.
3. The thighs should make a right or an obtuse angle with the body proper.
4. The lower legs should make a right or an obtuse angle with the thighs at the knee joints. They should never hold an acute angle as this keeps the muscles of the back of the thighs in a state of tension.
5. The feet should rest at right or slightly obtuse angles to the lower legs at the ankle joints.
6. The arm on the floor should rest a little forward of the chest which is balanced through its middle. The lower part of the arm resting on the floor may be extended or bent at the elbow joint. It should be relaxed and of no assistance in the body's support.
7. The top arm may rest at full length upon the middle of the upper side of the body or it may bend at the elbow with some part of the relaxed hand touching the floor.
8. Alternate between lying on one side, and then rolling over to lie on the other side.

Plays for Resting in Any Position

1. Resting Animals

   Because of the differences between the human body and most animals, it is not desirable to imitate the exact positions animals use in rest. There is enough similarity however, to use the child's dramatic interest in animals as an incentive for resting well. For the lying on the back, use pictures of bear and leopard cubs, who frequently take the position in play and for naps. For younger children, pictures of kittens and puppies will be equally good. For the face down position, the seal, alligator and fish are the closest to the human position in resting face downward. For resting on the side, domestic animals such as the cow, sheep, pig, cat or dog may be used.

2. The Cradle

   Images of floating on water or on a cloud can be used for relaxation on any of the resting positions. This verse can also be used to suggest ease and comfort while resting:

Be a cradle made of willow,
With your chest soft as a pillow,
And cuddle down into it.

Breathing in the Resting Positions

Our aim in breathing is to lengthen exhalation. Children who are less well coordinated are often unable to exhale easily. These children can be helped to exhale by practicing a muscle pattern which lengthens the muscles along the sides and down the back of the spinal axis. Exhalation and lengthening the muscles down the back of the spine work together. As you do one activity you are also doing the other.

Plays for Better Breathing in the Resting Positions

1. The Tail Image

   The feeling the child senses when he strokes a cat from its head down toward its tail can become a symbol or image for what his own spine can be like. The image can be applied in all positions by the teacher who encourages the child to think of the cat as she strokes down his back. The resting positions are a good place to begin. As the teacher traces down the back, the child lazily blows an exhalation through the lips. Eventually, the positions of sitting and standing can also be used. The child should be reminded of the idea frequently—every day if possible. Then he will form the habit of lengthening his spine downward as he releases his breath and starts to move.

2. The Tape Measure

   A tape measure to mark the distance down the back achieved in exhalation can be used as an incentive. Show the tape measure to the child and let him see a length of ten inches. Then, place the tape over the middle of his upper back and use the pressure of your finger to indicate the distance he will try to go in exhaling. As ten inches becomes possible for him, try fifteen inches and so on. The well known locations on the body, such as the waistline, the back of the knees or the heels, also serve well as goals.

3. Blowing an Instrument

   Blowing a whistle, horn or other musical instrument is very good for lengthening the exhalation phase of the breath. Encourage the child to think down the back as he blows.

4. Abacus

   Touch the spinous processes of the vertebra with gentle pressure down the back. Start at the lowest levels and move upward. At each level, the child imagines the bead of an abacus sliding downward.

5. The Train

   The child plays the part of the engine letting off steam. The child can hiss as the teacher slides her hands downward over the sides of his ribs to relax them. Eventually the child can be taught to cross his own arms over his chest and slide them downward over the ribs as he takes the hiss.

6. Teakettle

    Use the image of the simmering teakettle. Drink in the breath through the nose and then let off steam by slowly hissing the breath through the teeth.

SEQUENCING BASIC MOVEMENTS

When the children are familiar with most of the basic movements and resting positions, it is useful to combine them.

Play for Combining Several Basic Movements

Ponies

Let the child decide which color pony he will be today. First the pony backs a long way out of his stall [crawling backward]. Then, he pulls a heavy load up a hill, crawling very slowly [crawling forward]. When he comes to the pasture he is so tired and hot that he rolls on his back in the grass [backward roll - 1/4 way]. With all four feet straight up to the sky he rolls from side to side. He scratches his back and rolls to the left, and then he scratches his back and rolls to the right [sideways roll with arms and legs extended]. Finally, he rests [resting on the side] and breathes quietly.

Technique
for
Movement
Lessons

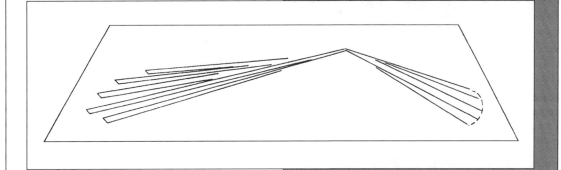

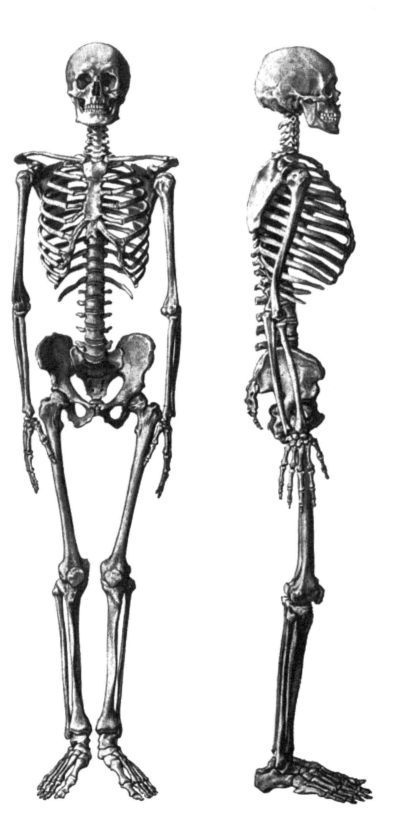

The Skeleton

Spalteholz-Spanner

GENERAL INTRODUCTION AND SPINAL CONSTRUCTION

Teaching Materials: Picture of the skeleton
Picture of the superficial muscles of the back
Bones - pelvis, femur and a few lumbar vertebrae
Design of the foot - top view

Demonstration 1:

We teach more efficient use of the body in movement. A simple understanding of levers and ful-crums can help us learn how to distribute weight through the bony structure.

> (Show picture of the skeleton.)

The bony structure consists of the spine with the skull, two lower extremities and two upper extremities. The heavier end of each of these five parts is located near the center of the structure.

> (As you speak, move pointer from the skull down through the spine.
> Then, move the pointer from the ends of the extremities toward the
> mid-line of the body.)

Demonstration 2:

> (Show the femur, pelvis and vertebrae.)

The extremities consist of straight levers. The spinal column has round or irregularly shaped levers called vertebrae. There are twenty-four of these vertebrae, which are like building blocks in the column we call the spine. The sacrum is the base of the column. The weight of the head and other attachments to the spine is lowered to the sacrum through the bodies of the vertebrae on the front side of the column. From the sacrum, the weight passes through the pelvis to the ischia in sitting. The ischia are two rounded bony masses or prominences at the lower end of the pelvis. Since the body rests on these in the sitting position, they may also be called sitting bones. The spinal column should be centered between the ischia.

Practice Movement A: Resting on the Ischia

With palms turned up, sit on the fingertips to experience the transfer of weight. Return hands to the lap and rock from side to side on the ischia.

Practice Movement B: Centering the Head between the Ischia

Combine the image of centering the head between the ischia with rocking very slightly from side to side.

Trapezius

Latissimus Dorsi

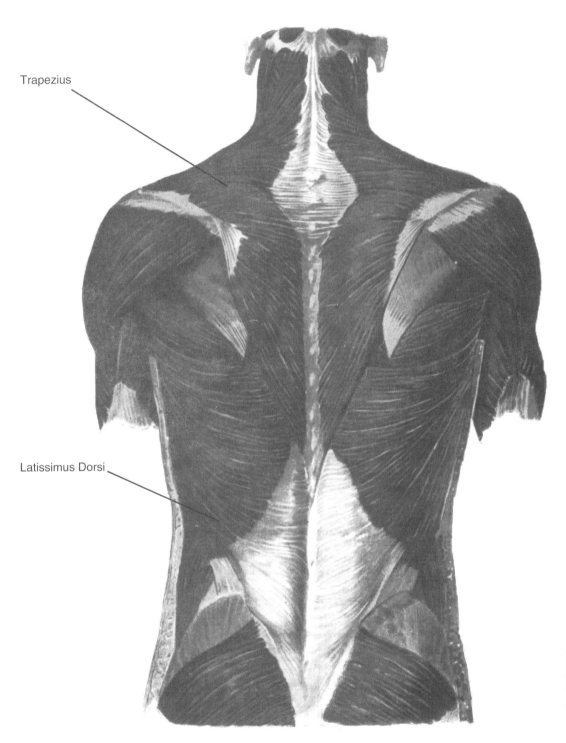

Spalteholz-Spanner

Superficial Muscles of the Back

Demonstration 3:

Lowering the weight through the spinal column may be disturbed by improper shoulder action.

(Show picture of the superficial muscles of the back.)

The trapezius and latissimus dorsi muscles of the shoulders and back have their inner attachments on the spinous processes of the vertebrae. The spinous processes are the little knobs we feel when we run our fingers down the mid-back line. These projections on the back of the spinal column are behind the round bodies of the vertebrae. Undue shoulder tension, pulling upward on these points, disturbs the lowering of weight through the vertebral bodies to the base of the column. We need to lengthen, relax or let go of these muscle lines, some longitudinally and some transversely, to enable the spine to distribute the weight well.

We will use "imagery" in learning to improve balance and acquire better habits of movement. In the first practice movement, the image or picture of rocking was used in balancing the weight of the spine and transferring it from one ischia to the other. In the next practice movement, we will use the image of lengthening the lower angles of the trapezius and latissimus dorsi muscles.

Practice Movement C: Relaxing the Shoulder Pull on the Spine

We use the table for some of our positioning and practice. The large horizontal resting surface allows the pupil to distribute the body weight more easily. The pupil is placed on the right side so the teaching may begin on the left side of the body. Generally, people are more active on the right side. This gives the right side greater control and therefore more tension. The left side should be stimulated to do more work. As the left side takes over more of the body support, the right side will begin to relax.

Place a pillow under the head and see that the back is aligned with the side of the table. The knees should be slightly flexed. Place a folded blanket between pupil's lower legs and feet. The teacher's fingers should be placed lightly over the lower angles of the trapezius and then the latissimus dorsi. The teacher's touch should give direction to the pupil and note response. Change from one area to the other in accordance with results.

Imagery: *Lengthening the lower angles of the trapezius and latissimus dorsi downward; the extension of their pointed ends.*

Practice Movement D: Aligning the Toes

Aligning the toes can help the pupil regain sensory awareness of action at the center of the foot. Thinking of action through simple lines will help the pupil relate the toes to the ankle.

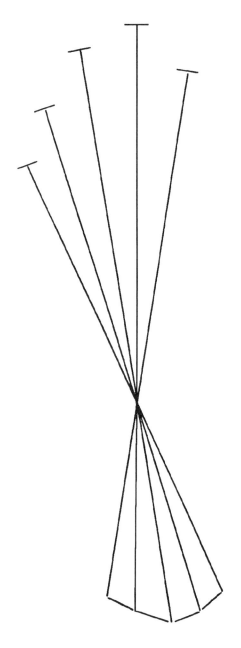

Foot Design - Top View

(Show foot design - top view.)

Support the pupil's foot with one hand. Run the fingers of the other hand lightly from the tip of the large toe to the ankle fulcrum. Request the pupil follow the movement of your fingers toward the ankle in his imagination. Continue with the other toes, one by one. Repeat the action with the first and second toes. Emphasize the idea of the weight moving in from the tip of the toes to the ankle.

Imagery: Train moving into station,
            boat moving into harbor, etc.

Have pupil change from the right to the left side. Repeat Practice Movements C and D.

Practice Movement E: Getting Off the Table

Explain the importance of using the imagery not only in rest but also as the pupil goes into movement. The pupil should move his knees close enough to the edge of the table, so his lower legs will swing down easily as his body comes up. The hand lying on top of the body can aid him by giving a little push on the table.

Imagery: As the pupil comes up to sitting, he
            can imagine lowering the weight
            through the round bodies of the
            vertebrae from head to ischia.

Demonstration 4:

The main objective of each lesson can best be learned through a pictorial illustration. Show the principle in an ideal manner, using something that would appeal to the pupil's age and interests, such as pictures of a Greek statue, a modern dancer or an athletic figure. The picture for this lesson should show ideal sitting or good alignment of the spine as it rests on the ischia.

SPINAL AWARENESS

Teaching Materials: Picture of superficial muscles of the back
                            Picture of pectoralis major muscle

Demonstration 1:

(Show the picture of the trapezius and latissimus dorsi muscles so the pupil may renew his concept of these images for the back. Turn to the picture of the pectoralis major.)

Point out the origin of the pectoralis major along the side of the sternum and the length of the collar bone. Describe how the muscle ends on a ridge on the upper arm bone. The pectoralis muscle in the front of the shoulder acts in the same way the trapezius does for the back of the shoulder. There will be better shoulder movement if the tonus of the pectoralis and the trapezius are more alike. The usual tendency is to keep the pectoralis muscle overly contracted, which disturbs structural alignment.

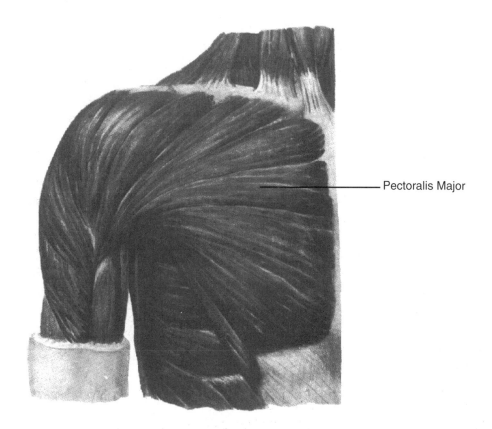

— Pectoralis Major

Spalteholz-Spanner

Pectoralis Major Muscle

Practice Movement A:

Review Resting on the Ischia and Centering the Head Between the Ischia.

Practice Movement B: Walking

Walk naturally around the room. Think of centering the head on its level between the ischia on their level.

Practice Movement C:

Lying on the table, review Relaxing the Shoulder Pull on the Spine.

Practice Movement D: Evening the Tonus Front and Back of the Shoulders

The teacher's fingertips are placed in the soft hollows slightly below the glenohumeral joint in the front of the body. The fingertips of the other hand are placed in the corresponding area in back and slightly below the glenohumeral joint. Adjust through sensory awareness until pectoralis and trapezius muscles seem more equal in tonus.

Practice Movement E:

Review Aligning the Toes. Have the pupil change from his right side to lying on his left side and repeat Practice Movements C, D and E.

Demonstration 2:

We will begin quarter-turn rolling by rolling from the back to the left side. This follows the pattern for development of the left side of the body that we are using for other movements. Unequal use of the body can best be corrected by strengthening the weaker side.

Practice Movement F: Rolling the Body a Quarter-Turn to the Side

The pupil rests on his back with the knees flexed and toes turned slightly inward. The arms rest at the sides of the body. He should begin by visualizing the lower angles of the trapezius and latissimus dorsi muscles extending downward. As he gets a little sensory awareness of lengthening the spine, he starts to turn the body toward his left. In completing the roll, he brings the right leg to a position of rest over the left leg. The return to the starting position should be slow and smooth. The pupil's right foot should move back a little to support the body as the movement begins. The thought of lengthening the lower angles of the back muscles continues until he has reached the starting position of lying on his back. Repeat this rolling action once or twice to the left side only.

THIGH FULCRUM AWARENESS

Teaching Materials: Bones - pelvis and femurs
Design of mechanical axis lines
Picture of temporalis muscle

Demonstration 1:

(Show the pelvis and thigh bones in the standing position.)

We have seen how the ischia receive the weight of the body in sitting. In standing, the tops of the thigh bones receive the body's weight. The femurs have heads shaped like golf balls. These femur heads fit well into socket cups placed deeply in the pelvis. Changing from a sitting position to standing does not alter the position of the ischia. In standing, the ischia become hanging protuberances beneath the thigh sockets.

(Show mechanical axis line design.)

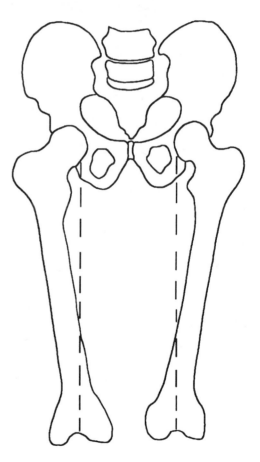

In standing, the counter-thrust to gravity is carried from the center of the foot to the thigh joint. The action follows a straight line called the "mechanical axis line," rather than the curve of the bone.

Practice Movement A: Sitting to Standing

The pupil moves forward on the chair seat, places one foot a little in advance of the other and rises to the standing position. The pupil should picture the action of a crowbar, prying up a heavy mass. The mass is the weight of the torso. The crowbar action occurs at the top of the mechanical axis lines. This image will help the pupil get a feeling of support at the top of the femurs rather than through the knees, lower legs or feet.

Practice Movement B: Standing to Sitting

The pupil places one foot a little behind the other and lowers to a sitting position. The pupil visualizes the crowbar action at the upper ends of the mechanical axis lines supporting the body weight as it is lowered to the chair. Repeat Practice Movements A and B, three or four times.

Mechanical Axis Lines

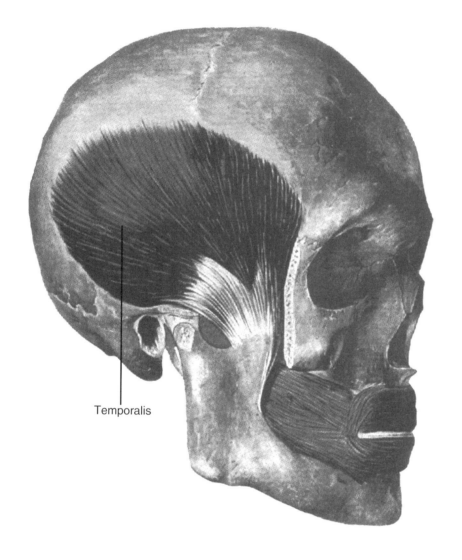

Temporalis

Spalteholz-Spanner

The Temporalis Muscle

Demonstration 2:

The center of action for the dance plié or thigh folding action is at the thigh joints. The body support should be sensed at the tops of the femurs as the movement takes place. The folding action will strengthen the psoas and iliacus muscles and relax their opponents, the gluteal muscles.

Practice Movement C:

Review Walking. Moving naturally around the room, the pupil imagines support on the tops of the femur bones.

Practice Movement D: The Dance Plié

The pupil imagines support of the body on the tops of the femurs as he practices a slight folding movement. He lets the knees, lower legs and shoulders relax as much as he can.

Imagery: Balancing on the tops of the thigh heads.

Practice Movement E:

Lying on the table, review Relaxing the Shoulder Pull on the Spine, Evening the Tonus Front and Back of the Shoulders, and Aligning the Toes.

Demonstration 3:

(Show picture of skull with the temporalis muscle.)

The temporalis muscle is a spherical muscle on the side of the skull. Notice that the perimeter of the muscle begins on the back of the head and extends around the side of the skull nearly to the eye socket. The temporalis muscle attaches to the jaw in front of its fulcrum. The jaw has its fulcrum in front of the ear. Place the fingertips of each hand over these joints and sense them by opening and closing the jaw. The temporalis muscle lengthens as the jaw drops and shortens to close the jaw. Hypertension of this muscle is common and most people need to recondition the use of it.

Practice Movement F: Expanding the Temporalis Muscle

With the pupil lying on the right side, the fingertips of the teacher's hand should lightly trace the extensive perimeter of the temporalis muscle. Begin with the area around the mastoid process and work forward to above the ear and then to the temple.

Imagery: Fan open the temporalis muscle.

The pupil turns and lies on his left side. Movement is repeated on the right side of the pupil's head. Review Rolling the Body a Quarter-Turn to the Side and Getting Off the Table.

PSOAS ACTION AWARENESS

Teaching Materials: Bones - pelvis and femurs
Picture of psoas muscle
Cloth pattern of psoas

Demonstration 1:

The psoas muscles suspend the thigh bones from the lumbar spine. From each side of the spinal column, they follow a diagonal path through the abdomen and pelvis. They pass over the front of the pelvic rim and fasten to the lesser trochanters on the inner, upper sides of the thigh bones. The lesser trochanters cannot be felt with the fingertips. The greater trochanters, on about the same level as the lesser trochanters, are near the surface of the body on the outside of the thigh.

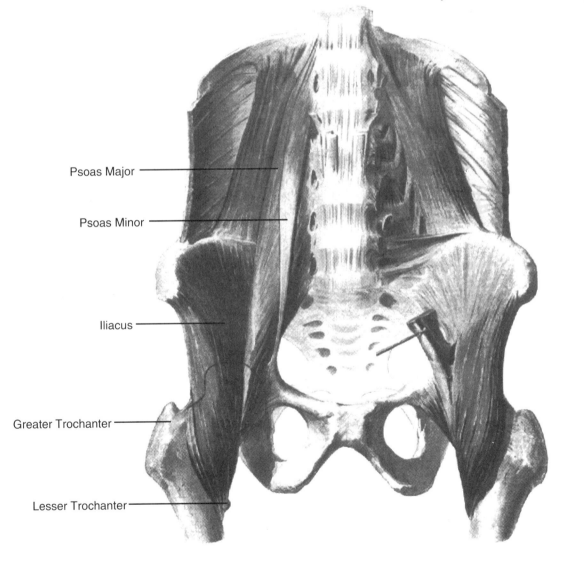

The Psoas Muscle

> (Fasten the cloth pattern of the psoas muscle to the top of the thigh bone. Articulate the femur with the pelvis. Place the upper end of the cloth pattern at the twelfth thoracic vertebra. The lower end will be at the little trochanter of the femur. Suspend the thigh bone through the cloth pattern and swing it slightly.)

This is the way the thigh lever moves in walking. We will practice the "psoas walk" to become aware of these muscles as they instigate forward movement of the legs.

Practice Movement A:

Review Sitting to Standing and Standing to Sitting.

Practice Movement B: The Psoas Walk

Start with the left thigh. Instruct the pupil to place the back of the left hand over the left side of the twelfth thoracic vertebra just above the waistline. [Tactile indication of the highest origin of the psoas muscle in the back of the body.] He then places the fingertips of the right hand over the pelvic rim to the left of the pubis. [Tactile indication of the insertion of the psoas muscle at the lesser trochanter deep in the thigh crease.] Thinking of the action of the cloth pattern of the psoas, he swings the left thigh forward, making a short step. He continues walking with the right side and then the left. The right comes forward a half-step to even the stance with the left foot, making three and one-half steps in all. He retraces his steps backward, beginning with the left thigh, taking three and one-half steps. Have the pupil move the back hand one-half inch lower and repeat the same process. He lowers the back hand again and repeats. Since there are six vertebrae involved, going forward and backward will take place six times.

Have the pupil reverse hands [so the right hand moves down the sides of the vertebrae and the left hand indicates the right lesser trochanter] and repeat the procedure on the right side. Have the pupil change to the left side. Repeat the practice on the left side again to strengthen the weaker muscles through additional practice.

Imagery: Visualizing action through the psoas muscles.

Practice Movement C:

Review Relaxing the Shoulder Pull on the Spine, Evening the Tonus Front and Back of the Shoulders, and Aligning the Toes on both sides. Review Rolling the Body a Quarter-Turn to the Side and Getting Off the Table.

Demonstration 2:

Present a picture showing good action of the psoas muscle, such as *Winged Victory.*

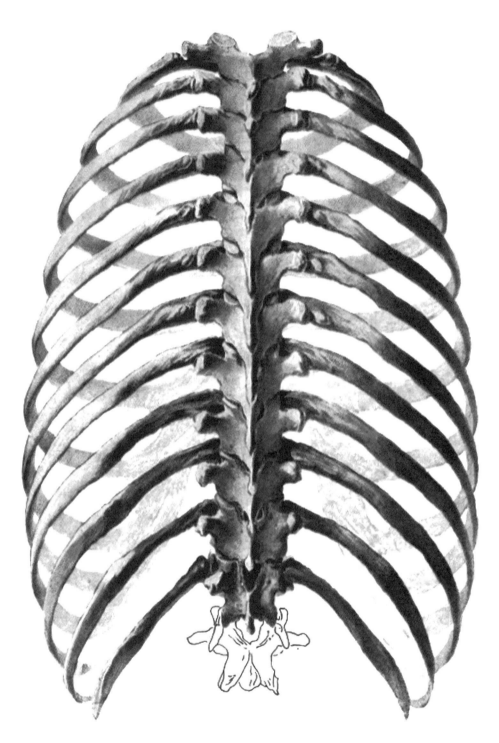

Spalteholz-Spanner

Thoracic Skeleton - Back View

RIB FULCRUM AWARENESS

Teaching Materials: Picture of thorax
                            Picture of thoracic vertebra with ribs

Demonstration 1:

(Show pictures of the thorax and thoracic vertebra with ribs.)

In these lessons, we have changed the habit of holding weight in the upper part of the spine by allowing it to pass down into the lower part of the spine. This lengthening action can take place more easily if we also sense the deep rib fulcrums on the sides of the vertebral bodies.

There are twelve ribs on each side of the spine. The head of each rib should be centered in its socket on the side of the spinal column. These articulations are in the sides of the vertebral bodies and intervertebral discs, almost two inches deeper than the surface of the body. The ribs are paired, right and left. The weight of each pair should be centered equally in their sockets in the column. This helps to keep the spine straight, rather than veering to either side.

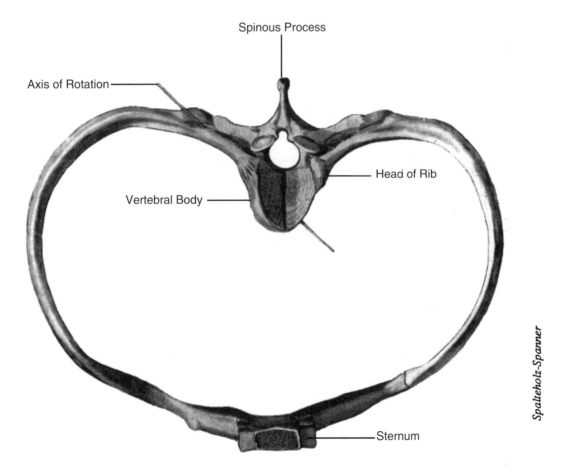

Thoracic Vertebrae with Ribs

Practice Movement A:

In standing, review The Dance Plié and The Psoas Walk.

Practice Movement B:

Lying on the right side, review Relaxing the Shoulder Pull on the Spine and Expanding the Temporalis Muscle.

Practice Movement C: Centering the Ribs at the Spinal Fulcrums

The teacher begins with the first rib on the pupil's upper left side. The teacher places the tip of the thumb or a fingertip of the right hand lightly over the area of the spinal fulcrum of the rib. The fulcrum is on the side of the vertebral body, deep to the teacher's touch. The teacher can only indicate the location by touching to the left of the spinous process.

Imagery: *The pupil visualizes the center of the head of the rib meeting the center of its spinal fulcrum, about two inches deeper than where he feels the teacher's touch.*

The teacher continues this process for each of the twelve ribs from the top to the bottom of the thorax. The teacher should stand toward the pupil's feet to give something of a diagonal thrust, upward and inward. The teacher numbers the ribs aloud, one through twelve, as he works at each level. This will help to give a better sense of location for each of the ribs, making it easier for the pupil to practice by himself.

The teacher should be careful not to drag his finger from one rib to the next. Touch lightly, feel the response. Pick up the finger from the pupil's body and place it over the fulcrum of the next rib. For the average adult the spacing between each fulcrum is about an inch.

Practice Movement D:

The pupil changes to the left side and repeats Practice Movements B and C.

Practice Movement E:

Review Rolling the Body a Quarter-Turn to the Side and Getting Off the Table.

Demonstration 2: Present a picture showing a well-aligned back.

THIGH ACTION

Teaching Materials: Pictures of psoas, iliacus and pectineus muscles
Cardboard clock face
Top view of pelvis

Demonstration 1:

The action of walking is the slight flexing of one thigh and then the other towards the front body wall. Continuous adjustment of the extensors of the lower back aids this flexion. In the back, through the extensors, the weight of the spinal column is continually seeking a lower level. In the front, the legs are being lifted from above. The deep abdominal (psoas), pelvic (iliacus), and thigh (pectineus) muscles draw the weight of the thighs up over the top of the thigh bones.

The psoas muscle suspension of the thighs from the spine, is like the manipulation of puppet strings from above the puppet. This action can be very powerful as the psoas muscle has multiple beginnings. Its spinal attachments cover the sides of the spine, from the inner ends of the lowest rib to the base of the spinal column. The psoas inserts into the lesser trochanter on the inner upper side of the femur.

The iliacus muscles line the inner bony walls of each of the ilia and insert into the inner upper surface of the femurs just below the psoas muscles. The fan-like action of these muscles helps to keep the pelvic mass spherical and guides the weight from the spine to the thigh heads.

The pectineal muscles reinforce the psoas and iliacus in pulling the thigh weight over the inner pelvic rim. They have their beginnings on each side of the pubic joint and attach to the inner upper side of the thigh bones, behind the iliacus muscles.

Practice Movement A:

Standing, review The Dance Plié and The Psoas Walk.

Demonstration 2:

(Show cardboard clock face superimposed on top view of pelvis.)

Awareness of the action of the iliacus muscle is best begun with an imagined circling movement. The circle can be compared to a clock face. 12 o'clock is in the front of the pelvis at the pubis, 3 o'clock is in the middle of the right inner pelvic rim, 6 o'clock is in the back of the pelvis at the sacrum and 9 o'clock is in the middle of the left inner pelvic rim of the pelvis.

Practice Movement B:

Lying on the right side, review Relaxing the Shoulder Pull on the Spine and Expanding the Temporalis Muscle.

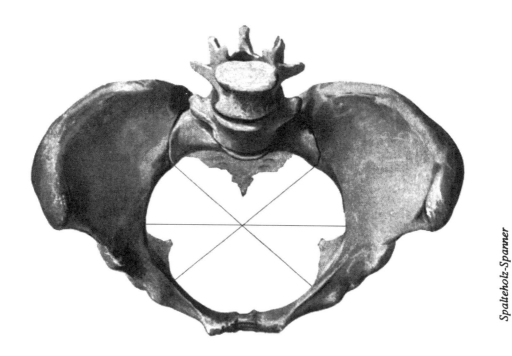

Top View of Pelvis

Spalteholz-Spanner

Practice Movement C: Circling through the Iliacus Muscles

Lying on the right side, the pupil visualizes a circle within his pelvis. The pupil should picture the hand of the clock in movement around the inner pelvic circle in the clockwise direction. The action moves from 12 to 3 to 6 to 9 to 12 o'clock. Repeating the visualization three to four times around the clock face is enough before a pause. Then, the image can be repeated.

Practice Movement D:

Lying on the left side, repeat the procedures in Practice Movements B and C. In Circling through the Iliacus Muscles, the movement will be in the counter-clockwise direction. The action moves from 12 to 9 to 6 to 3 to 12 o'clock. Repeat the circling three or four times and then pause before practicing again.

Practice Movement E:

Review Rolling the Body a Quarter-Turn to the Side. In the rolling movement, for every three rolls to the left make one roll to the right. Review Getting Off the Table.

Demonstration 3:

Present a picture showing well-aligned movement of the thigh in walking.

ATLANTO-AXIAL SOCKET

[Only fragments of the text and practice movements for this lesson were found in Miss Clark's records. However, students working with her during this period were able to supply information about the probable nature of the demonstrations and exercises.

Although the title of the lesson refers to the atlanto-axial socket, the text of this lesson probably introduced the articulation between the skull and the atlas, as well. In teaching head balance on the atlas, attention was drawn to the occipital condyles at the base of the skull. Their rocker-like action in articulation with the atlas was experienced in the movement of minutely flexing the head at the top of the spine, as if nodding the head "yes."

The awareness of the dens or odontoid process of the axis was emphasized in teaching the atlanto-axial articulation. The dens was compared to a finger pointing upward toward the center of the head, which could serve as its axis of rotation. Awareness of this articulation was practiced in small rotations of the head to the left and right, as if shaking the head "no."

The Practice Movement "Flexing Ankles and Turning Head," frequently cited in subsequent lessons, was probably introduced here. In the prone position, feet hanging over the end of the table, the student was to lift the head and upper thorax off the supporting surface by extending the spine. While maintaining this position the student then flexed the ankles alternately or rotated the head at the atlanto-axial socket. In turning the head, the student faced the table to avoid hyperextension of the cervical spine.

In another lesson fragment, the rectus capitis anterior and rectus capitis posterior muscles were discussed. These muscles, immediately in front of and behind the atlanto-occipital and atlanto-axial articulations, have diagonal designs similar to the psoas major and latissimus dorsi muscles. Thinking upward through the A-shaped design of the rectus capitis anterior muscles in the front of the spine was suggested as a means for reducing tension in the V-shaped rectus capitis posterior muscles in the back of the spine. Thus, thinking through the design of these muscles was another approach to improving the balance of the head and lengthening the cervical spine.]

SHOULDER ACTION

Teaching Materials: Picture of shoulder girdle and thorax - top view
Sternoclavicular design

Demonstration:

(Show top view of shoulder girdle and thorax.)

The center of the back body wall is a strong bony column, with weight descending from the top to its base. The ribs have sockets with the vertebrae of this bony column. The head of each rib should center in its socket on the side of the spine. Shallow articulations along the sides of the sternum are for the sternal ends of the top seven pairs of ribs. The sternal ends of the ribs in the front, help to brace the rib heads in the back at their spinal articulations.

The upper arm bone or humerus has a rounded head like the thigh bone, which fits into a shallow socket. The socket for the arm bone is on the side of the shoulder blade. The shoulder blade or scapula makes its joint with the collar bone or clavicle over the top of the socket for the arm bone. The collar bone meets the sternum at the sternoclavicular joint in the center front of the body. Through these many joints, the arm thrust enters the sternum and is taken by the ribs to the spine.

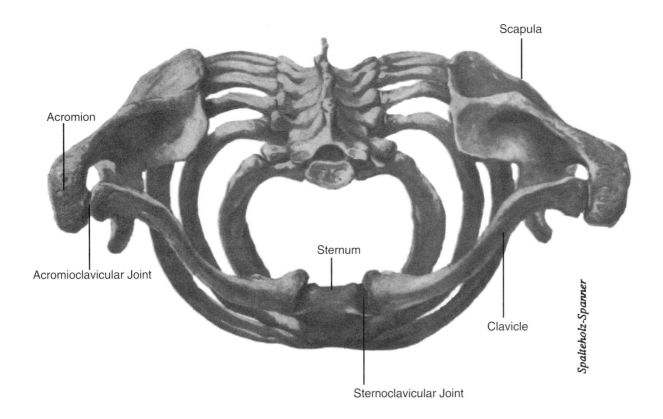

Bones of the Shoulder Girdle and Thorax - Top View

The average person is not sufficiently aware of these sockets. We need to allow our thoughts to center the bony heads (humerus and clavicle) at their sockets. These joints act as hubs for the wheel-like patterns of movement in the shoulders and arms.

Practice Movement A: Centering the Sternoclavicular Sockets

In standing, review The Dance Plié. Let the relaxation of the lower legs and thighs carry through to the thigh fulcrums. Gradually, become aware of the collar bone contact with the sternum. Let the relaxation of the arms and shoulders carry through to the sternum. Swing the arms easily with awareness of the sternoclavicular sockets.

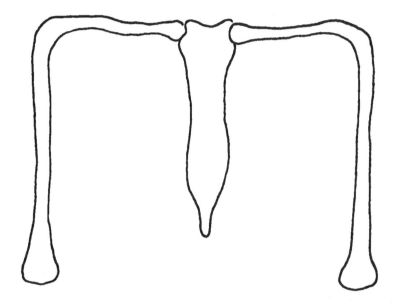

Sternoclavicular Design

Imagery: *Think of the inner ends of the collar bones as the inner ends of the arms.*

Practice Movement B: Circling the Ischia

Lying on the right side, the pupil will visualize circling around the left ischium. The circle will be much smaller than used in Circling through the Iliacus Muscles on that side. The direction for the circling around the left ischium will be clockwise. The pupil changes to lying on right side and repeats the procedure. The circles around the right ischium will be in the counter-clockwise direction.

Practice Movement C:

Review Centering the Ribs at the Spinal Fulcrums, Circling through the Iliacus Muscles, Aligning the Toes and Expanding the Temporalis Muscle on the right and left sides.

THIGH MOVEMENT

Teaching Materials: Picture of hamstring muscles
                                Design of biceps femoris muscle

Demonstration 1:

The thigh bones cannot center well in their sockets if the muscles on the back of the thighs are shortened. Imagery that will take us into slight flexion of the thighs can help us overcome the bad habit of holding the hamstring and gluteal muscles in the standing position. As we strengthen the psoas, iliacus and other muscles of flexion, the extensors of the thigh will tend to lengthen. The movement of shuffling the feet forward has been selected for practice with these ideas because most people find more can be accomplished through tiny movements than large ones. Small movements improve balance closer to the axes of the body and lower extremities.

Practice Movement A:

In the sitting position, review Centering the Sternoclavicular Sockets.

Practice Movement B: Shuffling

Without moving the torso, the pupil shuffles his feet forward two or three tiny steps. He should repeat this several times with a short pause between movements. Some pupils are aided by placing the palm of one of their hands over the abdomen, with the back of the other hand over the lower spine. This seems to help in establishing action in the psoas and iliacus group and relaxing their opponents, the gluteals and hamstrings.

Imagery: *The pupil pictures a statue resting on a pedestal and compares it with the torso resting on top of the thigh bones. Since it is easy to accept that the statue should be centered on its base, it is logical to follow through with the idea of centering the torso on the lower extremities.*

Demonstration 2:

(Show picture of hamstring muscles.)

It may be easier for a pupil to visualize the function of a single muscle, than the more complicated action of a group of muscles. The teacher should point out the inner and outer ends of the biceps femoris muscle. The first is on the ischium and the latter on the head of the fibula. To avoid confusing the pupil, the long head of the muscle is the one to mention. For our purposes, there is no need to call attention to the lower head of the muscle.

(Show biceps femoris design.)

The image of the biceps femoris muscle lengthening is helpful in improving thigh action. In this instance, the image for the muscle could be the draping of material in the shape of a festoon. The festoon droops loosely, rather than holding taut. As the biceps femoris muscle begins to relax, the upward pull on the fibula is released. The thigh bone moves toward flexion at the thigh joint and the fibula can center in its socket beside the knee. This stimulates awareness of the axis of the lower leg, which allows better coordinated movement of the foot.

Practice Movement C:
Lengthening the Biceps Femoris Muscle

Lying on the right side, the pupil pictures the path of the biceps femoris muscle from its attachment on the ischium to the head of the fibula. The teacher places the second and third fingers of his hand over the head of the fibula, where the lower end of the biceps femoris muscle is attached. The direction of the teacher's touch is upward towards the upper end of the muscle. The pupil imagines draping a paper or cloth festoon to give awareness of increased length for the muscle.

Practice Movement D: Swinging the Fibula
The pupil will allow the fibula to relax by visualizing it swinging slightly, forward and backward, from its socket near the knee.

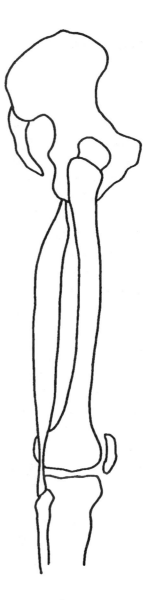

Biceps Femoris Design

Practice Movement E:
Lying on the right side, review Expanding the Temporalis Muscle, Centering the Ribs at their Spinal Fulcrums, Circling through the Iliacus and Aligning the Toes. Repeat Practice Movements C, D and E with the pupil lying on the left side. Lying prone, review Flexing Ankles and Turning Head. Review Getting Off the Table.

SPINAL AXIS MOVEMENT

Teaching Materials: Picture of anterior longitudinal ligament
Picture of the spine

Demonstration 1:

The vertebrae are united into a strong column by the anterior and posterior longitudinal ligaments. There should be good development of the short muscles between the vertebrae, so these ligaments are not under strain.

The anterior longitudinal ligament is on the front of the vertebral bodies, from the skull to the front of the sacrum. The posterior longitudinal ligament is on the back side of the bodies, in the front of the neural canal, from the skull to the back of the sacrum. In the practice movement, Flexing Ankles and Turning Head, the image of moving up the front of the spine (mid-sacral to lower lumbar) will strengthen the anterior longitudinal ligament as the pupil moves the legs or turns the head. Of course, all of the ligaments will be strengthened by the exercise, but only one is selected for imagining.

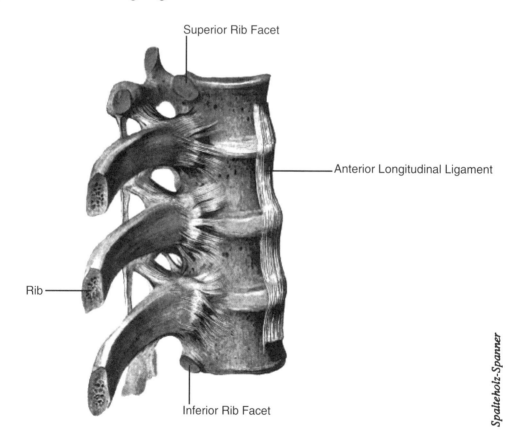

Spalteholz-Spanner

Anterior Longitudinal Ligament

Practice Movement A:

In the prone position, review Flexing Ankles and Turning Head. Imagine coming up the front of the lower lumbar spine through the anterior longitudinal ligament.

Demonstration 2:

Isadora Duncan said all movement should start from the center of the body. This is in line with the idea of lowering the weight toward the base of the spine as the beginning for any movement. By lowering the weight along the spine as a preparation for movement, the pupil gains good support at center for moving the thighs or other parts of the body.

The pupil started exploring this in the movement of Rolling the Body a Quarter-Turn to the Side. Now, he should be able to visualize a lengthening action between the vertebrae in the more tense areas of his spine as he practices rolling. In the next practice movement, the pupil will repeat Rolling the Body a Quarter-Turn to the Side. Movement of the arms will be added to stimulate deeper awareness of fluidity in spinal movement.

Practice Movement B: Rolling the Body a Quarter-Turn with Arm Action

Review Rolling the Body a Quarter-Turn to the Side. As the pupil rests on his back with the knees flexed, he should visualize lengthening down the spine. This is what he has been doing as he imagined extending the lower angles of the trapezius and latissimus dorsi muscles. As he gets a little sensory awareness of this, he starts turning the entire body toward his left. The pupil moves the feet in small steps in the process of the roll. This will allow him better centering of the thigh thrusts (crowbar action). The smaller the steps he takes, the better centered will be the thrusts. Repeat Rolling the Body a Quarter-Turn to the right side.

More extensive arm movement can now take place in the shoulder which is uppermost as the pupil turns in the roll. As the pupil starts the rolling movement to the left, direct him to allow the weight of the right arm to center at the right sternoclavicular socket. Trace up the front of the abdomen with the right fingertips and continue up the center front of the thorax. The right arm slowly comes to a position of rest over the side of the head. The hand will be on the floor above the head. Good timing will bring the completion of the shoulder movement at about the same time as the left thigh reaches the side lying position. As the right thigh completes its movement, resting on top of the left, the pupil should visualize the diagonal line of the latissimus dorsi muscle lengthening down over the lower end of the spine. Reverse directions for rolling to the right side.

Practice Movement C:

Review Getting Off the Table.

SHOULDER MOVEMENT

Teaching Materials: Picture of the serratus anterior muscle

Demonstration:

The muscle mass of the serratus anterior lies close to the ribs on the inner wall of the arm pit. The muscle attaches to the vertebral margin of the scapula. Notice the finger-like projections extending from the margin of the scapula to the first nine ribs. If the muscle is long and supple, these "fingers" will allow the shoulder to glide freely over the ribs, providing a wide range of movement at the sternoclavicular socket.

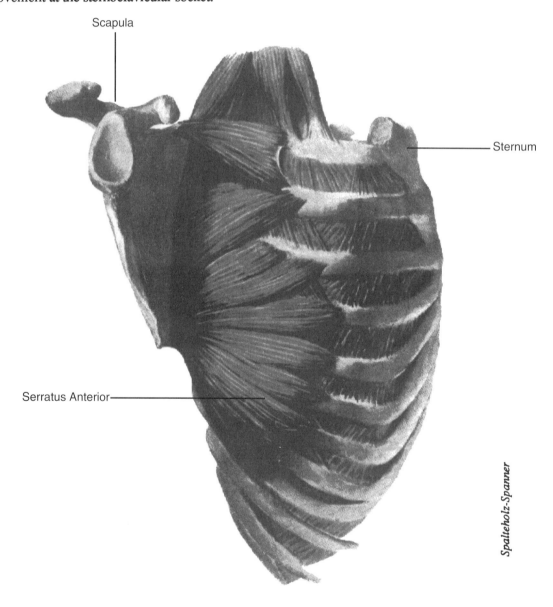

Right Serratus Anterior

Practice Movement A: Lengthening the Serratus Anterior Muscle

As the pupil rests on the right side, the teacher places a fingertip of his right hand at the upper vertebral margin of the shoulder blade. The teacher places one or two fingertips of his left hand on the upper part of the sternum. The first "finger" of the serratus anterior (upper boundary of muscle) lies on the curving line between the teacher's two hands. The pupil visualizes lengthening the line from the teacher's hand on the shoulder blade, around the body toward the teacher's hand at the top of the sternum.

The teacher moves his right hand down one-half inch along the margin of the scapula. His left hand may remain as before or be removed and replaced again at the upper part of the sternum. The pupil visualizes the second finger of the muscle lengthening toward the top of the sternum. The teacher moves his right hand down another half-inch along the margin of the scapula. His left hand can be removed from the front of the pupil's body, touching the sternum only as necessary to aid the pupil in visualizing the remaining fingers of the muscle. The right hand will continue down the margin of the scapula beside the spine, indicating seven more fingers for the muscle. This will end at about the level of the tenth rib. Count the serratus fingers one by one as the pupil visualizes expansion at each level.

Imagery: *To expand or relax the serratus anterior muscle, the pupil will imagine lengthening its "fingers," one by one.*

Pupil changes to lying on the left side and repeats the practice movement. Review Getting Off the Table.

Practice Movement B: Sliding Hands Over Thighs

In the sitting position, the pupil will slide the open palms over the tops of the thighs from the knees to the body. Pause with the fingertips over the thigh fulcrums. Continue the touch over the right thigh fulcrum as the left fingertips slide down the back of the left thigh toward the knee. The body rocks to the right ischium to do this. Then, from the top of the left knee, the left hand slides back over the top of the thigh to the left thigh fulcrum.

To repeat the action on the other side, the pupil will place the fingertips of the left hand over the left thigh fulcrum. The pupil's right fingertips will slide down the back of the right thigh towards the knee. The body rocks to the left ischium to do this. From the top of the right knee, the open palm of the right hand will slide back over the right thigh to the thigh fulcrum. Repeat the movement from the beginning a few times on each side.

Practice Movement C:

Review Centering the Sternoclavicular Sockets in the sitting position and Sitting to Standing.

FOOT AWARENESS

Teaching Materials: Bones - skeleton of the foot
                                 Foot design - side view

Demonstration 1:

In the first lesson, we worked with aligning the toes and regaining sensory awareness of the center of the foot through imagery which was viewed from above the foot. In a side view, the foot is seen as hollowed out in the center, like the hand.

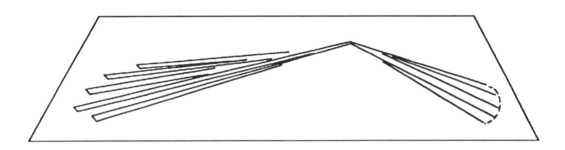

Foot Design - Side View

The hollow of the foot is formed by some of the small tarsal bones and the front of the heel bone. Maintaining the hollow shape at the center of the foot is aided by the image of Swinging the Fibula. This image also helps to relax the muscles of the lower leg and the Achilles tendon. As the calf muscles become easier, so will those on the back of the thigh. The gluteal area will also ease its tension.

Practice Movement A: Thinking Up the Front and Down the Back of the Femur

The pupil begins by standing, thinking of balancing equally on the tops of his femurs. In this position, he should picture moving upward over the front of the left thigh along the mechanical axis of the femur. This action should carry him over the top of the head of the femur. From here he will proceed to visualize down the back of the leg along the back of the mechanical axis. As the body balance becomes centered over the left thigh the pupil should swing his right thigh forward a short step. The process is then repeated on the right side to swing the left thigh forward. Repeat alternately for several short steps.

Demonstration 2:

> (Show the intermetatarsal articulations and the metatarsophalangeal articulations on the skeleton of the foot.)

The intermetatarsal articulations include two sets of side by side joints, those between the heads and bases of the metatarsal bones. The gliding movement between the bones is an important function of the transverse arch. There is a spreading of the arch when weight is upon it and a return to its plantar concavity when the weight is taken off.

The metatarsophalangeal articulations include the joints between the heads of the metatarsal bones and the bases of the proximal phalanges. The centering of these articulations will aid the hollowing of the foot, relaxing the downward pressure on the joints. These articulations should be related to similar joints in the hands, noting the angle of the knuckles on the top of the hand.

Practice Movement B: Metatarsophalangeal Joints

With the pupil lying on his right side, the teacher touches the undersurface of the metatarsophalangeal joint of the little toe. The pupil should think of upward movement there instead of downward. As he senses this and relaxes the downward pressure, the teacher continues on to the metatarsophalangeal joint of the fourth toe, then on to the third, second and first toes. The whole process can then be repeated. Depending upon the condition of the pupil's foot, one of the toes may be singled out for special emphasis. End by returning to the third toe, as the center of the foot. Ideally the second toe would be sensed as the center of the foot. For most people, the center is more easily accepted as the third toe. Gradually, the pupil can be guided to shift awareness toward the second toe as center.

Imagery: *Imagine the metatarsophalangeal joint being like the peak of a knuckle on the top of the hand.*

Practice Movement C: Intermetatarsal Articulations

Lying on the right side. By clasping the left foot very gently the movement between these side-by-side articulations can be felt.

Practice Movement D:

On the right side, review Lengthening the Biceps Femoris Muscle, Swinging the Fibula, Lengthening the Serratus Anterior Muscle and Rolling the Body a Quarter-Turn to the Side with Arm Action.

Repeat Practice Movements B, C and D with the pupil lying on the left side.

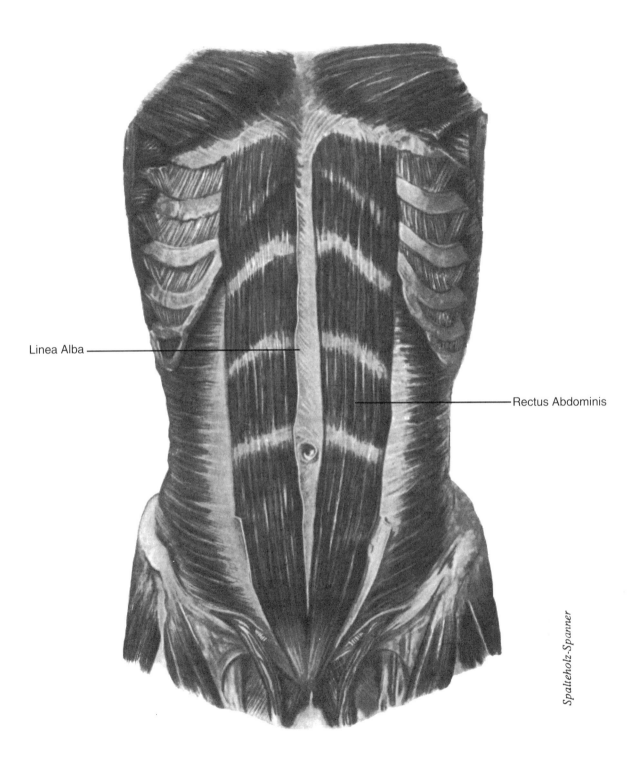

Linea Alba

Rectus Abdominis

Spalteholz-Spanner

Rectus Abdominis Muscles

ABDOMINAL ACTION

Teaching Materials: Picture of rectus abdominis muscles

Demonstration:

It will be easier to lengthen the spine if the tonus of the surface abdominal muscles is improved. This can be easily done through the simple image of decreasing the width of the rectus abdominis muscles.

(Show picture of rectus abdominis muscles.)

The rectus abdominis muscles lie on either side of the mid-front line of the abdomen. They extend from the pubis (mid-front of the pelvis) to the lower sternum and the costal cartilages between the sternum and the front ends of the fifth, sixth, and seventh ribs. Each of the muscles is subdivided into four sections. Visualizing the narrowing of the middle section of each muscle, toward the mid-front line, will begin to decrease the downward pull on the sternum. With more length in the mid-front of the body, more lengthening of the spine is possible in the back of the body. This brings about the relaxation of muscles which maintain overly pronounced spinal curves and promotes better use of the diaphragm.

Practice Movement A:

Review Sliding Hands Over Thighs, Sitting to Standing, Thinking Up the Front and Down the Back of Femur and The Psoas Walk.

Practice Movement B:

Lying on the right side, review Centering the Ribs at the Spinal Fulcrums.

Practice Movement C: Decreasing Width of the Rectus Abdominis Muscles

Working first on the left side of the body, the pupil should visualize the narrowing of the middle section of the rectus abdominis muscle toward the mid-front line of the body. The teacher may apply a gentle pressure here, indicating the direction inward. The tip of his thumb is placed about an inch to the left of the center of the pupil's abdomen. This will be just above the level of the umbilicus.

Practice Movement D: Review Breathing along Inner Walls of the Nostrils.

Lying on the Left Side - Review Practice Movements B, C and D.

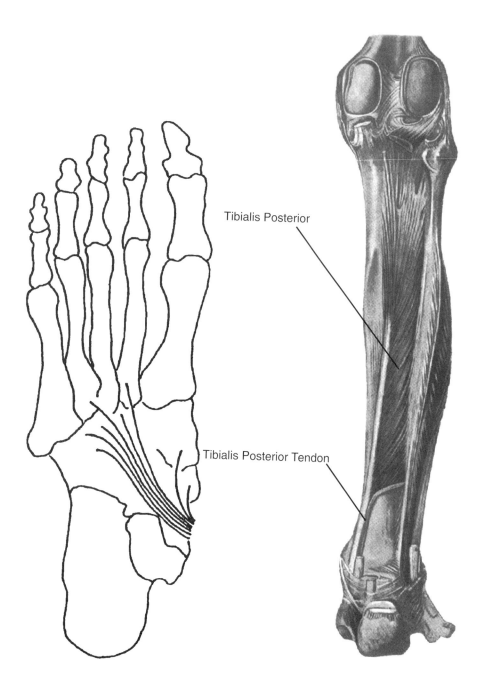

Tibialis Posterior

Tibialis Posterior Tendon

Spalteholz-Spanner

*Dorsum of Foot with Tibialis
Posterior Tendon
(redrawn after Spalteholz)*

Tibialis Posterior Muscle

FOOT MOVEMENT

Teaching Materials: Bones - tibia, fibula and foot skeleton
Pictures of the tibialis posterior muscle

Demonstration:

As the pupil relaxes the superficial muscles of the lower leg, he will become aware of the separateness of the lower leg bones. It is similar to the feeling of the bones of the lower arm. The images of Swinging the Fibula and Lengthening the Biceps Femoris Muscle have been helpful in this. Now, the pupil can become aware that the space between the bones of the lower leg is filled by the tibialis posterior muscle. The tibialis posterior muscle begins just below the knee. The muscle ends in a thin tendon which divides into eight tiny slips attaching to bones around the arch of the foot. Deepening the center of the foot relates to the action of the tibialis posterior. Inward rotating movements circling the center of the sole of the foot will strengthen the action of this muscle.

Imagery: *The pupil will visualize movement around a tiny circle at the center of the foot.*

Practice Movement A:

Lying on the right side, review Centering the Ribs at Spinal Fulcrums, Decreasing Width of the Rectus Abdominis Muscles, Circling through the Iliacus Muscles, Lengthening the Biceps Femoris and Aligning the Toes.

Practice Movement B: Circling the Center of the Foot

Lying on the right side, the pupil will visualize making a circle, no larger than a dime, around the center of the foot. This movement is in the same direction as the circling for the iliacus and ischia on that side of the body. On the left foot, the movement will be clockwise. Later, when the pupil works on the right foot, the direction of the circling will be counter-clockwise.

Practice Movement C: Breathing Along the Sides of the Spine

After a review of Lengthening the Serratus Anterior Muscle, the pupil practices Breathing Along the Inner Walls of the Nose. Then, he can continue to think along the inner wall of the left thorax. Although the action is actually beside the spine, the pupil will obtain a better result by thinking of the inner wall of the thorax, as he did with the nostril.

Lying on the Left Side - Repeat Practice Movements A, B and C.

LENGTHENING THE SPINE

Teaching Materials: Design for the ligamentum sacrotuberosum

Demonstration:

The ligamentum sacrotuberosum, aids in anchoring the weight from the spine to the pelvic area. The two parts of this ligament begin on the sides of the sacrum and unite to insert into the ischium. A side view of the ligament would show its diagonal path moving forward from the sacrum toward the ischia.

The axis of the body should be centered between the ischia. However, if the spinal curves are overly contracted, the ischia will be held up in the back. As the pupil learns to give the muscles around the spine greater length, the ischia will drop under the center of the body. This helps to center the thighs in their sockets above the ischia.

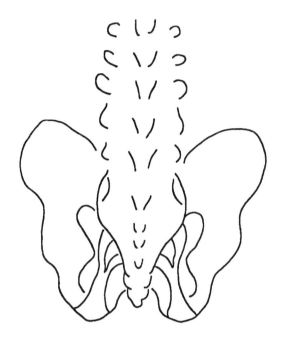

Ligamentum Sacrotuberosum

Practice Movement A:

Review Sitting to Standing, Standing to Sitting and The Dance Plie'.

Practice Movement B:

Lying on the right side, review Centering Ribs at the Spinal Fulcrums, Circling the Ischia, Lengthening the Biceps Femoris, Aligning the Toes, Metatarsophalangeal Joints and Circling the Center of the Foot.

Practice Movement C: Lengthening the Ligamentum Sacrotuberosum

With the pupil lying on the right side, the teacher touches the mid-sacral area, a tiny bit to the left of center. The pupil will visualize lengthening the ligamentum sacrotuberosum from the left side of the sacrum toward the left ischium. The direction is downward and slightly forward.

Practice Movement D:

Lying on the right side, review Breathing Along the Sides of the Spine.

Lying on the left side, review Practice Movements B, C, and D.

SHOULDER MOVEMENT

Teaching Materials: Side view of the latissimus dorsi muscle

Demonstration:

(Show latissimus dorsi muscle.)

In this lesson, the pupil will become aware of the insertion of the latissimus dorsi muscle on the underside of the humerus. The latissimus dorsi inserts on the arm bone, not far from the gleno-humeral socket. Thinking along the outer border of the muscle is one way of lengthening the spine. Sensing the connection between the arm bone and the sacrum will improve the centering of the humerus in the arm socket and the balance of the shoulders.

Practice Movement A: Inhalation and Inward Rotation of the Arm

While standing easily, the pupil should think of the inner end of the latissimus dorsi muscle on the underside of the upper left arm. His left arm can then swing upward in a half circle in the direction of inward rotation to bring the hand over the head.

   The pupil can inhale during the movement and the arm should remain over head until the inhalation is completed naturally. Thinking down the outer border of the muscle toward the sacrum, the pupil lowers the arm, completing the circle.

   Repeat the movement with the right arm in its direction of inward rotation. Repeat a few times, alternating arms.

Practice Movement B:

In the sitting position, review Sliding Hands over Thighs and Centering at the Sternoclavicular Sockets. In standing, review Thinking Up the Front and Down the Back of the Femur and Shuffling.

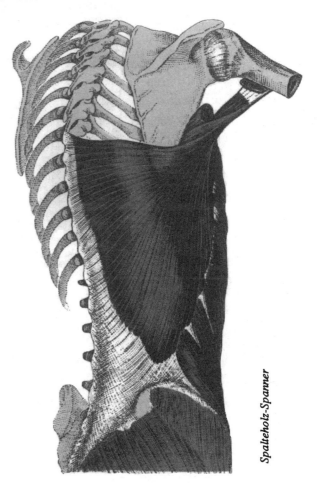

Spalteholz-Spanner

Side View - Latissimus Dorsi

CENTERING TO MOVE

Teaching Materials: Bones - the skull
                                  Picture of the skeleton

Demonstration:

Mabel Todd used the word "centering" to describe the integration of the body. By centering, the body prepares to move as a unit with its weight controlled deep within itself, where its strongest muscles lie. The basic images of the thigh thrusts and lengthening the spine have started the centering or integrating action. Imagery of "diagonal lines" should develop another level of awareness.

The diagonal lines pass from the center of the right thigh socket to the center of the left atlanto-occipital socket and from the center of the left thigh socket to the center of the right atlanto-occipital socket. The two lines form a very slim "X" crossing the axis of the body.

(The teacher should show the occipital condyles of the base of the
skull and trace the diagonal lines on the picture of the skeleton.)

Notice that the diagonals pass behind the sternoclavicular socket. The wrong pattern is to think of a wide X, as if the glenohumeral sockets began the diagonals, rather than the occipital condyles. Use of narrow diagonal lines in action brings about better awareness of control of the body at center. Whether body action is tiny or large, light or powerful, the movement will be rhythmical and enjoyable, if it is well integrated.

Practice Movement A: The Diagonals

Lying on the right side, the pupil will visualize a diagonal line from the center of his left thigh socket to his right occipital condyle. First, the teacher's touch will be just above the left greater trochanter. After allowing a few minutes for imagining the thigh thrust projecting through the neck of the femur into the inner rim of the pelvis, the teacher can suggest that the diagonal passes close to the side of the sacrum.

Then, the teacher should touch lightly near the right mastoid process. Working with the upper part of the diagonal, the pupil can picture the movement reaching the side of the atlas, near the rectus capitis anterior muscles. The pupil should repeat the visualization of the lower end of the diagonal.

Practice Movement B:

Review Lengthening the Biceps Femoris Muscle, Circling the Center of the Foot and Breathing along the Sides of the Spine.

Repeat Practice Movements A and B with the pupil lying on the left side.

AXES OF THIGH MOVEMENT

Teaching Materials: Picture of adductor magnus muscle

Demonstration:

The pupil has been lengthening the biceps femoris muscle on the outside of the thigh for several weeks. This has encouraged the muscles on the inside of the thigh to increase their tone or strength. The pupil is now ready to begin active consideration of these inside muscles.

Turn the picture of the adductor magnus sideways to show that it is shaped like a very broad triangle. The base of the triangle extends from the knee to the pubis. The apex or top of the triangle is in the middle of the femur. The upper side of the triangle goes up from the apex toward the pubis. The lower side of the triangle extends downward from the apex to above the inner knee.

Practice Movement A:

Lengthening the Adductor Magnus Muscle

Lying on his right side, the pupil visualizes a lengthening action along the upper side of the triangle from its apex towards the pubis. The teacher places his middle finger lightly on the back of the pupil's left thigh, near the apex of the triangle. Because of the location, the teacher should not fumble or be concerned about the accuracy of the position. If the teacher is casual about the procedure, it will help the pupil. Accuracy comes with experience. The pupil visualizes the lengthening of the upper side of the triangle from the apex toward the pubis.

Practice Movement B:

Review Centering the Ribs at the Spinal Fulcrums and the Diagonals. Repeat Practice Movements A and B as the pupil rests on the left side. Review Getting Off the Table.

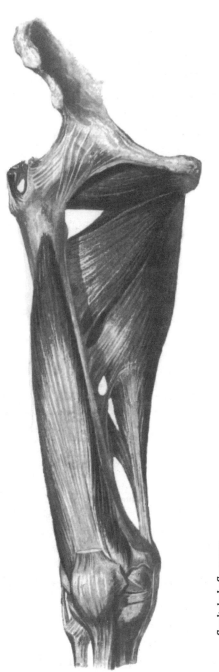

Spalteholz-Spanner

Adductor Magnus Muscle

STERNAL SUSPENSION

Teaching Materials: Picture of sternocleidomastoid muscle

Demonstration:

The pupil has learned how the shoulder thrust enters the sternum by way of the collar bones and is taken by the ribs to the spine. The sternum hangs like an ill-shaped star in the center of the front body wall with its base or largest end upwards. Expansion and relaxation of the serratus anterior muscle through the lengthening of its muscle "fingers" toward the mid-sternal line helps the suspension of the sternum. Now, the pupil can become aware of the way the head suspends the sternum.

The sternocleidomastoid muscles suspend the sternum from the sides of the head just behind the ears. The inner fork of the muscle, the one to the sternum, is the most important pathway to sense. If the outer fork of the muscle is shortened, the best use of the sternoclavicular fulcrums is hindered. The shoulders are pulled up and the thorax depressed, which unseats the balance of the head. Thinking up along the inner fork of the muscle heightens the top of the sternum. The shoulders can then gain greater range and ease of movement.

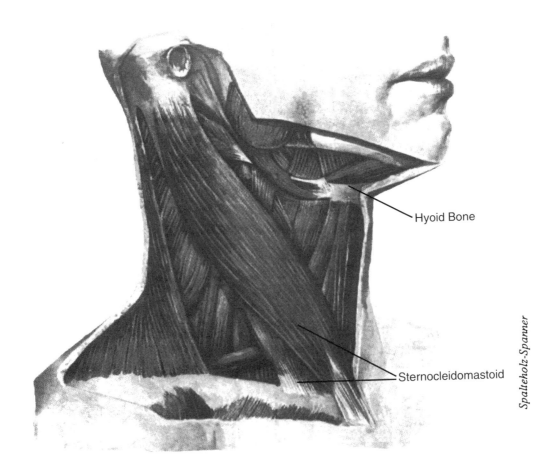

Hyoid Bone

Sternocleidomastoid

Spalteholz-Spanner

Sternocleidomastoid Muscle

Practice Movement A: Circling the Sternoclavicular Socket

In a sitting position, move near the left side of the chair so the left arm hangs straight down at the side of the body. Place the right fingertips over the left sternoclavicular fulcrum. Think around the rim of the fulcrum or socket in the following direction: up the front, continue towards the back, down the back side and then forward to where you started. Circle three times on the left side. Then, as rhythmically as you can, swing the left arm over the left thigh, visualizing movement taking place at the sternal fulcrum.

Change to the right side of the chair with the right arm hanging down in a relaxed manner from the shoulder. Repeat the circling as described above using the left fingertips over the right sternoclavicular fulcrum. Following the circling, swing the right arm to a position of rest over the right thigh. Visualize the movement of the arm taking place at the sternoclavicular fulcrum.

Imagery: *Picture the top of the sternum as a floating member in the thorax.*

Practice Movement B:

In the standing position, review Inhalation and Inward Rotation of the Arm and Thinking Up the Front and Down the Back of the Femur.

Practice Movement C:

Lying on the right side, review Lengthening the Serratus Anterior Muscle. As the pupil reviews Lengthening the Serratus Anterior Muscle, the teacher will emphasize the relationship between lengthening this muscle and the suspension of the sternum.

Practice Movement D: Relating Exhalation to Narrowing the Rectus Abdominis Muscles.

Lying on the right side, the pupil should direct his attention to visualizing the narrowing of the mid-section of the rectus abdominis muscle toward the mid-front line of the body. The teacher may apply a gentle pressure here, indicating the direction inward, with the tip of his thumb placed about an inch to the left of the center of the pupil's abdomen, just above the umbilical level. As the pupil reviews narrowing the mid-section of the rectus abdominis muscles, instruct him to notice the rhythm of his usual exhalation. This should be related to narrowing the rectus abdominis without any conscious change of the breathing rhythm in length or effort.

Repeat Practice Movements C and D with pupil lying on the left side.

PUBIC FULCRUM AWARENESS

Teaching Materials: Picture of the psoas, iliacus and adductor muscles
Bones - pelvis or model of the pelvis

Demonstration:

In improving pelvic action, the thrusts from the thigh heads through the pelvis are very important. The thrust from the thigh bone goes to the center of the thigh socket in a one-way thrust. From the thigh socket, the thrust becomes a two-way action. Part of the thrust goes to the pubic fulcrum in the front of the pelvis. The other part of the thrust goes to the sacroiliac fulcrum in the back of the pelvis. This design is similar to the thrusts at the sternal and spinal ends of the ribs in the thorax.

The individual is usually more aware of the sacroiliac fulcrum in the back of the pelvis and the pubic fulcrum in the front may be overlooked. This can be the result of gluteal tension or the image of the body as a flat structure rather than a round one. In this lesson, the pupil will learn that the pubic fulcrum plays a part in the process of lengthening the spine.

Applying the pattern of imagery the pupil has learned in the thorax to the pelvic area seems to be a successful way of improving pubic fulcrum awareness. In doing this, the pupil must learn to visualize the sacral and coccygeal spine apart from the ilia. The pupil will also think of the sacral and coccygeal vertebrae as separate units like the thoracic vertebrae.

Practice Movement A:

Lying on the right side, review Centering the Ribs at the Spinal Fulcrums.

Practice Movement B: Centering the Pelvic Ribs at the Pubic Fulcrum

Lying on the right side, the pupil visualizes the left ilium as if it were formed of five separate ribs. Each of these imaginary ribs is fastened to one of the five sacral vertebrae. The pupil starts with the middle or third sacral rib. As he pictures the sacral rib, he circles the inner pelvis from the sacrum to the pubic fulcrum. The third sacral rib is nearly level from front and back. As he proceeds to the fourth sacral rib, he will need to think upward as the rib circles to the front of the pubis. With the fifth sacral rib the inclination upward is even further. The same imagery is very effective when applied to the coccygeal vertebrae. With the coccygeal ribs, the curve to the front is more acutely upward.

In guiding this procedure, the teacher touches the mid-sacrum and goes to the level of the fifth sacral vertebra. The finger touch is kept lightly there while the pupil visualizes the coccygeal ribs.

Repeat Practice Movements A and B, lying on the left side.

SPINAL-RIB THRUST DIAGONALS

Teaching Materials: Picture of thoracic vertebrae with rib

Demonstration:

Practice in centering encourages the pupil to move with an awareness of the axis within the body. For many people, the tendency is to hold at the sides of the body and ignore the axis. This weakens the action of the psoas, iliacus and adductor muscles in maintaining the axis.

The place to change one's structural alignment is at the fulcrum, rather than the middle of the lever. In the pelvic imagery, the pubic fulcrum is emphasized. In this case, the narrowing in the front allows the spine to lengthen downward. This centers the thigh bones in their sockets and lessens the pelvic tilt. In the thoracic imagery, the spinal fulcrums are emphasized. Here the narrowing in the back allows the spine to lengthen, and the sternum to slip upward in the front of the thorax.

(Show picture of the thoracic vertebrae with rib used to introduce *Rib Fulcrum Awareness*.)

Notice that the axis of rotation for the rib points toward the sternal socket of the opposite rib along a diagonal line. In this lesson, the pupil will visualize the spinal end of the rib thrusting diagonally through the body to the opposite sternal socket in the front. This imagery will gradually lessen the depression of the chest and give greater ease, as well as improved symmetry.

Practice Movement A: Rib Thrust Diagonals

The teacher's procedure is similar to the procedure used in the practice movement, Centering the Ribs at the Spinal Fulcrums. Lying on the right side, the pupil will imagine the vertebral sockets of the ribs on the left side of the spine. The pupil begins by imagining a diagonal thrust given by the head of the rib to the center of its vertebral socket in the back of the body. The pupil follows the thrust through the body to the opposite fulcrum in the front on the right side of the sternum. The diagonal thrusts for the first few ribs will be at the same level in the front and in back of the rib cage. Because the lower ribs must come up from their vertebral sockets to meet the sternum in the front, the pupil will think of those thrusts slanting upward as they move through the body.

Practice Movement B:

Lying on the right side, review Breathing Along the Inner Walls of the Nostrils. As the teacher touches the side of the sacrum, introduce the idea of Breathing along the Sides of the Spine at the level of the sacrum.

Change to lying on the left side and repeat Practice Movements A and B. The rib thrust diagonals will move from each vertebral socket on the right side of the spine to the sternal socket of the opposite rib on the left side of the sternum.

Part III
The
Manuals

The Children's Book

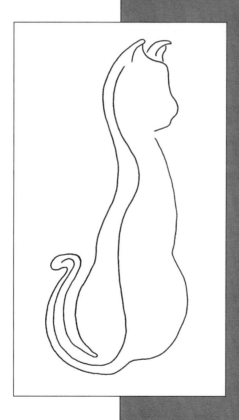

[The table of contents for *The Children's Book* also included the lesson titles listed below. These lessons were not available to the author.

HOW DO WE SIT? TOUCHING THE SPOTS

How do we sit?

We balance on the sitting bones at the lower end of our bodies. We have two sitting bones, a left one on the left side of our bodies and a right one on the right side of our bodies.

Look at the spots in the circle. What do you think they are for?

The two spots you see on the drawing are to show you where your sitting bones touch the chair.

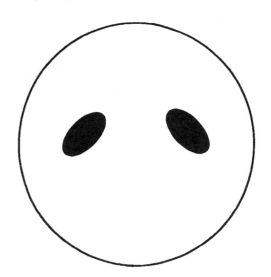

The spot on the left side is for the left sitting bone.

The spot on the right side is for the right sitting bone.

Touch the left spot with your left fingertips. Then, touch the right spot with your right fingertips.

Are you ready to find your sitting bones?

If you are, you have already begun to think of how your sitting bones touch imaginary sitting spots on your chair.

Let's start by sliding your left fingertips between your body and the chair seat. Use your fingertips to find the sitting bone that touches the left sitting spot. Then do the same on your right side by putting your right fingertips under the right side of your body. There you will find the sitting bone that touches the right sitting spot. Now, place both hands in your lap and look straight ahead with your eyes.

Are your heels resting on the floor?

When they are, you are balancing on your two sitting bones.

HOW DO WE STAND? FEELING THE ACTION

How do we stand?

We balance on our thigh heads at the tops of our leg bones.

Stand and walk forward slowly, in tiny steps. Let your arms hang with the palms of your hands on the front of your legs. Walk again in tiny steps.

Can you feel your legs push your arms as you take a step?

Of course you can. You feel the leg action under your palms.

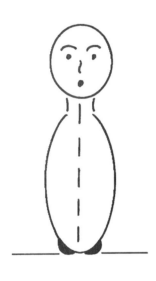
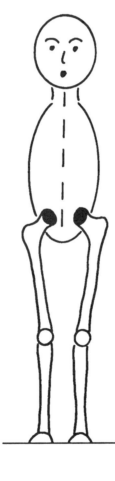

What you might not know is that the tops of your legs are just below your elbow level. This is where you balance when you are standing.

The sitting places, called the sitting bones, are on the first floor of the body. They rest on the ground like a house does.

The standing places, called the thigh heads, are on the second floor of our bodies. They are higher in our house and we go up to them.

It's a fun game to play.

Sit down on the first floor of your body. Stand up on the second floor of your body.

Repeat this a few times.

THE CAT'S CENTER LINE – TRACING IT OUT

Would you like to move as easily as a cat?

It will help you to learn, if you play this game a few times every day.

Look at the picture of the cat. What is the longest line you can see in the picture?

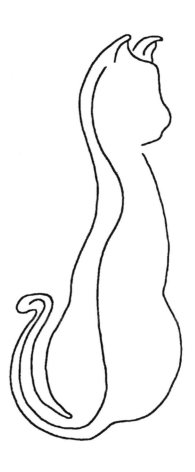

It is the one that goes from her head to the end of her tail. The cat has a long center line which begins just below her nose level, travels down the middle her back and ends at the tip of her tail.

Can you think of another name for the cat's center line?

The cat's spine would be a very good answer.

Can you tell me how to stroke a cat's back? Where does a kitty like to have you put your hand first in stroking her back?

The answer is gently over the shoulders. Then you stroke **down** her back, toward her tail. This makes her feel very comfortable and happy. A cat knows who her friends are by the way they touch her.

How does the kitty thank you?

She p—u—r—r—s.

Since there may be no kitty for you to stroke, let's play a tracing game with a kitty picture. Tracing is like stroking except that you will use your fingertips instead of your hand. At the top of the next page you will be looking at a picture of the kitty's left side.

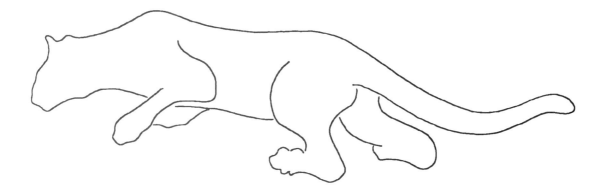

Have you found it? This picture is for tracing with the left hand. You can start by placing the middle fingertip of your left hand over the top of the kitty's head. Follow the line to the end of the kitty's tail. Why don't you repeat it once and then give a friend a turn.

Do you suppose the kitty will turn around for us so we can see her right side and trace down her center line with the right hand?

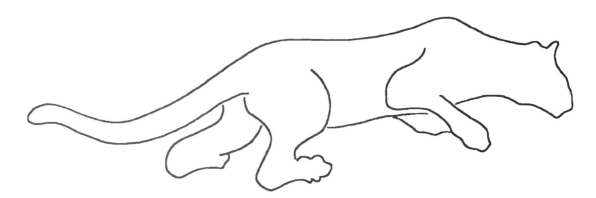

Oh, there she is, ready to have her back stroked.

Place the middle fingertip of your right hand over the kitty's head and softly feel along to the tip of the tail. Take a second turn and then share the picture with a friend.

YOUR OWN CENTER LINE – TRACING IT OUT

The cat's center line is very long and her tail helps to make it so. This is why cats can balance on almost anything. A cat likes to balance. It seems that she is playing a game when she is walking and balancing through her long center line.

Boys and girls can play a game like this, too. We might call it an imagining game. The best way for boys and girls to find the center line is to remember the center line of the cat.

Can you tell me where the cat's center line begins?

It begins at the nose level.

In what direction does the line go from the nose level?

It goes down through the middle of the cat's back into its tail.

Look at the picture on this page and notice where the boy's center line begins.

It starts at the top of his spine just below nose level.

Where does his center line end?

In standing you can think of the center line lengthening all the way to the floor like the tail of a cat. In sitting you can imagine it dropping down to the floor from between the sitting bones.

Let's try an experiment.

Sit on your sitting spots. Place the fingertips of one of your hands over your nose and the fingertips of the other hand, at the same level, on the back of the head. Your center line begins in between, at the center of your head.

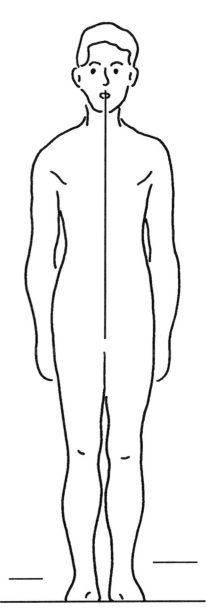

Now, let both hands relax in your lap. The line is now ready for you to follow down through your back. You can trace it in your imagination.

When you stand, you will change from the support of the sitting bones to the support of the thigh heads. Again, place the fingertips of one of your hands over your nose and the fingertips of the other hand, at the same level, on the back of the head. Feel the beginning of your center line. In your imagination, trace the line down your back beyond the sitting bones to where your imaginary tail might end.

The
Center
Line
goes
Down
from your
Nose
through
your
Back
to let you
Balance
on your
Thigh Heads
when
you are
Standing.

When you are ready, take a walk around the room. Use the idea of a long center line to help you balance as you walk. When you are back beside your own seat, stop and wait for a signal before you sit down. The signal is an idea: think of your long center line as you sit down.

Would you like a second chance to try to sit down better?

> Good. Stand on the other side of your chair. Think again of your long center line being like the cat's. Very slowly, think of moving down through your center line as you sit.

Do you know how to tell if your body really enjoys having a long line as you sit?

> Your heels will be resting on the floor.

YOUR LEG LINES COME FROM THE CENTER LINE

This is another imagining game.

Close your eyes and pretend you have a long tail like a cat. You can choose to be any kind or any color of cat, as long as you have a long tail.

The muscles on the backs of the legs will help us do this. When we imagine a tail like the cat's, dropping down to the floor, the backs of the legs can let go toward the heels.

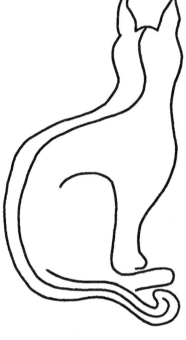

The cat can keep her balance easily when washing herself with her tongue. Her back muscles are so long and elastic that she can lift first one leg to be washed, and then the other, all the way up to her mouth. She does this so easily, without losing her balance,

up   her
goes   back
leg   goes
because as her   down.

This is a good stunt for boys and girls to try.

Sit on your sitting spots and then lift each leg, one at a time. Think of moving the top of each leg towards your head. Let your sitting bones go down in back like the cat. Move your haunches easily, thinking up and down in a vertical line. Keep the rhythm going down the back into your imaginary tail and breath easily.

Remember: Lower body down—raise leg up.

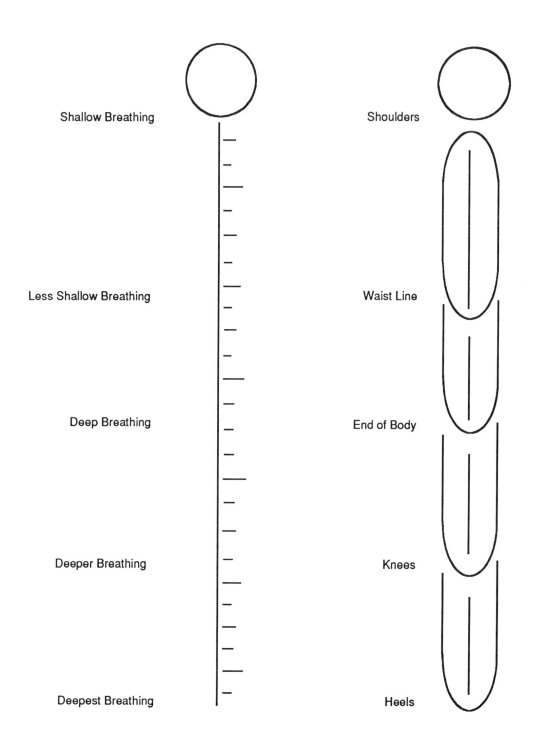

Shallow Breathing

Less Shallow Breathing

Deep Breathing

Deeper Breathing

Deepest Breathing

Shoulders

Waist Line

End of Body

Knees

Heels

Breath Inching Down the Line

YOUR OWN CENTER LINE – BREATHING WITH IT

Do you like to do experiments?

Good. It will be fun to work at some together.

Experiment 1: In this experiment, you will let out your breath as you think down your center line. Begin by sitting on your sitting spots with the heels resting softly on the floor. Follow the center line down through your back by tracing it in your imagination. Let go of your breath or exhale as you trace the line.

Give yourself a good chance to do this experiment by repeating it two or three times. As you trace the center line, let the breath go out very slowly.

You also can try thinking of the line first on one side of the body and then on the other. Trace along the left side of the line first and then on the right side. Notice if it is easier on one side than on the other.

Experiment 2: This experiment is to see how many inches you can move down through your center line as you let out your breath. We will use a tape measure to see the number of inches your breath travels down your line as you exhale.

(The teacher of the class or an adult in the home should take a tape measure and unroll it a little way, four to six inches. Hold this for the children to see.)

Your teacher will measure down the center line of each of the children, one at a time. She will start with someone who looks ready to do it—

someone who has taken the time,
to think of a long center line.

(The teacher places the tape along the child's spine from the base of the neck to between the shoulder blades. The end of the tape is the goal for the child's exhalation.)

Next, you can try breathing ten to twelve inches down the center line. Another day, try fifteen inches down the line. Every day think of letting the breath go down the line a few inches further.

YOUR TOE LINES LEAD TO THE CENTER OF THE BODY

Lie on your back and place your feet on the seat of a chair. The position is shown in the illustration below.

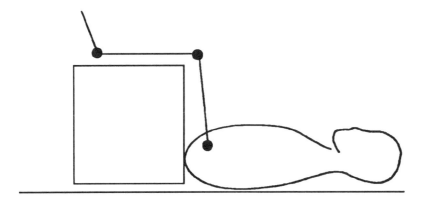

Where do you think your leg weight goes when you are lying this way?

Beginning with the toes, the weight rolls down through the foot, lower legs and thighs toward the center of your body.

Would you like to play a game that relates your toes to your center line?

Good. Our game begins with the large toe of the left foot. Think of action moving along a line from the tip of the large toe to the ankle. From the ankle the action moves along the center of the lower leg toward the knee. Finally, from the center of the knee imagine movement down the thigh toward the thigh head. You can pretend this action is like the movement of a tiny auto traveling toward a garage in the center of your body.

Next, another auto starts down the second toe line toward the center of your body. Then, a third car travels along the third toe line, followed by a fourth car on the fourth toe line, and a fifth car on the fifth toe line. All the cars go through the center of the ankle and the center of the knee toward the head of the thigh bone at the center of your body.

With all the cars driven into the garage, you can close the garage door. Close the back of the garage by letting your breath go down the center line until it reaches the end of your spine. Now, draw your left foot toward you, bending your knee as you go. When your foot is to the edge of the chair, pick up your leg and place it back where you started.

Now, play the game with the right toes in the same way.

STAND AND WALK – TALL

Since your spine is your body center, your back muscles should equal the length of your front ones and your front muscles should equal the length of the back ones. Here are some experiments to help you in this.

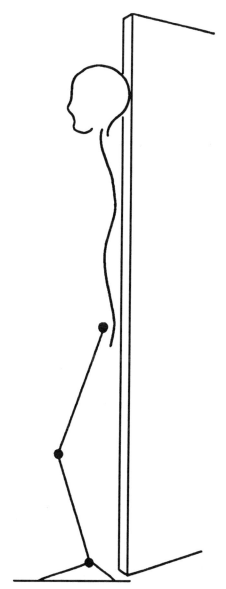

Experiment 1: In this experiment, you can learn to stand tall by spacing your spinal bones along the edge of a door. The narrow door edge is a reminder of your center line— the spine. Let's start at the base of the spine with the lowest of the spinal bones, the sacrum. Your sacrum is also the largest and longest of your spinal bones. It is cone shaped and points down toward the heels of your feet. Think of its shape and then place it at the door edge. Then slide the sacrum down the edge of the door and slip back up. Your toes should be farther ahead than your nose, and your arms should hang at the sides of your body.

Experiment 2: When *Experiment 1* becomes easy, you can add more of the spinal bones to the sliding action along the door edge. Not all the bones will touch the door. The back of the waist and the back of the neck should not touch the door edge. Finally, place the back of your head along the edge of the door. Slide it down and slip it back up along with your spinal bones.

Experiment 3: Take the thought of the door edge with you as you walk away from the door. Balance your head over your sacrum and walk tall.

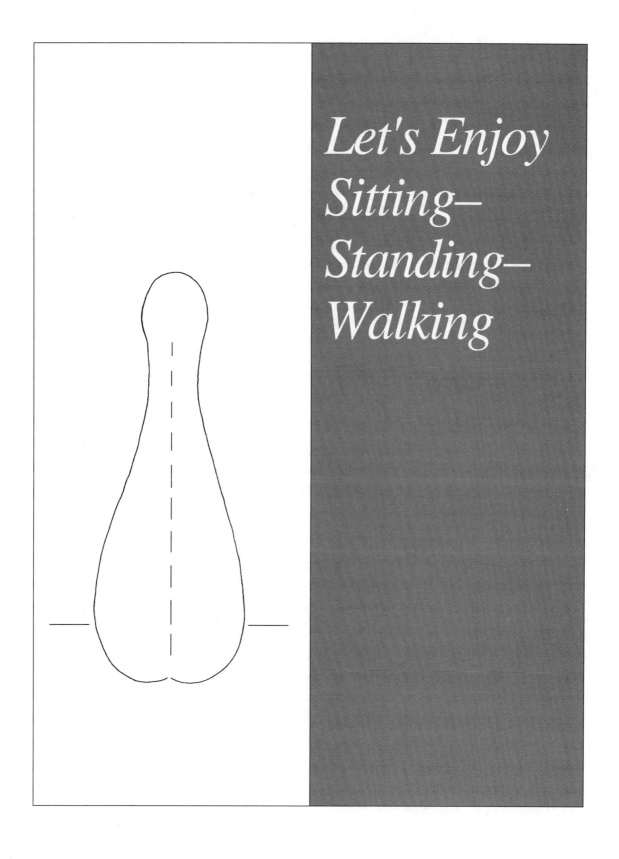

Let's Enjoy
Sitting–
Standing–
Walking

INTRODUCTION

Nature never meant movement to be a harsh discipline. As animals run and birds fly, they exhibit such joy and satisfaction in body action. Joy in movement should help us in living, as it does for the animals.

We can have more pleasure in movement if our body structures are not pulling us in opposing directions. In a well-aligned body, the weight is evenly balanced right and left, and front and back of a center line. Many people make the mistake of allowing their muscles to pull the weight of the pelvis and legs up the back of the center line. This habit throws them off balance and they begin to drop their heads and abdomens down the front of the center line. The result is a hump on their backs and a hollow in their chests. These people might use their bodies better if their early environment had been better shaped for development. Heredity and personality factors also play a part in forming movement patterns.

One way to improve the way we express ourselves through posture and movement is through better sensory awareness. The five senses—sight, sound, smell, taste and touch—have considerable influence on the use of the body and its healthful upkeep. This manual makes greater use of the tactile sense in building awareness than other approaches to this subject.

Supporting structures receive the first attention in the construction of buildings. Similarly, the supporting structure of the human body deserves first attention in the study of body alignment. Our habits of living and working today demand activity of the shoulders, arms and hands which tend to make the body top heavy. This would not happen if the body axis or core were well supported in sitting and standing. All aspects of body balance and movement can be performed best with well-aligned support through the lower body and legs. Therefore, directions for better aligned movement of the legs and spine are emphasized in this manual, while shoulder movement has been purposefully left out.

The tactile and other senses can help us learn the art of movement. Just as a juggler balances his moving objects in time and space, we can learn to bring our body weights into better balance and rhythm. Gradually, a little sensory awareness can put more enjoyment into the ordinary daily living of us all.

HOW IMAGERY WORKS

These lessons have been planned in an orderly way so you may gain the benefit from them as easily and quickly as possible. Be satisfied to study the first lesson before proceeding to the next. Take the lessons in order, in the same way you climb the steps on the stairway, to be assured of better body alignment upon reaching the end.

As you follow the instructions, and frequently read them over, your mind gathers data that readily passes from the conscious to the subconscious. If you have the patience to work with it, this knowledge will gradually help you change your habits of daily living. One wave of the magic wand will not do it. However, if you continue to wave the wand somewhat as a cat does its tail, very casually and rhythmically, a lot will happen.

Let's take a specific case. The image of a continuing vertical line through the center of the body is very important because it gives a center for all action. This idea may not make sense to you at first, but try to stick with the image and let your imagination run free. As you work through the lessons, a word or picture may suddenly bring to light something that has not meant anything at all to you before. Your emotions will clarify themselves and you will find yourself able to move more easily than you ever could before.

While muscles act in groups, the image of a single muscle pair is often used to indicate the direction for the imagery. A good example of this is the psoas muscle pair which illustrates the path connecting the thigh to the spine so perfectly. By using the psoas muscle design as imagery, we avoid the confusion which might occur in a beginning pupil's mind if several muscles were mentioned at one time.

Similarly, people generally have a better understanding of action in one area of the body than in some of the others. Transplanting an idea from the better known area of action to the less well known, has proven very helpful. A good illustration of this principle is the use of imagery for hand action to improve foot action.

Directions are given for practice with the left side [non-dominant] of the body first, and then repeated for the right side [dominant]. As a general rule, the right side is more difficult to change because it is used more than the left side. Start practice with the left side, and the right will automatically begin to adjust and bring about a better balanced relationship between the two sides. Then, when the practice is directed to the right side, less attention will be needed to make them equal. Don't try to save time by doing the two sides together. There is no need to push this type of study. It will develop as you feel ready. Muscle functions better when coaxed than when driven.

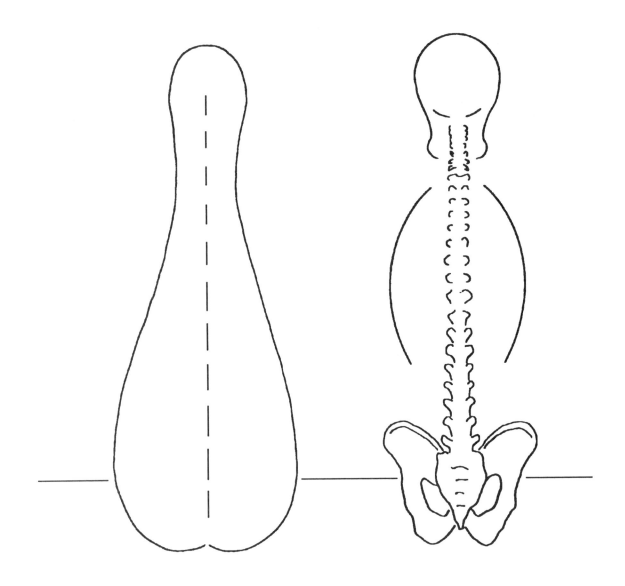

*A Tenpin Balances
Through Its Center Line*

*Body Axis in Balance
on the Sitting Bones*

SITTING WITH A CENTER LINE

The bony structure has the spinal column as its center or core. At the base of the column, the spine joins the two pelvic bones. Each of the pelvic bones contains a deep socket for the right and left thigh bones. These are called the thigh sockets. Beneath each thigh socket are the rounded rocker-like bony projections called the tuberosities of the ischia or the **sitting bones**.

In sitting, the body rests on the sitting bones. Your body is well balanced when you rest equally on them. The imagery of a **center line** is helpful in carrying out this principle of even balance in the human body.

Notice in the illustration how a tenpin balances equally around its center line. As you are sitting, the core of your body is the part of you that corresponds to the center line of a tenpin.

Let's start using this imagery. Sit in a chair that allows you to rest the center of your feet on the floor directly under your knees. Relax and begin to think of a center line passing through the middle of your body, from the center of your head to the lower end of your spine. As a next step, visualize a center line passing through the center of a tenpin. Imagine you are like a tenpin having no shoulder weights. Free yourself by imagining you have no left shoulder weight and then by imagining you have no right shoulder weight.

At first, this may seem difficult to accomplish. Try it a few minutes at a time as you have the opportunity. Some people notice immediate relief from strain. Other people take longer to realize they can rest more easily on their sitting bones if they allow their shoulders to relax.

The next thing to be observed in a tenpin is the flow of weight through its center line from the head to the base of the pin. There is no obstruction to the smooth easy flow downward through the middle of the pin. Neither should there be any obstruction in the passage of weight down through the center line or core of the body.

Your feet should feel light. The weight of the knees should fall toward the body through the front of the thighs. This brings the thighs to a right angle, or less, with the long center line. Maintaining a right angle between the thighs and the center line through the body, helps the spine to be easy and relaxed.

You **rest** when you sit with a long center line.

REST AS YOU SIT

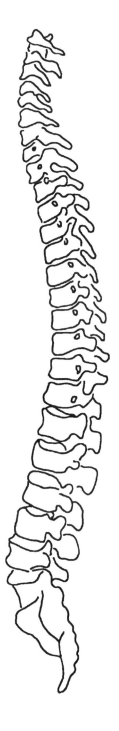

The spine assembles twenty-four units called vertebrae to make a long column. The spinal column is united with the thigh bones at its base and balances the head at its top. The weights of the head and other attachments to the spinal core, like the shoulders and ribs, are lowered to the base of the column through the round vertebral bodies on its front side. The intervertebral disks unite the vertebral bodies and form one quarter of the column's length. The pelvic bones join the sacrum at the base of the spinal column to form a somewhat spherical mass. The joint between the two pelvic bones and the sacrum is called the sacroiliac.

In the last lesson, you learned to balance on the two sitting bones. Comfortable sitting depends more on the proper positioning or alignment of the sitting bones than on any other single factor. Awareness of these sitting bones helps to relax the muscles around them. The whole structure becomes unbalanced if more weight is placed on one sitting bone than on the other, or if the weight is maintained in front or in back of the two sitting bones. The first practice movement will help you learn more about the feeling of balance on the two sitting bones.

Movement 1: In the sitting position, place the tips of your fingers under each sitting bone. Just use the fingertips, otherwise the seat of the chair may strain your fingers. Make a tiny rocking movement from the tips of the fingers of one hand to the tips of the fingers of the other hand. Remove your fingers and place your hands, palms down over your thighs. Repeat the rocking movement from one sitting bone to the other, two or three times. The image of the center line of the body should stay with you as you sway from one sitting bone to the other.

On the backs of the vertebral bodies are projections called spinous processes. These processes end in the little nubs we feel as we run our fingers down our mid-back line. The spinous processes are as long as the round bodies, measured from front to back. The spinous processes of the spinal column are for the attachment of spinal extensor muscles. It is good imagery to think of these muscles pulling downward on the rear projections of the vertebrae from the column's base.

Everyone is familiar with smoothing down the muscles over the spine of a pet animal. The child learns, quite early, the direction the cat or dog enjoys is toward the tail. The cat purrs its gratitude and the dog wags its tail for the same reason. It is the relaxing or lengthening of the spinal muscles on the backs of the vertebrae that feels so good. It allows the spinous processes of the vertebra to move ever so slightly toward the tail. The second practice movement will help you with this feeling.

Movement 2: As you sit, balance your head in the center line. In your imagination follow the action of the spinal extensors, dropping the spinous processes down the back, from the base of the back of the head to between the two sitting bones. Rock slightly sideways from the right sitting bone to the left sitting bone. Your head should be centered between the two sitting bones.

The bony structure is designed to support the body weight. The muscles are made to move the bones.

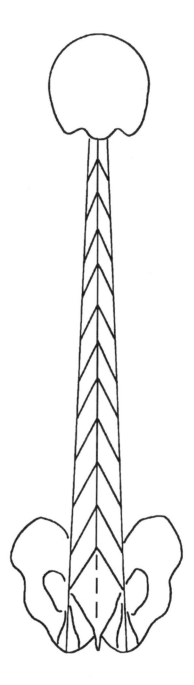

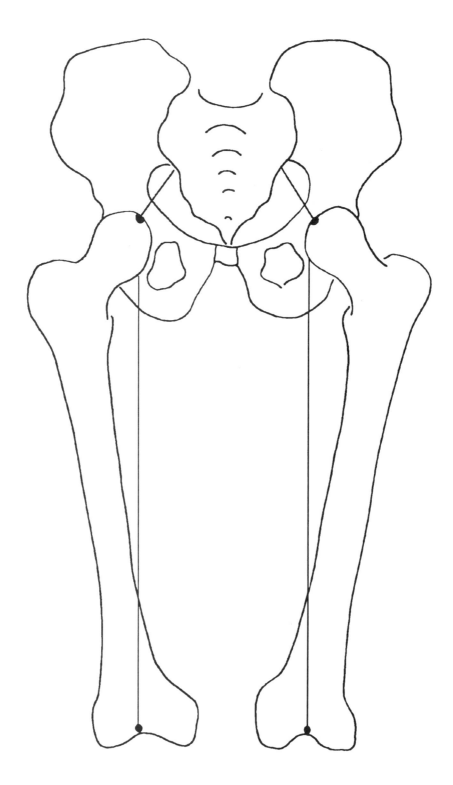

Front View of Pelvis and Thigh Bones

STANDING WITH A CENTER LINE

Above the sitting bones, is the **deep** socket for each thigh head. In this tunnel-like socket, you stand upon the heads of the femurs. For balance when standing, the general pattern is the same as in sitting. Just as you imagined a center line when you were sitting, so do you imagine a long center line when you are standing. Remember how you relaxed as you thought of the weight passing down through the middle of your body. Similarly, the best way to stand is to continue this imagery by sensing the flow down the back of the center line.

Question: How did you begin to let this line of movement flow when you were sitting?

Answer: By alternately relaxing each shoulder and letting the sitting bones come to rest under you. When you stopped trying to draw your weight up, you began to sense your sitting bones. This awareness started the flow down the back of the center line.

Question: How can I keep the sense of a flowing line when I stand?

Answer: You can start with a review of the first practice movement from the previous lesson. When you feel the two rounded sitting bones, gently rock sideways from the fingertips of one hand to the fingertips of the other. Remove your hands and relax them in your lap. Rock again, very slightly, back and forth from one sitting bone to the other. Now you are able to feel the parts of the sitting bones which are near the surface of your body. The sitting bones do not change position when you stand. They don't need to. The weight of the body is focused on the tops of the thigh bones while you stand.

Find the heads of the thigh bones in the illustration on the facing page. Then you can locate your own thigh heads before standing. Although you cannot touch the thigh heads, you can indicate their location in the thigh creases, where your thigh folds toward the front of the body.

As you sit, your knees should be near each other. Place your middle fingertips over the exact centers of your knees, left hand—left knee, right hand—right knee. Keep the distance between your right and left fingers the same as you trace up the front of your thighs. **Lightly** place your fingertips into your right and left thigh creases. Here, at the top of **straight** lines from the centers of your knees, is where you stand.

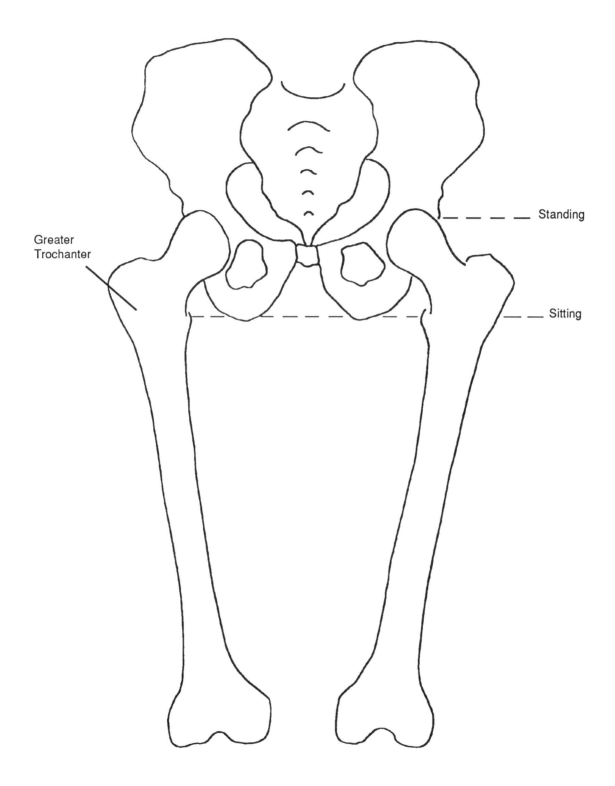

Greater
Trochanter

Standing

Sitting

I Sit Below Where I Stand – I Stand Above Where I Sit

REST AS YOU STAND

In the sitting position, we are balancing on the sitting bones. Changing from the sitting position to a standing one does not alter the position of the ischia. When we stand, the femur heads take over the body weight and the ischia becoming **hanging** protuberances in about the same position they were in sitting. In this way, the pathway for the passage of weight remains much the same in the two positions. A simple sing-song can help you recall this. It would go something like this:

> I sit **below** where I stand,
>
> I stand **above** where I sit.

In the illustration, notice the thigh bones have necks which extend diagonally from their bony heads to the sides of the thigh bones. Here at the sides of the body are what might be called **false** heads of the femurs. These false heads (greater trochanters) are for the attachment of muscles. They may give us the impression of support because we can feel them.

In the last lesson, you learned we are unable to touch the actual heads of the thighs with our fingers. To indicate the location of the heads you drew straight lines from the knees to the thigh creases. The line of thigh action does not follow the bone to the false head. Instead, it travels from the center of the knee joint to the center of the thigh joint. In this way, the femur heads can take over the weight without disturbing the circular base of the pelvis. You can improve the support of the pelvis by thinking of balancing on the **true** heads of the thigh bones and letting go of the false heads.

Now again, with your fingertips, touch your knee centers. Drag your hands over the surface of your thighs in straight lines toward their heads. Lightly change the position of the hands to rest them in your lap. Relax the shoulders and sway a bit from one sitting bone to the other. Let the upward thrusts through the center lines of the legs to your thigh heads lift you onto your feet. Then, think of the feeling of a long center line as you rest in standing.

> You **rest** when you stand with a long center line.

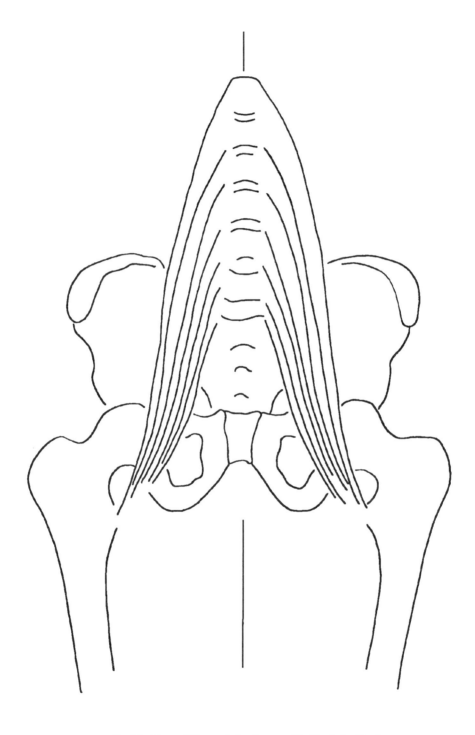

Inside Front View of the Lower Half of the Body
Showing the Psoas Muscles from the Sides of the Spine to the Thighs

WALKING FROM YOUR AXIS IS A GAME

Question: Why do some people become so tired when walking?

Answer: Because these people are thinking of their feet instead of the use of the psoas muscles above the thigh socket. Walking easily and well depends upon good use of these deep abdominal muscles.

As a child, you may have placed your hand above your elbow to feel the contraction of your biceps muscle. This was evidence of how strong you were getting. Try it, first with one arm and then the other. Feel the biceps muscle action **above** the elbow joint swinging the lower arm upward. Look at the illustration. Like the biceps, the psoas and allied muscles swing the thighs from above the thigh joint. This action lifts each thigh forward and you find yourself walking. The child learns to use these muscles in crawling and walking on all fours. You can become more aware of this action through imagery.

In walking there is a play between the spine and the upper thighs. Look at the illustration and notice that the psoas muscles form a bridge between the upper part of the thighs and the spine. We will call this design the "traffic bridge." Let's locate each end of the bridge, working with the left side first.

Place the right fingertips at the center of your left thigh crease in the front of the body. This is the lower end of the bridge. Place the back of your left hand on the left side of your spine just above your waistline to indicate the upper end of the bridge. Relax your shoulders and start walking forward easily. Think of the muscle action passing upward, from your right hand in the front to your left hand in the back. To work with the right thigh action, use the fingertips of your left hand in the right thigh crease in the front of the body. Place the knuckles of your right hand on the right side of your spine at waist level. Relax your shoulders and start walking forward as easily as you can. Think of the muscle action passing upward, from your left hand in the front to your right hand in the back.

A good image to follow is of traffic moving up a bridge, as you swing one leg and then the other in the walking pattern. Take time to notice the action above the thigh joint. This takes strain out of the leg muscles and makes the feet feel as light as they did when you were sitting.

At first, taking **very short steps** will make it easier for you to feel the psoas muscle action. It also helps the image of the long center line stay with you. The spinal muscle action **down the back** of the center line contributes to the psoas muscle action **up the front** of the line. If you can feel this, you will be able to sit as you walk.

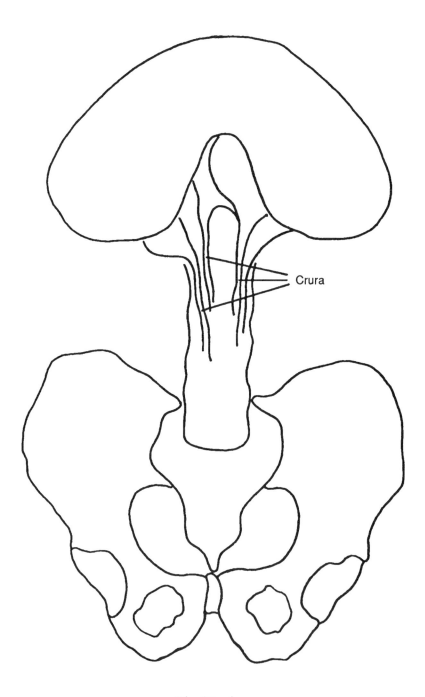

Crura

The Diaphragm

THE SECRET OF BREATHING

Question: Do you breathe along the center line?

Answer: Yes, the secret of breathing lies in moving down in back and up in front of the central axis. Breath is channeled into the body primarily through the diaphragm, the muscle lying at the heart of the muscular system. The diaphragm works best with a lengthwise image. Good use of the breath in speech and song demands a long axis.

Question: Is the diaphragm attached to the spine?

Answer: Yes. The least understood part of the diaphragm action is between its center and the lower spine. In the illustration you see slim, tentacle-like attachments on the front of the spine. These are called "crura" which means **legs**. The crura reach down from the lower rib level to the middle of the lumbar spine. With the help of the muscles of the traffic bridge, the crura help the diaphragm to cling low on the spine on inhalation.

Nature has provided two familiar muscle responses to help us maintain a long center line in breathing. One response is called the yawn, and the other is the sigh.

Question: What do these responses do?

Answer: The yawn and sigh act as muscle barometers for the breath. Without being aware of it, you can shorten your breathing over a period of time. This can happen in a rapid or prolonged buildup of physical or emotional tension. When you have built up tension to an uncomfortable level, you may have the desire to yawn or sigh. Nature takes you into a deeper exhalation, which starts you on the way to better relaxation. The action of the diaphragm must be increased to channel oxygen into your circulatory system. You yawn at the theatre, not so much because you are bored, but because fatigue or emotion have interfered with your breathing. Your muscular system will function naturally to do this, if you are not holding it taut.

Question: Is there a "best" way to yawn?

Answer: Yes, let the yawn start by traveling down the back of your center line. Gradually, the awareness of it should go deep into your thighs, in the direction of your heels. This will help you relax the muscles in back of the legs, if you have been unconsciously holding them too tightly.

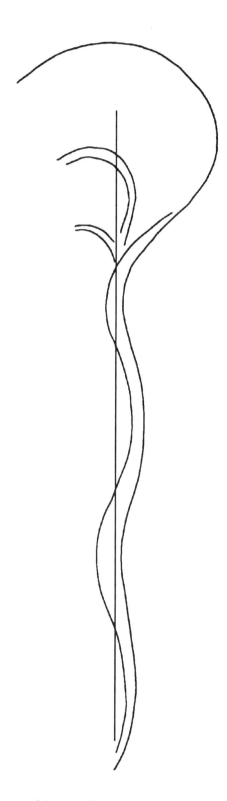

Abstract Design of the Head and Spine Indicating Breath Rhythm

A sigh produces somewhat the same result, but is usually less noticeable. Watch a baby or a dog yawn. The relaxation of the jaw is not what they are really after. It happens as a by-product. Their yawns channel deep into the pelvis and thighs. For animals and young children, yawning is an enjoyable experience they like to prolong. Try thinking of it in this way and feel how it lengthens both the spine and the rib case.

Question: Having relaxed down in back of the center line, what should I do next?

Answer: Nature can help teach you the next step if you will consistently follow through with a period of letting yourself yawn at least once a day. The way to accomplish this with the greatest enjoyment and benefit is also the most courteous. It involves what we have just discussed, put in the following order:

1. As the yawn starts, slowly allow the lower jaw to soften and fall away. This begins the lengthening of the center line of the neck and the upper back.

2. Follow the center line down through the spine into the lower back and pelvis and into the backs of the thighs. The longer the line becomes, the longer the breath which follows it.

3. Close the jaws as silently and slowly as possible. Your ability to do this, without making it evident, will gradually increase.

A prolonged yawn down in back of the center line should be followed by a slow release up in front of the line. Thus inhalation follows exhalation. Remember, the greatest muscular effort involved is in the diaphragm, near the center of your body. It is not at the nose level. The air flows through the nose channels but the nose should not act as a pump. It is merely a bed through which the stream flows.

Sensing the action below the waistline, in the lower back and pelvis, builds awareness of the crura of the diaphragm. The crura seek the center of your body just as the roots of the plant seek the center of the earth. Both seek life and need this action to fulfill their functions. This cannot be done well if the jaw and facial muscles are held tensely. So relax the jaw, neck and shoulders by visualizing the deepening action along the center line into the lower body. Gradually, your breathing will lengthen and become stronger.

You need a long axis, I need a long axis—everyone needs a long axis in breathing.

Take Time To Breathe.

SITTING DOWN AND GETTING UP

The sitting action is an incomplete movement. It is really a **half squat.** The squatting action brings more muscles into play. Try the squat. If you allow your thigh and knee joints to fold sufficiently, you will see how it helps lower your body weight through your center line. It forces you to keep the thigh joints flexible and get more action into the upper part of your legs. Chairs allow you to be careless in this because you are unconsciously planning to move just a short distance to the seat.

Picture a juggler as he goes into action. He starts an object moving and then follows it with another one, timed in good rhythm. He can keep two or more objects in the air by properly timing the distance between them and understanding the effect of gravity on each. You have bones in your body with which to carry out the same trick. Let's start with the center line as it is the body's lead off in launching any movement.

Movement 1: Use a simple wooden chair or bench. It will give greater freedom of movement while you are learning a new habit. Stand in front of the chair. Picture the center line. Place the heel of one foot two or three inches nearer the chair than the other. Imagine the sitting bones leading you down to the chair. Give them the go signal. When you are seated, slide back in the chair by relaxing the left sitting bone and placing it back a bit. Then, relax the right sitting bone as you place it back a bit. Continue to slide back until you are comfortably seated.

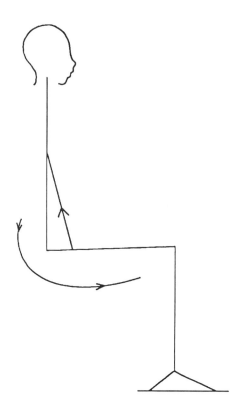

This pattern of movement uses your deep abdominal muscles close to your center line. It will flatten your abdomen and slim your figure.

Movement 2: To stand up, imagine the center line lengthening down. Relax the shoulders and rest your hands in your lap. Relax the left sitting bone. Think up into the traffic bridge as you lift the bone and place it forward a trifle. Relax the right sitting bone. Think up into the traffic bridge to lift the bone and place it forward. Continue until you are near the edge of the chair. Then, place one heel two or three inches back of the other. Balance your head in the center line as it takes the lead in going up. Think up through the traffic bridge and give your thighs the go signal, as you rise to your feet. This movement is difficult until your legs have the power to boost you from below. Before the legs can take over the booster thrust, the sitting bones must relax under you.

ANKLE ACTION

The middle lines of the thighs continue all the way down through the ankle bones. Of course, the lines also pass through the knee joints. You have learned to become aware of the muscle bridge which swings the legs from the spine. There are also muscles which swing the lower legs from above the knees. All these muscles should be well relaxed to allow the lines to pass through the leg joint centers.

Question: Is there an image to help me in this?

Answer: Observe the movement of children. They enjoy a continuous play between the heel and the toes at the ankle joint. It is like the game of seesaw. The following movement can assist you in a better understanding of the flexion of the foot in walking.

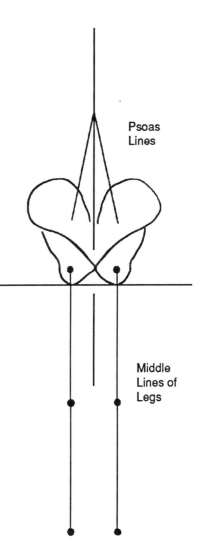

Psoas
Lines

Take the sitting position on a firm low seat and adjust your body along a long center line. Place your left leg out in front of you with a slight bend at the knee. The back end of the heel bone should rest on the floor with the front end of the foot sticking up. Either end of the seesaw is now in position and ready to move.

Think up on the left psoas muscle and let this action flex the toe end of the seesaw upward. The farther the front of the foot can easily come towards the front of the leg, the farther down the heel can seem to drop below the ankle. Return to position by softly and slowly letting the toes droop and curve. This will allow the weight to remain in the center of the seesaw. Change to the other foot and repeat the instructions.

Middle
Lines of
Legs

The foot can also play a seesaw game in walking. Walk, swinging your leg with its middle line continuing all the way down through the ankle bone. The slower and softer this movement is, the easier and more centered will be the flexing of the ankle. The difference between youth and age shows up here.

Stay young and walk with a flexing ankle.

THE DANCE PLIÉ

The plié perfects the art of balancing the body on the tops of the thigh bones. For this reason we should think of the plié as primarily **thigh socket** movement. The knee and ankle follow along but are secondary to the action which takes place at the thigh socket.

The spine starts the plié by lengthening. As the spine lengthens, the psoas muscles transport you up through the traffic bridge. Then the legs progressively fold and unfold at the thigh, knee and ankle joints.

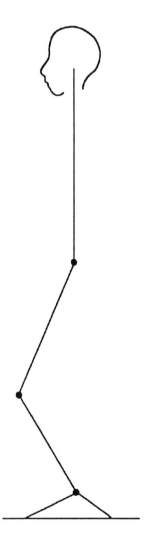

The plié can carry the body from standing erect all the way down to a position of squatting. Let's begin to use the pattern with a focus upon the slight flexion of the thighs in the beginning of the plié.

1. Stand with a long center line and awareness of your thigh heads. Start folding at the front of your thigh sockets with a tiny sitting movement. Pretend you are going to sit down, but then come up by using the path through the traffic bridge. Continue this pattern of starting to sit and then coming back up, for a few repetitions. Rest by discontinuing the exercise for a moment.

2. After practicing the very short distance down and up for a few weeks, gradually increase the distance you go. Judge the depth downward according to the height to which you are carried upward, through the imagery of the traffic bridge.

The plié action is the basis of the powerful crouch and spring action of many animals. The dancer also uses its strong dynamic possibilities in propelling the body into space. This power is built up along the center line. The movement in the plié action can be adapted to a rhythm using the following jingle:

Sit low through the body,
Stand high through the thighs.

Sit low on the sitting bones,
Stand up through the bridge.

CIRCLING THE AXIS –THE VERTICAL POSITION

Question: What does turning around a center line do for the body?

Answer: It gives you more awareness of your center line—the axis from which you move. The most efficient and beautiful movement comes from an awareness of its source along the axis of the body.

Movement 1: Take an easy stance, balancing on the tops of the thigh heads. The circling movement begins at the mid-pelvic level. This is where the psoas muscles lie close to the lower spine. Think of your center line as stationary and begin revolving around it from the right to the left. To make the turn, you will be alternately lifting your left foot and then your right foot off the floor.

At first, it will be a little difficult to get into the rhythm. Turn **slowly** and get the form of the movement first, then your subconscious control will take over. Recall your imagery of thinking up on the psoas muscles on either side of the spine. Then your feet will **follow**, rather than lead, the body as it turns on its axis. After turning around the axis two or three times, walk ahead a few steps taking the center line with you.

To turn from the left to the right side, start by thinking of your center line as stationary. Turn your body slowly as you alternately lift your feet off the floor. Think up into the traffic bridge so your feet will follow and not lead. Turn two or three times and walk a few steps forward, taking the line with you.

If you are quite dominant on the right side, you will need to do more turning from the right to the left (counter-clockwise) than from the left to the right (clockwise).

Movement 2: The action of walking is the slight flexing of one thigh and then the other towards the front body wall. Continuous adjustment of the extensors in the back of the spinal column, aids this flexion. The weight through the spinal column is continually seeking a lower level, while the legs are being lifted from above. Let the weight go down between the sitting bones if you can do it easily. Take very short steps to keep the image of the center line more vivid.

CIRCLING THE AXIS – THE HORIZONTAL POSITION

By turning around your axis in a horizontal position, you learn to use more sockets or fulcrums in the turn. The baby practices this action by rolling on the floor. The proportions of the young child or baby are well suited for rolling all the way over. However, the adult body usually does not benefit from a working on a complete turn. The adult can benefit more from rolling a quarter-turn from a position of resting on the back to a position of resting on either side. This action brings the rib and sacral sockets into use along the sides of the spine.

When lying on the floor a small pillow may be used to align the center of the head and the vertebrae of the neck with the rest of the spine. The size of the pillow should depend on the head size and the shoulder adaptability. The pillow should be used for the head only. It should not be placed under the shoulders as this disturbs their alignment.

Movement 1: First, it is necessary to lie on the floor in a way which allows the spine its greatest length. This requires some flexion of the thighs.

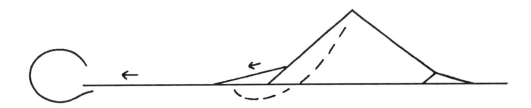

Starting Position on the Back – Profile View

Look at the illustration above. Allow the soles of your feet to rest on the floor with the toes slightly turned in. Your arms should rest at the sides of your body. Center your head in relation to your sitting bones.

Visualize a long axis lengthening down the back. A good image for lengthening the axis is the cat's tail. Roll to your left with the pelvis, thighs, ribs and head turning in unison to the position of resting on your left side.

Rest for a few moments and then return slowly to the starting position of lying on your back with the knees flexed. Repeat this slowly a few times. When done well, this rolling action brings about better alignment through the spinal structure, and makes you more aware of long, lithe lines. The exercise builds better alignment and therefore better movement, as it does for the baby.

Movement 2: When the image of lengthening the axis down the back is familiar, add thigh movement. As you roll to the left, the left thigh should move to the front of the axis. As you finish the turn, the left thigh will approach a right angle with the body. When you reach the side position, place the right thigh, leg and foot over the left thigh, leg and foot. Rest for a few minutes in the position shown in the illustration below.

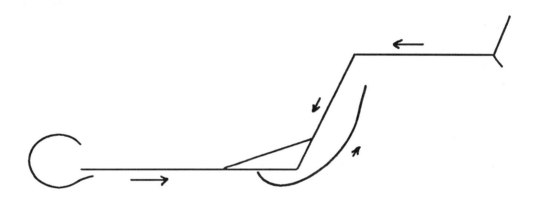

Lying on the Left Side – Bird's Eye View

Movement 3: Return to your back by following these directions:

Visualize the lengthening of the axis or tail down the back. Let the right foot drop back onto the floor behind the left foot. Again, visualize the lengthening of the axis or tail. Use the right thigh and foot, as well as your left thigh and foot, to help you to maintain your axis as you slowly turn back to the starting position. When you reach the starting position, check that your feet are parallel. You should end the movement with the feet a few inches apart and toes slightly turned in. Center your head in the axis line. After a short rest, repeat the quarter turn roll to the left three or four times.

After a few sessions or more of practice in turning to the left, begin making a turn to your right side. For this you will simply reverse the directions. As you practice, compare the two sides and use your judgment in alternating them. For instance, you might turn one time to the right and two times to the left side. As you compare the two sides for ease of movement, your sensory awareness will begin to become your teacher.

MORE SITTING AND STANDING EXERCISES

Question: Why do some people become uncomfortable while sitting?

Answer: Their chairs are probably not well suited for their proportions. Chairs should allow you to balance on your sitting bones, and help you lengthen the central axis. The angle made by the body and the thighs in sitting should be a right or an acute angle. Oblique angles do not allow the structure to balance well and should be avoided as much as possible. Sitting at a right angle will probably be most comfortable at first. Gradually, you will find it more comfortable to use chairs which allow an acute angle.

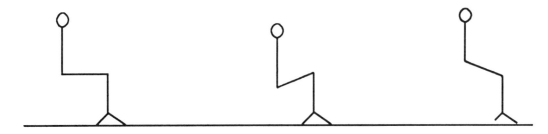

Right – Acute – Oblique Sitting Angles

The muscles which aid the lengthening of the central axis are strengthened as you learn to get along without the support of the back of the chair some of the time. The chair back can be used when you are tired or ill, when it is comforting to rest into its support. However, the chair back should not be substituted for one's own axis. It should remind you of your axis rather than interfere with the use of it. If you are too tired to sit well, you should probably lie down.

Cutting off the legs of a chair you use frequently, may be helpful. Using a firm pad or cushion under the sitting bones will also allow you to be more comfortable. When in a public building or conveyance, the body can adapt to the proportions of a larger chair by practicing the lengthening the center line. Relax the muscles on the back of the thighs and lower legs to allow the heels to rest on the floor, if possible. If the proportions of the seat in relation to your body are within reason, you can be comfortable for a while.

Question: Why do some people find standing difficult or tiresome?

Answer: These people are not aware that the main part of the body has a **single** track system for its support, while the legs have a **double** track system. In the illustration for the lesson on *Ankle Action* you saw the way the two systems merge through the pelvis. The baby learns to merge the double track system of his legs with the single track system of his body by rolling and crawling. Movements to help the adult merge the two systems are given on the next page.

The imagery for these movements should be practiced first in the sitting and lying positions. As the imagery becomes more familiar, apply the directions while standing or walking.

Front of Body

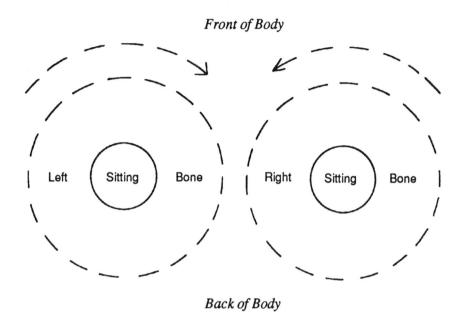

Back of Body

Movement 1: Look at the illustration. Start on the left side with your left sitting bone. In your imagination, think clockwise around the bone, or around the spot on the chair where the sitting bone rests. As you do this, you are visualizing a circle from the front of your left sitting bone toward your center line. Proceed slowly around the circle until you have completed it and are back to where you started. Repeat imagining two or more times around the circle.

Change to your right sitting bone. In your imagination start thinking counter-clockwise around the right sitting bone. As you do this, you are visualizing a counter-clockwise circle from the front of your right sitting bone toward your center line. Proceed slowly towards the back and then go on to the outside of the circle. Then you will be back where you started. Repeat two or more times around the circle.

Movement 2: *Movement 1* can be varied by using the imagery of skywriting by a plane.

Movement 3: A clock face makes good imagery for the same movement. In your imagination follow the hand of a clock as it goes from 12 to 3 to 6 to 9 to 12 etc., on the left side of the body. For the right side of the body you will follow the clock hand from 12 to 9 to 6 to 3 to 12 to 9, etc.

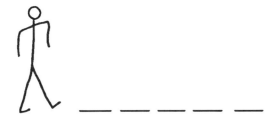

Some people walk at their Foot Level—
they shuffle along on their feet.

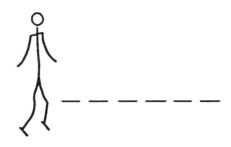

Some people walk at their Knee Level—
they have found little use for their thighs.

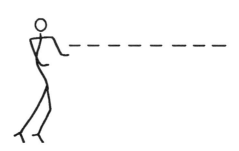

Some people walk at the Shoulder Level—
holding themselves up by their arms.

MORE WALKING EXERCISES

Question: Why do some people enjoy walking and others find it hard work?

Answer: The people who tire easily are walking the hard way. Look at the illustration. Some people walk thinking of the action at the foot level. Others emphasize awareness of their knees or shoulders as they walk. All three of these patterns **walk the body apart**. Walking up the front of the axis **integrates** your thigh and spinal muscles together.

Other people have the habit of pushing from behind rather than folding in the front. There are muscles in the front of the pelvis and thigh as well as on the back of it. Unless you realize the thigh is more easily worked from the front, you may overdevelop the muscles on the back of the pelvis and thigh. This weakens the action of the psoas and allied muscles and interferes with easy folding forward movement of the thigh in walking.

Movement 1: Sit, thinking of your center line. Slide both hands over the top of the thighs from the center of the knees to the center of the thigh sockets. As the right hand holds its position with the fingertips over the right thigh socket, slide the fingers of the left hand down the underside of the left thigh to the knee. You will need to rock your body sideways to your right to do this. Move the left hand over the top of the knee and slide back over the front of the thigh to the left thigh socket. Steady your body here for a moment on the two sitting bones. Then you can slide the fingers of the right hand down the underside of the right thigh to the knee. In doing this, the body will rock to the left. Slide the right hand over the top of the thigh toward the thigh socket to complete the movement. Repeat the exercise slowly a couple of times. Feel the sense of direction the fingers are conveying to the muscles of the thighs. The hands should communicate a sense of aliveness to the muscles which makes an image for their action.

Movement 2: Stand with a long center line. Fold at the front of each thigh socket with the lower leg and foot relaxed. As you fold each thigh think of the suspension of the thighs from the spine through the psoas muscle. You can imagine this muscle action being like the manipulation of puppet strings from above the puppet. Become accustomed to thinking **up** as you fold, whenever you can. Gradually, you will be able to increase the time spent with the imagery. Before you know it you will begin to actually enjoy walking with your deep abdominal muscles.

MORE SITTING DOWN – GETTING UP EXERCISES

It is easier to sit down or get up if the thigh, knee and ankle joints center one over the other. The middle line of the leg is a good image to follow in doing this. In sitting down or getting up, the movement at one joint should carry the impulse to the others in sequence. The first impulse in sitting down or getting up should come from deep in the abdomen where the thigh is slung on the spine. Better awareness of the way this impulse begins action at the level of the thigh socket, allows flexibility of the lower leg and ease of movement at the ankle. The following movements will help you to become more aware of integrated action of the thigh, knee and ankle joints. These exercises will build the coordination you need for ease in sitting down and getting up.

Movement 1: Elevating the Lower Legs and Feet.

This technique requires relaxation down the back of the center line, while muscle action is moving up the front of the center line. The cat is a good example of this. As you stroke the cat along its spine to its tail, the suppleness you feel is like the flow of a stream. This makes an excellent image to hold in mind for good muscle action.

Place a chair on a rug. The chair is for elevating your lower legs and feet. Place a medium sized pillow on the rug about where your head will come when you are on your back. Sit on the rug in front of the chair and put your feet up on the seat of the chair as easily as you can. Lie back and rest your head on the pillow. With your heels and lower legs resting on the chair seat, take hold of the chair legs and pull the chair toward you.

As you lie on the floor with the lower legs in the chair, align your body with the same imagery you have used in sitting. Five to ten minutes in this position with the feet elevated is enough at the start. It can bring about change for the body in many ways although it seems to be a very mild exercise. The position of the legs makes it easier to let the weight of the thighs fall toward the center line. It is also easier to sense greater depth in the thigh sockets. As a result, the muscles in front of your center line are called into action and those in back of the line stop putting on the brakes.

Movement 2: Drawing the Legs over the Chair Seat

Let's see what you can do with movement up the front of the center line.

Review the diagram of the psoas muscles. Notice the lower end of each muscle is on the inside of the thigh bone just below the thigh socket. The upper end is beside the center line at about waist level. In *Walking from Your Axis is a Game*, you used the image of traffic moving up a bridge for swinging the thighs alternately forward from this muscle.

As you think from the lower end of the left psoas muscle to its top, draw your left heel over the chair seat toward your center line. This should happen very, very slowly. When your left heel reaches the chair edge visualize traffic pouring through the left psoas muscle bridge to draw your leg toward your chest.

Place the heel back into its first position on the chair seat. Start dragging your right heel over the chair seat toward your center line in the same way you did for the left. Watch the traffic pour upward through the right psoas muscle bridge to draw the right thigh toward the chest. Return the heel to its first position on the chair seat. Alternate the two sides in the movement two or three times. Use discretion and proceed slowly. The movement is very beneficial if done in this manner.

Movement 3: Movement for Tying the Shoes

Many men instinctively use the following folding movement in tying their shoes. It is a wonderful exercise for keeping the leg joints supple. Because it is a daily necessity, it does not become boring and is not easily forgotten.

When you have put on your shoes and are ready to tie them, stand to the side and a bit to the rear of a chair. Give yourself enough room to swing the leg next to the chair directly forward. Visualize the action high in the psoas muscle and swing your leg up, allowing the knee to softly fold. When the foot is on a level with the chair seat, drop your foot onto the chair. The inner edge of the shoe should be parallel with the edge of the chair seat.

With the foot resting on the chair seat, you are ready to go into the squatting or plié action on the standing leg. Do this by lowering the body. Think of the center line and the balance of your head. When you have a nice awareness of this, lower the line toward the floor. Your position is now low enough to put your hands in place to tie your shoes. To tie the other shoe, stand to the side of the chair facing in the opposite direction and follow the same instructions.

Tying your shoes in this way everyday will be very rewarding in keeping the joints supple and in maintaining good body alignment. It relaxes the muscles in which most of us are overly contracted and strengthens those that are weak.

MORE BREATHING EXERCISES

Using the breath to the best advantage in speech and song is dependent on balancing your head well. You have learned the muscle action determining the rate and volume of breathing takes place low on the spine. Now you can become aware of the resonant chambers at the upper end of the spinal instrument. The head is like an expanded vertebra sitting at the top of the spine. To unite the head with your spinal column, imagine the center line of the head rests on the center line of the spine.

If you begin thinking through the head, using the center line image, you will be surprised at how much lighter and smaller it will seem. This will give you more of the awareness the dancer experiences in balanced movement of the head. In gaining the concept of a center line, it is helpful to make use of the sense organs such as the nose and eyes.

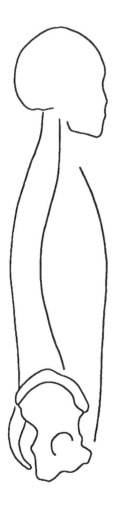

Movement 1: Sit and imagine lengthening down in back of the central line. Close your eyes and very **lightly** touch the eyelid of the left eye. If the eyeball feels hard and tense, think of softening the eyeball. When you are able to feel the eyeball quite relaxed, change to the right side and repeat the directions with the right fingertips touching the right eyelid. Use the image of a small wet sponge to help in relaxing the eyeball. When the eyeball is well relaxed, it may feel like the eyelids are larger and longer. In your imagination, see them as curtains or draperies falling down very softly over the eyes.

Movement 2: Lightly touch the side of the left nostril with the fingertip of your left hand. Soften this outer left side of the nose by lightly touching its surface near the tip of the nose. This is where the adult's nose tends to be overexpanded. The baby is extremely soft and relaxed in this area. He allows the inflow of air to take a central path through each nostril. Directing the air flow against the outer wall of the nostril is a poor pattern learned later in life.

The partition at the center of the nose acts as the inner wall for each nostril. Softening the outer wall of the nostrils encourages muscle action to become stronger in your lower spine. Soften the outer walls of the nostrils to allow exhalation to travel even deeper down in back of your center line. This strengthens the action of the diaphragm and lets inhalation travel up the front of the line.

MORE EXERCISES FOR FOOT AND ANKLE ACTION

As you continue to think of action in the psoas muscles you will feel your movement higher in the body. The feet will relax and let the long levers of the thighs and lower legs swing from their upper ends. The following exercises will help you balance the lower legs and feet.

Movement 1: Swinging the Fibula

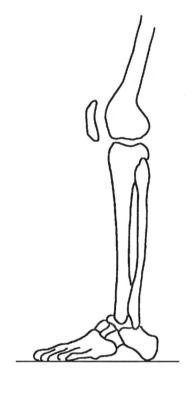

In the illustration you can see the little outer bone of the lower leg (fibula) has no part in the knee joint. Knowing this will help you balance the thigh bone over the large lower leg bone (tibia). The socket for the fibula is on the outer surface of the tibia, one to two inches below the knee. The lower end of this little bone on the outside of the ankle should not be held rigid. Visualize it as relaxed, and free to swing about like your little finger. This will allow you to be more conscious of the line through the middle of the leg.

Lie or sit in a well-adjusted position. Imagine a rhythmical swaying of the fibula forward and back from the head of the bone, a little below the knee joint on the outside of the lower leg. The action of a pendulum in slow motion is a good image to have in mind. The sway forward needs the greatest attention since the muscle pull in this direction is weaker than the pull backward on the bone. After imagining the sway forward, simply imagine the bone returning to position.

Gradually, this exercise will help relax the calf muscles and strengthen the muscle action on the front of the leg. As it becomes more familiar, use it in any position or as you walk.

Movement 2: The average person uses his hands enough to keep the palms soft and supple. As you observe your palm, you will see crinkles or puckers in its surface. Thinking of the sole of the foot being more like the palm of the hand can improve your posture. Use the image of a soft hollow in the center of the left foot, at the front end of your heel bone. This will relax and lengthen the Achilles tendon in the back of your ankle. Repeat the imagery for the right foot.

Movement 3: Another approach is to think of puckering or crinkling the under surface of the large toe joint. First, touch the under surface of the thumb and soften it. Think of the softening extending into the hollow of your hand. A similar softening of the area beneath the large toe can be extended into the hollow of the foot. This softening action can also be imagined under the joints of the other toes. Time spent coaxing the action into the sole of the foot, will be very rewarding. It soothes the nerves and adds to one's comfort.

MORE PLIÉ EXERCISES

In the foregoing lessons you have been adjusting the bony weights of your body. First, you relaxed the sitting bones lower on the axis and centered the head higher on the axis. Letting go of the breath down the back helped you learn to lengthen your axis. Learning to use the thigh bones in a better way aided the support of the center of the body when standing and walking.

Movement 1: In the illustration, notice there are no hinge or folding joints in the upper half of the body. The first folding or hinge joint is at the thigh joint. Here, either half of the body has been designed to fold on the other. The body can fold on the thighs or the thighs can fold on the body. The vertebral column is not designed for folding. The lower half of the body has our folding joints. The habit of folding the spine gradually weakens the structure. Fold at your thigh, knee and ankle joints, not in your back. Following this rule, in all of your movement, will strengthen your whole body.

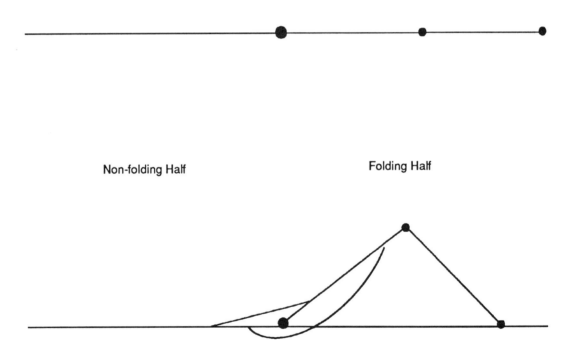

Non-folding Half   Folding Half

Movement 2:   Standing with the feet parallel is the natural position in which the thigh, knee and ankle joint areas can be at rest.   When the foot is turned outward, the top of the thigh bone is also turned outward.   The body structure cannot balance as well in this outward rotated position.   To offset this strain, dancers should practice some of their pliés in the parallel position.

Although the plié is an action of all three of the folding joints, the action at the knee and ankle joints is usually the most familiar.   You will do well to concentrate more upon the tiny folding action which takes place at the front of the thigh joints.   Focus upon lengthening the center line will help you balance the action of the three folding joints.

Movement 3:   The body should breathe freely as it moves, **combining** breath and movement. We should not inhibit one to do the other.   Breath and movement can happen in unison because they follow the same path—the path of the axis or center line.   Letting out the breath as you start the plié will help you coordinate breath with movement.

Start to exhale down the back of the center line as you go into the thigh folding action.   Follow the flow down the back of your center line and into the leg axes as well as you can.   With each plié, you will exhale at an increasingly longer interval.   Prolong the exhalation, and inhalation will automatically become longer.

In time, you will begin to feel the way exhalation helps to lengthen your spine.   The action flows down to the level of the sacrum and into the muscles in back of your leg axes.   As a result, your legs fold at the front of the thigh sockets.   Continue to let your breath go down in back of the line as you lengthen it.   When the breath goes low enough you will discover you float upward through the thigh sockets to the psoas muscles above them.

Movement 4: Try what you did in *Movement 3* along with this jingle for your imagery:

Sit low on the sitting bones—stand up through the bridge.

As you exhale, sit low on the sitting bones.   As inhalation starts, stand up through the psoas bridge.   Be sure to take your thinking all the way up to the upper end of the bridge.   Three repetitions at the start is enough. Practice can be increased as you improve.

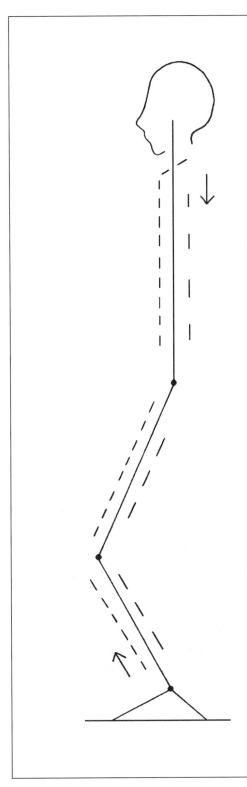

How To Live In Your Axis —Your Vertical Line

INTRODUCTION

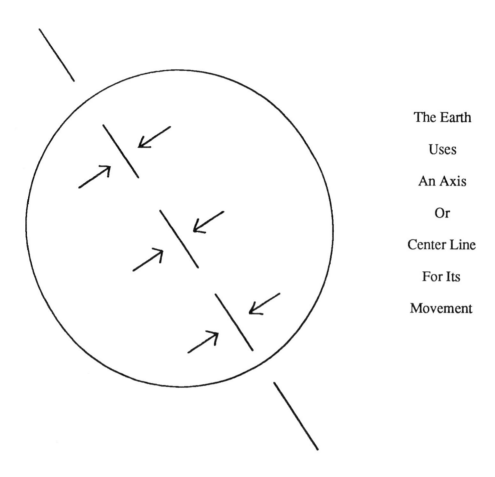

The Earth

Uses

An Axis

Or

Center Line

For Its

Movement

Like the earth, we also have a center line or axis. We should learn to balance along that center line. Body movement travels up and down the axis, along with the breath.

An observation of children would show them to be quite aware of their axes which brings skill and ease into their actions. Children often shake their heads or nod them up and down, experimenting with the balance of the skull on the central axis. They use the plié to remind themselves of the axis when learning to stand. They roll, turn somersaults and move in lots of ways that bring the axis into play.

In contrast, the average adult seems to carefully preserve his axis from participation in full body movement. Movement is confined within the arms and legs instead of flowing through them from the axis. The axis may be pulled upward by intellectual factors or outward by the emotional. Gradually, all these factors shorten and distort the axis.

Have you ever thought of your axis as a part of you? Do you use your axis as a means of action as readily as you use an arm or foot? Since your axis lies deep within the center of your body, it may escape your thought in your usual activities. If the axis is forgotten in breathing, you may lose awareness of expanding the spine and ribs downward on exhalation. Then the leverage for expanding the ribs up the front on inhalation is lost. If you forget your axis in the simple movement of getting into and out of a chair, you may depend too much on your arms and legs. This is where the movement of the plié can help you. It develops the muscles along the axis that lower you down or take you up through the center of the body.

You can bring the axis into greater use through simple visual imagery. Imagery can help you to be more aware of the central role of the axis in all movement. The images and exercises in these lessons have been planned to follow each other as well as possible. In the beginning, you will probably find one lesson is as much as you can handle at one time. When you are familiar with two lessons you will be able to combine them. As you learn to understand the design and purpose of the lessons, you will see how they work into a coordinating pattern for the body at rest or in motion.

You can learn anything if you begin slowly and confidently. However, if a lesson is difficult, do not struggle with it. Try to see something easy in the movement and practice this a bit. Read the lesson over to find another easy part to add to the familiar one. Remember movement belongs to your unconscious mind. When you try to do a new action consciously the mind rebels until it begins to come easily. Don't expect too much of yourself all at once and stay relaxed about it. Just think of the image as you practice the action and your unconscious mind will catch on.

You can slowly bring better awareness into your habit patterns by turning your attention to the imagery presented in this manual every day. Enjoy practicing anytime, anywhere. Take tiny moments of rest instead of longer breaks and think of the imagery. Soon, you will find you have less fatigue and better concentration. Eventually, even when you are not consciously trying to improve, you will start to experience deeper breathing and better form. Little gleams of light will dawn on you, as you work, play and rest.

BALANCING DOWN THE BACK OF THE CYCLE – THE PLIÉ

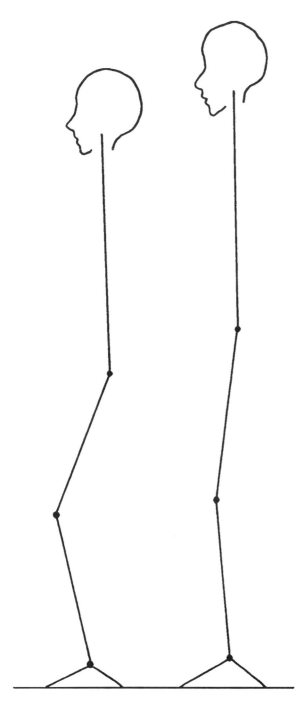

Stand and begin lowering your body along a center line. This is best done through a slight sinking of your body toward your heels. Return to the standing position and repeat the up and down movement several times.

Where along the center line are you holding your weight?

The center of weight should not be felt between the shoulders. If you feel yourself holding there, let your arms hang free. Put all your attention into letting the body sink through the action of the muscles close to the back of the center line. Then follow the rhythm of the movement down toward the middle of your pelvis.

As you continue to lower and raise your body, keep thinking down the back of your center line. After a little practice, you will begin to feel the mid-sacral area which is the base of the spine. As you become aware of this base, you will feel your thigh heads supporting it. This support comes to your thigh heads from the center of your feet through the middle lines of the legs. When you have found this balance you will feel the center of weight in the middle of the pelvis.

EXHALATION COUNT STRENGTHENS DOWN THE BACK ACTION

Breathing exercises can be practiced while sitting, standing, lying on the side or on the back. It is important to get the sitting bone level fixed in your mind as a goal for your usual exhalation. Let's begin working with your lower back vertebrae in breathing. Then the goal will be close enough to insure reaching it.

Exercise 1: Gently blow an exhalation through your lips. Repeat the exhalation, but this time do not center your attention on your lips, cheeks or chest. Instead, imagine the blowing starts from the middle of your first lumbar vertebra and continues down your center line toward your sitting bone level. Pause and breath easily.

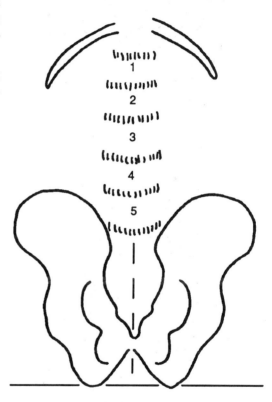

Continue by imagining the breath at the second lumbar vertebra. Take a gentle blow down the line from the middle of that bone toward the sitting bones. Rest again for a moment and continue with the middle of the third lumbar vertebra, the fourth, and finally the middle of the fifth lumbar vertebrae as your goals.

After your practice at each level, return to a more natural breathing pattern for a moment. If you are blowing easily, you will create action down through your lower back muscles.

Exercise 2: Try yawning and notice how it helps you relax your cheeks, lips and chest. If you tend to yawn wide and shallow, change to yawning narrow and deep. Then, return to the blowing exercise. See if you can produce a very slight blow from your lower back as you would a narrow yawn. Humming or vocalizing can also be used to lengthen your exhalation. Combine with the plié you practiced in the previous lesson.

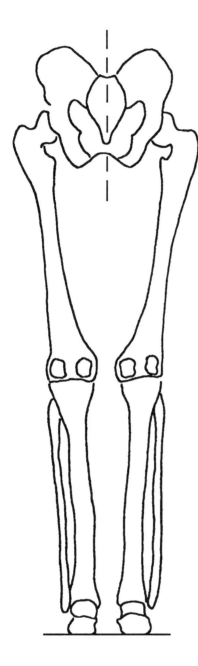

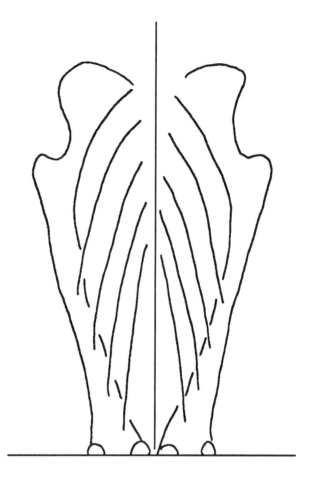

Back View – Bone and Muscle Designs

RHYTHM CONTINUES THROUGH
YOUR LOWER BACK AND THIGHS

The average person holds too much tension in the muscles behind the sitting bones and in the back of the thighs. These muscles should relax to allow the body to balance well in sitting or standing. Look at the illustration of the muscle design through the back of the pelvis and thighs on the opposite page. Your balance will improve as you think of lengthening along these muscle lines down the back of the thighs.

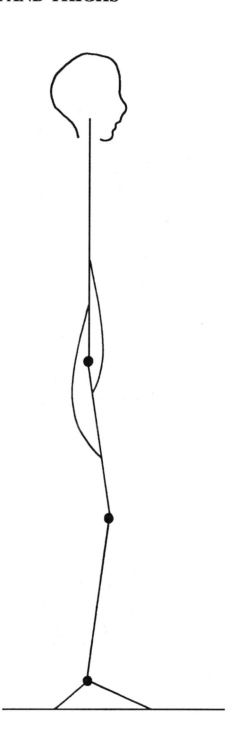

Exercise 1: Stand and start the movement of the plié again. As you slowly move down the center line, visualize the weight passing down through the lower back vertebrae into the sacrum. When you feel the weight on your thigh heads, think of them supporting your spinal column. You should not try to gain your balance by holding the sacrum up. In the illustration on this page, you can see how the bone support slants a little backward from the knee centers toward the center of the spine.

Exercise 2: Let the muscle action flow down the entire length of the spine into the back of your thighs. Think of lengthening along the thigh muscle design. As the large muscles through the back of the lower spine, pelvis and thighs become active and stop holding, the weight will pass more easily through the bones.

Exercise 3: Walk by folding one thigh forward and then the other. You will find you can gain leverage to do this more easily by lengthening the spine downward. As this action becomes familiar, think down the back of the thighs toward the heels. This idea should make it easier to flex the knees and move up the through the support of the thigh heads into the pelvis.

BALANCING THROUGH YOUR AXIS

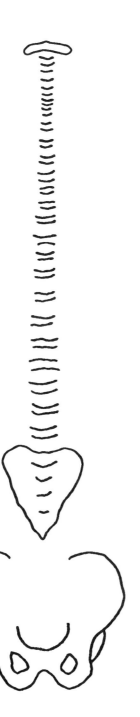

Sit in a chair that allows the knee ends of your thigh bones to be a little higher than the pelvic ends of the bones. Your heels should rest on the floor.

Look at the drawings of the spine and the pelvis. Notice that the two drawings can be combined as one.

Exercise 1: In your imagination, fit the sacral end of the spine down through the space in the back of the pelvis. Picture the image once again and raise your left thigh toward your head. Return to position.

Again imagine the spine sliding downward through the open space in the back of the pelvis. Picture the image again as you raise your right thigh toward your head. Return to position.

Alternate the two sides a few times in practice.

Exercise 2: Seeing the space the lower spine fills in the back of the pelvis also helps in breathing. Think down through the space as you easily exhale. Think up through the thigh sockets as you easily inhale.

Balancing through your axis takes place as you think of weight sifting down through the space in the back of the pelvis on exhalation. Think of support rising up through the thigh sockets as you inhale.

WALKING INTO YOURSELF – ACTION IN THE PSOAS MUSCLES

Many of us have shortened the spine for so long that we have lost the lovely feeling of the forward swing of the thigh in walking. What can we do about getting it back?

The muscle to imagine in walking is called the psoas. Study the design of the muscle on this page. The psoas raises the upper thigh toward the body to carry you forward into space. The ease with which your thigh comes up also depends upon the relaxation of the opposing muscles. As you know, these are the muscles lengthening down the spine and back of the pelvis and thighs. If you are not well relaxed in these, it is like putting on the brakes when you want to go. The tension of these muscles holds you back and you only half go.

An interesting image to use is the action of closing a jackknife. The handle of the knife can be your spine and the open blade, your thigh. The blade working at the hinge will remind you that your movement should begin at your **thigh socket**. To feel this happening it is helpful to see the spine slipping down through the space in the back of the pelvis as you did in the previous lesson.

To really enjoy walking, your deepest abdominal muscle, the psoas, needs its "go" signal. This starts the muscle action up the front of the body. There is no need to make a conscious effort to pull up through the superficial abdominal muscles. Instead lengthen down through the back lines and roll the thigh balls upward. With the support of the thigh heads, the psoas muscles will draw the action up the front to balance the pelvis.

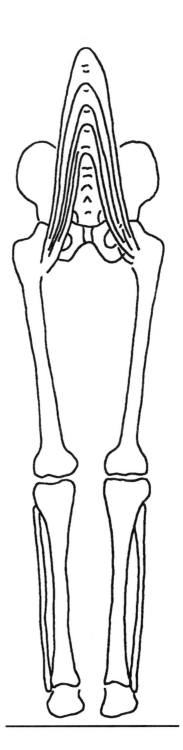

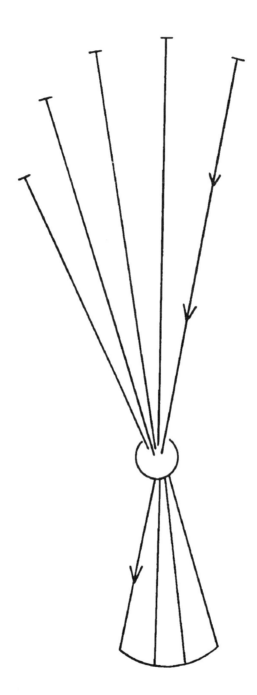

Abstract Design of the Axes of the Toes for the Left Foot

THE CENTER OF YOUR FOOT

The tibialis posterior muscle, helps support the long arch in the center of your foot. It is almost as long as your lower leg and loosely unites the two lower leg bones, the tibia and fibula. The muscle is too deep to feel with your fingers, but you can run your fingertips along the outer border of the fibula from top to bottom.

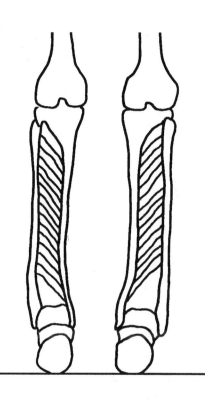

Exercise 1: Sit and begin to feel for the rounded head of the fibula on the outside of the knee and a bit below it. Let your fingertips slide straight down the outside of the bone toward the ankle. Near the ankle you will feel the rounded lower end of the fibula. If you think of casually swinging the lower end of the bone forward, as if it were the end of a branch swaying in the wind, you will feel a release of tension. The tibialis posterior muscle is then free to **draw up** on the inside or center of the foot. Change to the other leg and repeat the exercise. Practice in any position will help to trigger this muscle into its arching action.

Exercise 2: The strength of the hollow or arch of your foot depends on the release of your heels. Stand to experiment with this action. At first, place one hand on the back of a chair for the exercise. Keeping the feet parallel, support the body with the heels only. Change the support of your body from one heel to the other a few times.

When the movement is familiar, let go of the chair and take a few steps forward. Notice how letting the heels sink down, lengthens the muscles on the back of your legs. Releasing the heels encourages the muscles in the center of your legs, including the tibialis posterior, to draw up into the arch of the foot. Let the first three toes droop closer to the front of the ankle as you walk on your heels. Practice walking this way a few minutes a day, without your shoes, to strengthen your foot arches.

Exercise 3: Study the abstract design of the axes of the toes on the opposite page. In the sitting or standing position, imagine movement along the line from the large toe toward the outside of the heel. Just think of the movement. Keep your feet parallel as you practice.

THE OUTSIDE OF THE ARM FALLS AWAY

The outer lower arm bone or ulna should not be held up with muscle tension any more than the outer lower leg bone. Arm movement follows the same pattern you learned for the body and legs.

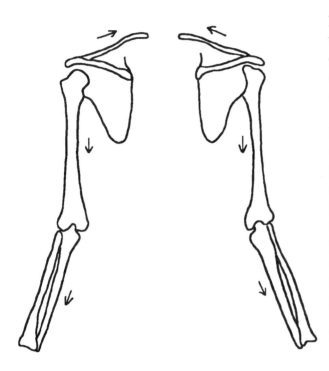

In the previous lesson, you thought of the fibula swinging from its upper end on the side of the tibia. Now you can do the same with the ulna on the outside of the lower arm.

Exercise 1: Sit and center yourself with your hands over your thighs, palms down. Place one lower arm over the other. Let your right hand feel along the outer edge of your left arm from the shoulder to the point of your elbow. Trace down the outer border of the lower arm to the tip of your little finger. Let the ulna hang from its joint at your elbow.

Repeat the exercise on your other side.

Exercise 2: As you repeat *Exercise 1*, find the little round end of the ulna bone just above the wrist. This is where the bone is sometimes held too rigidly. The wrist centers in the end of the other lower arm bone, the radius, on the thumb side of the arm. Think of lengthening the outer lines of your arms to lower your little fingers. This will relax your wrist. Repeat the exercise by finding the lower end of the ulna bone on the right arm. Think of letting the outside of the lower arm fall away to relax the wrist.

Exercise 3: Combine *Exercise 2* with the plié. You will find the image of lengthening down the outside of the arm will help you to lengthen down the back of the spine on exhalation.

THE SHOULDER BLADES STEER THE COLLAR BONES INTO THEIR STERNAL SOCKETS

Few people are aware of the articulations between the shoulder blade, collar bone and sternum. As you become more aware of the bones and their joints you will see how the shoulder blades steer the collar bones into the sternum.

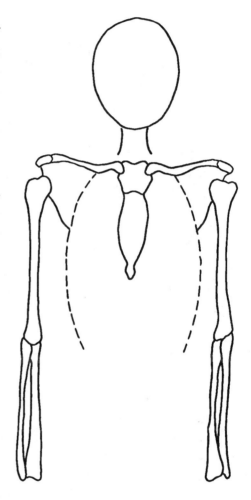

Exercise 1: Sit close enough to the left side of your chair to allow your left arm to hang straight down without touching the chair. Lightly place the fingertips of your right hand over the area where your left shoulder seam meets its sleeve. Let your left shoulder blade slide forward and backward as you explore the area with your fingertips. Soon you will feel the head of the shoulder blade (acromion) meeting the **outer** end of the collar bone. This is the location of the acromioclavicular joint.

Slide your fingers along the collar bone to a position over the top of your sternum on its left side. This is where the **inner** end of your left collar bone meets the sternum. This articulation is called the sternoclavicular joint.

Exercise 2: With the left arm hanging down at your side, slide the left shoulder forward and inward slowly and rhythmically. Picture the head of the shoulder blade leaning against its collar bone. Imagine the shoulder blade action **steering** the collar bone into the sternum. Repeat the exercise once on the left side.

Change to the right shoulder and go through Exercise 1 and 2 as you did on the left side. Then you can alternate the movement between the two sides in your practice. A catchy phrase to think to yourself could be:

My shoulder blade steers my collar bone, my arm trails along on a lower level.

RAISING AN ARM BEGINS ALONG THE SIDE OF YOUR AXIS

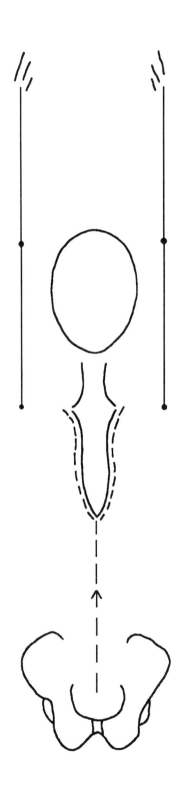

Exercise 1: Sit in balance with your hands at rest in your lap. Slide the fingertips of your left hand lightly up the front of your mid-front line from your abdomen to your neck. Place your hand back in your lap. Repeat the movement up to your neck again, thinking the direction upward along with your finger touch.

Change to the fingertips of your right hand and trace lightly up your mid-front line in the same way. Slide your right hand up to your neck again, thinking the direction upward along with your finger touch. Alternate the hands as you repeat the movement a few times. If you are thinking the direction **up the front** very easily, you may begin to feel the action continuing well up into the neck and then **down the back.**

Exercise 2: Stand to practice the arm movement once again. The fingertips of the left hand trace upward along the mid-front of your body as you practiced in Exercise 1. This time, let the arm continue to extend straight up toward the ceiling. Think of lengthening down the back of your center line to steady your arm in its upward course. As you unfold the arm over your head, you could imagine the arm being propelled by the lengthening of the lower back.

Exhale down the back of your center line as you lower your arm very slowly back to position. Repeat the exercise once with the left arm. Change to your right arm and follow the same pattern on the right side of your body. Alternate between the two sides in each practice session.

THE SHOULDERS AID THE WEIGHT TRANSFER

A short cut to better shoulder action is the image of the center line extending up over your head. Using a yardstick helps to create a vivid image.

Exercise 1: Stand and place a yardstick over the front of your body. Hold the lower end of the stick against your abdomen with your right hand. The other end of the stick will go up along your nose and above your head. Slide the fingers of your left hand upward along the yardstick. Let the arm continue straight up toward the ceiling as you did in the previous lesson. Think down behind your axis as you lower your arm as slowly as you can. Repeat once on the same side. Change to the right arm and go through the directions. Alternate between the two sides until you have the idea well in mind.

Exercise 2: Now you can use the image of a yardstick for your axis line in the center of your body. Study the design on this page. Picture the yardstick as your axis and raise your left hand up your mid-front line. As your arm extends toward the ceiling, picture your hand sliding along the imaginary yardstick. When the arm unfolds above you, let the fingers open out like a fan in space. The little finger will be in the front and the thumb toward the back. As you lower the arm into position, the fingertips will trace behind the yardstick image. The fingers gently bend and relax together as you think of the closing of the fan. Repeat on the left side.

Change to the right arm and follow the same pattern. Alternate the two sides a few times in each practice session.

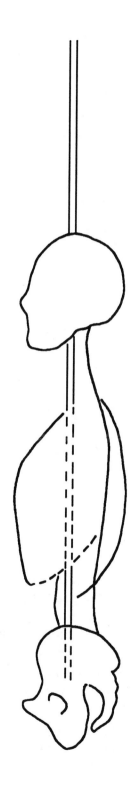

RAISE THE TOP OF THE STERNUM IN THE FRONT
TO LOWER THE SHOULDER BLADES IN THE BACK

Balancing the shoulders begins with balancing the body from beneath the shoulders. The foundation of a structure determines the set of the roof. We know the foundation for the shoulders is at the sternal sockets. This lesson should help you place the sternal sockets at a higher level. As you practiced the exercises in the two previous lessons, you might have realized that moving **up the front** helps to relax the forward pull on the shoulders.

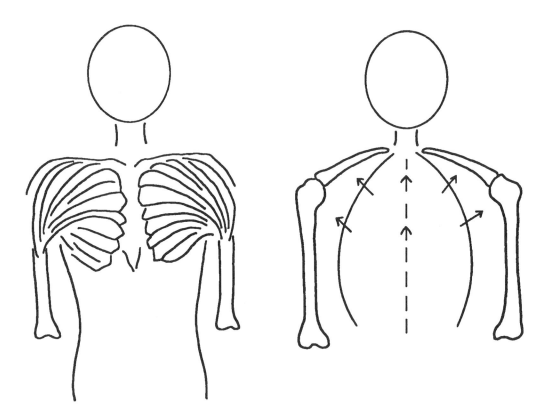

Exercise 1:   Look at the illustrations above. The muscles of the front of the chest (pectoralis major) are shown along with lines of movement you can think for them. Stand and slide the left hand fingertips upward along the mid-front of your body. As you reach the side of the sternum, picture the pectoralis major expanding upward under the collarbones. Let the hand continue to slide straight upward toward the ceiling. Lengthen down the back of the center line to steady your arm in its upward course. Lower your arm slowly to the starting position. Change to the right side and follow the same pattern.

Exercise 2:   Note that expanding the chest muscles takes place along the body of the sternum. Imagine action up along the body of the sternum toward its head (manubrium). The tail-like end of the sternum (xiphoid process) should remain relaxed.

THE SHOULDER BLADES SERVE AS FLOATING RAFTS

Ease in moving **down the back** depends upon this relaxation of the shoulders and the spinous processes of the vertebrae.Imagining your shoulder blades sliding down the back of your center line will help the head of the sternum move up in the front line. In this lesson, you can imagine the shoulder blades as **floating rafts** which convey action from up the front of the body to down the back of the body.

Exercise 1: Stand and raise your left arm up the front with the image of the yardstick along your center line. Notice how your left shoulder blade begins sliding down your back as your arm moves up over head. When you have reached the top and fanned your hand open, think down the back of your center line as you lower your arm to your side. Repeat on the left side to deepen awareness. The muscle action moves up the front, slides **over the top** of the shoulder blade, and then down the back into the center line.

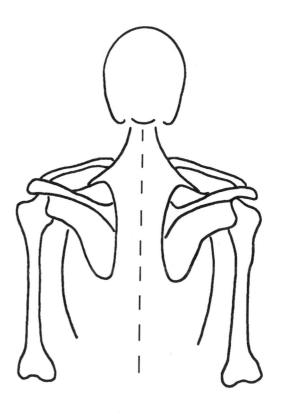

Change to the right arm and follow the same pattern. Alternate the two sides a few times in each practice session.

Exercise 2: Review *The Outside of the Arm Falls Away*. Stand and repeat the exercise above. Combine the image of releasing down the back of the arm toward the little finger with the image of lengthening down the back of the center line.

Exercise 3: Repeat *Exercise 2* with the breath as you are ready to do it. Tie the images from both lessons in with exhalation. Let the shoulder blade and outside of the arm slide down your back as you exhale. Then you can think of expanding the chest muscles up the front on inhalation.

LOWER YOUR SACRUM IN THE BACK
TO RAISE THE FRONT OF THE PELVIS

By now, you may have noticed that the image of sliding your shoulder blades down your back lengthens your lower back, too. The trapezius muscles pass the shoulder action down to the latissimus dorsi muscles. The latissimus dorsi muscles steer the action and weight of the arm down the back into the gluteus maximus muscles. The illustration below shows how you can use these muscle patterns as images. The action lines through the trapezius, latissimus dorsi, and gluteus maximus muscles can be compared to the flow of small streams into larger ones.

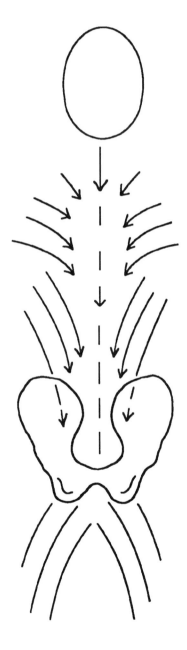

Exercise 1: Stand and raise your left arm up the front. Let your shoulder blade slide down your back along your center line. When your hand has reached the top and fanned open, begin to exhale, very slowly. Imagine the back muscle designs leading the shoulder blade and arm down the center line toward the sacrum. Repeat the exercise on the left side. Continue the flow through the back of the pelvis toward the heels.

Change to the right side and follow the same pattern for sliding the right shoulder blade down the back. Slow exhalation helps the arm movement and strengthens better breathing. Alternate the sides in your practice.

Exercise 2: Combine your awareness in the exercise above with the imagery of the pectoralis major. As you slide up the front, picture the pectoralis major muscle expanding upward **under** the collar bones. This can be combined with inhalation. Then picture the shoulder blade, as a floating raft, sliding down to your heels as you practice exhalation.

BALANCING THE BODY ALTERNATELY ON THE TOP OF EITHER THIGH

The muscle lines from the upper ends of the thighs should relate to the spine. If we can recognize this principle in our balance and movement, order can be maintained for supple action of the joints. Getting hold of the muscles on the inside of the thighs (adductors) takes you up through the psoas to the sides of the spine.

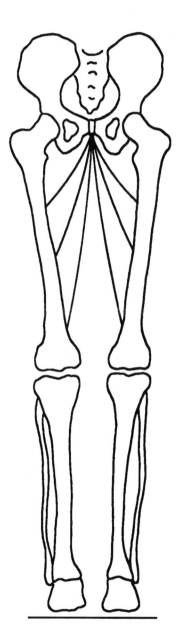

Exercise 1: Stand and think of supporting your body on the tops of your thigh bones. Begin to plié with softly flexed thighs, knees and ankles as you think upward through the psoas muscle lines. Balance your body with the image of flow through the back muscles down toward the sacrum.

Having sensed the weight of the body on the tops of both thigh bones, slowly take the weight off the top of the left thigh bone and place it all on the top of the right thigh bone. Return to balancing the body on the top of both thigh bones. Exhale easily as you unfold the legs and think down the back. Plié again and slowly shift the weight onto the left thigh bone. Return to balancing the body equally on the tops of both thigh bones. Exhale easily and unfold the legs.

Exercise 2: In your practice of the plié, alternate between balancing equally on both thigh heads and balancing on the right side or the left side. This will help you get the use of the muscles on the inside of the thighs. Using the muscles on the inside of the thighs, takes you up through the thigh sockets to the sides of the spine.

CROSS PATTERNING – THE OBLIQUE LINES INVOLVED

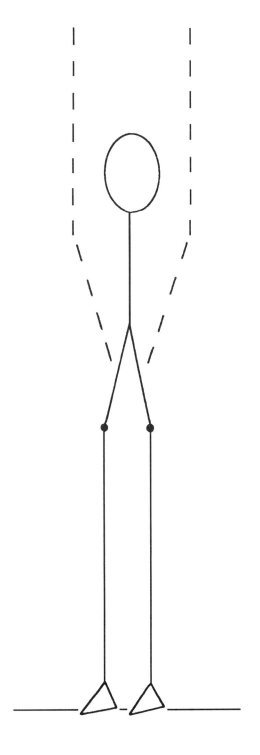

Front View

Cross patterning brings the oblique lines of the body into play. The axis of a round body also needs oblique or diagonal lines to give it support.

Study the illustration on this page. Notice how the axes of the legs turn toward the spine making an "A" shaped design pointing up the front.

Exercise 1: Stand and start your left hand in its upward course along your axis line. When your hand has reached your waist, go very slowly to give yourself time to visualize. Imagine picking up a line from the front of your right thigh. The line moves diagonally up through the front of the body to the spine at the level of your lowest rib. Continue up the center front and unfold the arm toward the ceiling. When your hand has reached over head, begin a slow exhalation and lower the arm weight down the back of your center line. Repeat the exercise again on the left side.

Change to the right arm and the left leg. Start your right hand in its upward course along your axis line. When your hand has reached your waist go very slowly so you can think of the imaginary line from the left thigh. See the line moving diagonally through the front of your body to the spine at the level of your lowest rib. Continue up the center front and unfold the arm toward the ceiling. When your hand has fanned open, begin a slow exhalation and lower the arm weight down the back. Repeat the exercise on the right side. Then alternate the sides in your practice.

CROSS PATTERNING – USING AN ARM WITH THE OPPOSITE LEG

Crossing and recrossing the axis through imagery of oblique or diagonal lines develops the muscles close to the spine and lengthens them. Look at the illustration. Notice how the axes of the arms turn toward the spine and form a "V" shaped design down the back. You can combine this image with the "A" pattern from the previous lesson.

Exercise 1: Stand, balancing equally on the two thigh bones. Lightly place the palm of your left hand over the front of your right thigh. As you begin raising your left arm, think of an imaginary line from the front of your right thigh socket up to your spine at the lowest rib level. Tracing the diagonal up the front of the abdomen can be used to establish a feeling for the pattern. Continue to trace up the front, reach over head and fan your hand open.

See all the energy that came up the front, beginning to fall down the back in a diagonal pathway. Use your slow exhalation to follow the diagonal down the back from the left shoulder to the sacrum. The passage of weight continues into the back of the right thigh, lower leg and heel, as your arm returns to your side.

Change to the right arm and trace an imaginary line up the front from the left thigh toward your spine at the lowest rib level. When your hand has fanned open, exhale and imagine the weight falling down through a diagonal line from your right shoulder to the sacrum. The outgoing breath continues down the back of the left thigh and lower leg toward the heel. Alternate between the two sides a few times in each practice period.

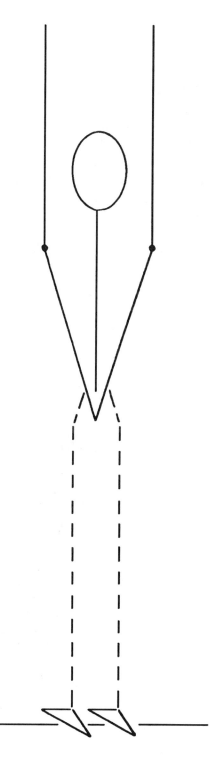

Back View

FOLLOWING THE HAND PATH TO THE SHOULDER AND LOWER BACK

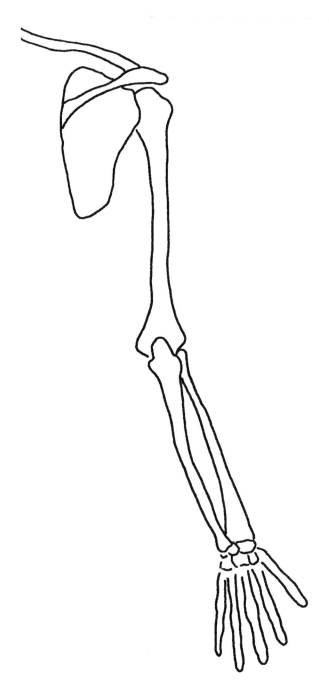

Your practice of the exercises in *The Outside of the Arm Falls Away* helped you center the hand in the wrist. Now, you can learn to center the hand along the length of the arm axis as the arm moves up and down through the oblique or diagonal lines.

Exercise 1: Begin to draw up the front of the right thigh with the left hand as you did in the previous lesson. As you trace up the front, imagine the base of the thumb being drawn up the **inside** of the arm toward the elbow. Continue to think through the arm to the shoulder as the arm reaches over your head. Think of the little finger line growing longer as you breath easily. Inhale once again. As you exhale, imagine the weight of the arm flowing down with the shoulder through the diagonal channel in the back of the body. Return your arm to your side and rest.

Change to the right arm and trace up the front of the left thigh. Imagine the base of the thumb being drawn up the inside of the arm toward the elbow and shoulder. As the arm goes up over your head, think of the little finger line growing longer. Inhale once again. As you begin your exhalation, imagine the weight of the arm flowing down through the diagonal lines in the back of the body. Complete the movement by allowing the ulna to hang free at your side. Alternate the two sides in each practice session.

INHALATION – UP THE FRONT FOLLOWS
EXHALATION – DOWN THE BACK

Holding the arm over your head while taking a complete breath, exercises the intercostal muscles between your upper ribs. Because the shoulders are not pressing down on the upper ribs, the breath gives an uplift to the chest and corrects the daily drag downward. The sternum leading up the front is established by the structure. The intercostal muscles of inhalation also point upward which makes good imagery to follow. The intercostal muscles of exhalation point downward in the back.

As the next step in breathing, you can combine the directions up the front and down the back with attention to the central axis of the body.

Exercise 1: Imagine the lower body as a balloon from the waist level to the ischial tuberosities of the pelvis. Work with the image of this long cylindrical balloon collapsing as the air goes out of it, and expanding as it refills. Keep the action vertical and close to the center line.

Exercise 2: Next imagine the balloon in the lower body is divided into four quarters. There are two long quarter sections toward the front of the body and two long quarter sections in the back. Think of action in each of the sections as follows:

Picture the left side in the back emptying and collapsing downward on exhalation. Imagine the left side in the front filling and expanding upward on inhalation.

Picture the right side in the back emptying and collapsing downward on exhalation. See the right side in the front filling and expanding upward on inhalation.

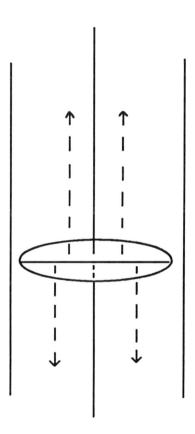

Repeat the sequence from the beginning two or three times. Gradually, you can increase the time of your practice and cross pattern between the two sides.

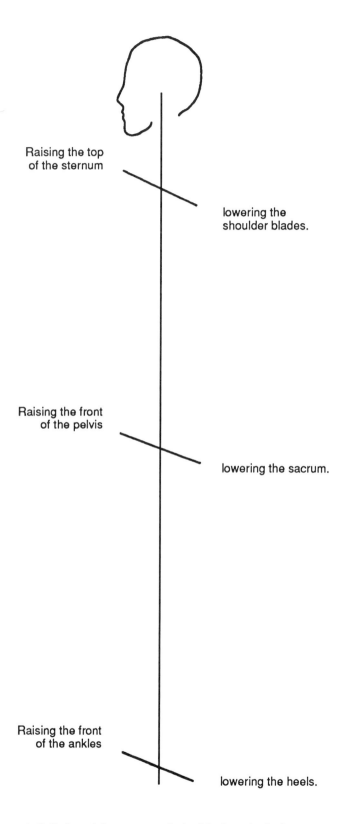

Raising the top
of the sternum

lowering the
shoulder blades.

Raising the front
of the pelvis

lowering the sacrum.

Raising the front
of the ankles

lowering the heels.

A Split Level Structure – Quite Modern in Style

LOWER YOUR HEELS IN THE BACK LINE – COME UP FROM YOUR TOES IN THE FRONT LINE

The heel of your foot rests on the floor. The ankle bone rides on top of the heel. No muscles attach to the ankle bone. The trick of balancing the ankle depends on the fair play of action between the front and back of the entire body—head to your heels and toes to your head.

Exercise 1: Stand with the palms of your hands resting over the front of your thighs. Let go of the breath or let yourself go into a long yawn. A prolonged exhalation creates action in the muscles down through the back of your spine and prolongs their relaxation too. Casually take a few short steps and feel movement passing upward under your hands as you walk. The illustration shows a path you can think of by following the arrows. The action up the front of the legs continues up the front of your body. From the level of the sternum you can think over the shoulder structure to move down through the mid-back lines again.

Exercise 2: Allow the arms to rest at your sides and continue to walk slowly. Thinking up the front through the foot takes you from the toes to the ankle. The down the back action helps the heels drop low enough to make ankle flexion easy. Seesaw play between the toes and heel as you walk can be fun. It gives normal ankle action and keeps the ankle bone in balance on the top of the heel bone. Letting the large toes fall toward each other will help you toward this goal.

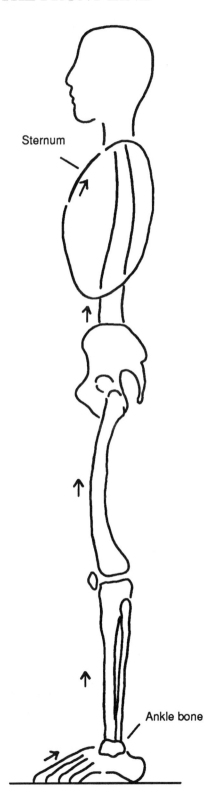

Sternum

Ankle bone

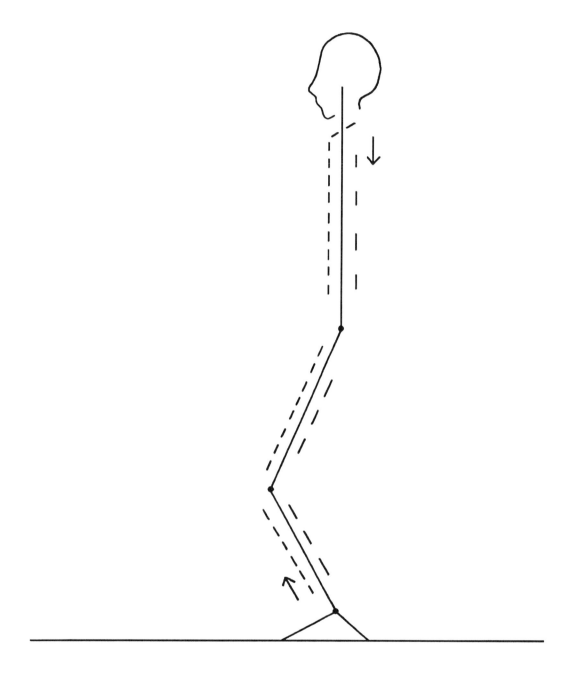

From Up the Front to Down the Back of the Body

THE BODY CYCLE – SUGGESTIONS FOR FURTHER PRACTICE

Some of the exercises you have practiced in this manual can become an entirely new experience with a change in position. You can increase your progress and pleasure in the lessons if you will review them lying on the floor. Lying down gives your spine better leverage and puts your shoulders at ease. After practicing on the floor you will find that when standing and walking, your shoulders and arms feel light. They feel this way because they are balanced. You have brought the many muscles of your back into greater action and given badly needed relief to your chest and abdominal areas.

Rolling can also be used in reviewing the lessons. Rolling is nature's first lesson in walking. Walking principles are easier to grasp when you are relaxed in a horizontal position.

Exercise 1: A long thin pillow can be used in supporting the head in relation to the spinal vertebrae as you rest on the floor. The rolling pattern should begin with the path of the psoas muscle which you used for walking in many of the lessons. The psoas and allied muscles draw the thighs upward giving a flexed position at the thigh joints and knees. This makes it easier for the muscles in the back of the body and thighs to relax. As you slowly turn onto your left side, think of the head of the thigh bones following the diagonal path upward and inward toward the center line. When you have reached your left side place your right thigh, lower leg and foot over your left thigh, lower leg and foot.

Take a few moments to exhale and inhale to restore your awareness of your center line. Place the right foot on the floor a little behind the left and think of the diagonal lines moving upward. Use the support of the right foot to aid you in returning to the starting position on your back. Rest again thinking of the diagonal lines down the back. Repeat the action to the left and then practice rolling to the right. Alternate the left and right sides in your practice.

Exercise 2: The rolling action can be combined with previous exercises for the arms. Start with *Raising an Arm Begins Along the Side of Your Axis*, and *Raise the Top of the Sternum in the Front to Lower the Shoulder Blades in the Back* when you roll. As you become accustomed to combining arm action with rolling you can add other imagery as well as cross patterning.

Lengthening the spine should be combined with everything you do in movement—walking, sitting down, getting up, or going up and down the stairs. In all of your movement, think of backing down the spine. **Down into the roots—up into the sunlight**, is the law for all axial bodies. It is the pattern for breath, communication and movement.

Body Proportion Needs Depth —Front to Back

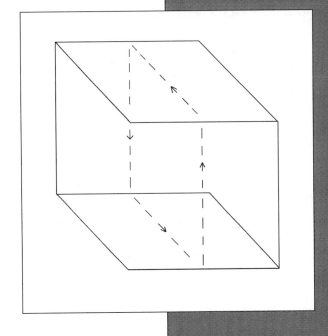

INTRODUCTION

The body is balanced through many different joints. Centering each joint is like playing a game of seesaw on the playground. There is a child on one end of the lever and a child on the other end. If they are playing fair, they will both enjoy the seesaw balance around the fulcrum. The muscles in the body use a similar play of balance around the joints.

Our goal is to find balance around the centers of each of the major joints. Usually people think along the surfaces or edges of the body rather than into their axis centers. You can develop awareness of your axis centers if you remember the body has **depth**. Although the body and its joints are more round than square, the design of the cube can help you realize the depth of the body. You can apply it to the body as a whole or to the smallest units of action, the joints.

The lessons in this manual really do not teach anything new. Babies inherit knowledge of how to balance the body and develop their manner of movement on their own. Their limitations lie in the environment provided and their structural inheritance. What the well-aligned person has already developed, is stressed in these lessons. This information can help you improve, if you can learn the way a child learns, through observation and visualization.

In teaching facts, information is grouped together so the relationship of the parts to the whole can be fully explained. However, in these lessons you will be learning by visualizing, which involves a different kind of organization. In working with imagery, success seems to lie in dealing with "crumbs of knowledge." Only what you actually use in movement will be explained, which eliminates a lot of non-essentials. A variety of images for many joints will be presented. Both the mind and the body like some variety in the "food" taken into the system.

As you gain better awareness of action at one joint, you will find that awareness affects other joints through unconscious reactions. In working with imagery, there is no need to try to create a muscular response within the body. Just hold the image in mind—see it—and it comes to pass. You defeat your purpose if you tense your muscles to bring it about. You cannot make it happen. Of course, you must really desire to accomplish what you visualize or picture. If you do, you can become what you think about.

Some of the exercises use imagery to direct a line of thrust from the center of one joint to another. Before you can do this easily through visualization, you can touch the surface of the body as close to the center of the joint as possible. Your touch should trace the line of direction the image describes very precisely. People use their hands and fingers to support the head or brace the tense and aching parts of their bodies. You can use your own touch to teach yourself good balance.

BODY PROPORTION NEEDS DEPTH

Many of us know that we move at the joints. However most of us do not realize we should balance at the center of each joint. How do you find the bull's eye center of the joint? By allowing balanced play in the ligaments and muscles in front, in back and on both sides of the joint. Thinking of the shape of a cube in the joints allows you to know where the front of the joint leaves off and the sides begin. It gives a back, a top and bottom to each joint. Cubes at the joints are our smallest units of action.

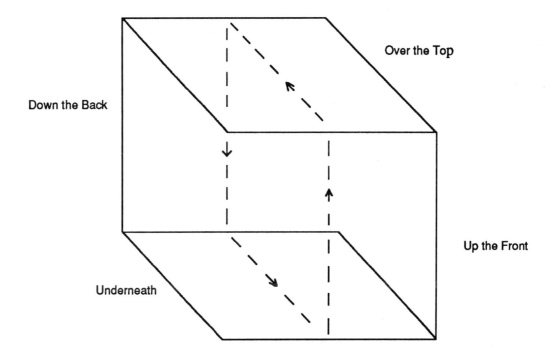

The cube design can also be applied to the body as a whole. You have a right side and a left side. Equal weight brings even balance between the two. You have a front and back side. Thinking up the front and down the back brings them into balance. You also have a central line or axis through the middle of the body. Extend your central line into a vertical plane from **front to back** to discover the depth of the body.

Why not think of extending a horizontal plane from side to side? Because you have probably already overdone that idea and given yourself too much width. For most of us, breadth from side to side has been overemphasized. Length has suffered as a result. Depth from front to back has been neglected. Begin to think more of the body's depth, the **over the top** and **underneath** portions of the body cycle. This idea will help you move more easily through your central axis and become more familiar with the centers of your joints.

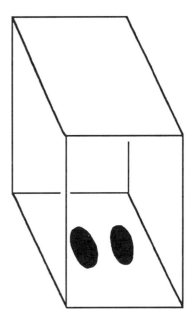

In sitting,
contact with
the chair or
bench is at the
bottom of a box.

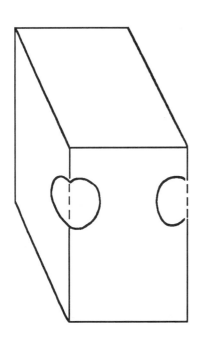

In standing,
contact with
the thigh bones
is on the upper
front surface
of a box.

STREAMLINE YOUR STRUCTURE
IN SITTING AND STANDING

Many of us tend to stand, sit and walk at the sides of the body. We are not as familiar with the central line up. The sitting bones are located where they can serve us best, at the lower end of the body. One of the reasons there are two of them, is that the weight of the spine can be more securely supported with two supports than with one. This happens if you use them alike. If you favor one more than the other or use one differently from the other, your structure gradually becomes unbalanced. You know what becomes of buildings and bridges that are not supported equally on all sides.

Exercise 1: Study the cube design for sitting on the opposite page. The sitting bones are in the same plane, front to back. Each of the sitting bones is also placed the same distance from your central line. Take time to become aware of the sitting bones and see if you are balancing equally between them. After a few periods of feeling this out, the underside of your thighs will feel more relaxed. Sitting well on your sitting bones is the first step in streamlining your body and preventing joint and circulatory difficulties.

Exercise 2: In standing, the body uses the thigh sockets which are located above the sitting bones. The thigh socket placement may be more difficult to sense. You cannot feel the sockets with your fingers because they are buried deep in the pelvis. You can learn to be aware of the thigh sockets by imagining that the inner pelvic area is like a cube.

Look at the illustration of the cube design for standing on the opposite page. The cube represents the **inner** pelvis. The breadth and depth of this cube would be about the same size as the inner pelvic rim. The sides of the pelvis, where you put your hands on your hips, are outside the dimensions of the cube.

Notice that the thigh sockets are placed where the side planes of the inner pelvis turn into front plane. This makes the distance between the thigh sockets only slightly wider than the distance between the sitting bones. Think of this as you stand on the tops of your thigh bones. It will help you to stand more easily.

For streamlining the structure, most people need to shrink their body width between the right and left sides of the pelvic cube. This will allow expansion of the distance between the front and back sides.

HOW ALIVE ARE YOUR FEET?
BEING ALIVE MEANS ACTION IN THE JOINTS

The joints are where the action is in your feet. You should know the beginning and end of each foot bone and how their sockets relate to one another. You can start by learning more about the ankle and heel bones.

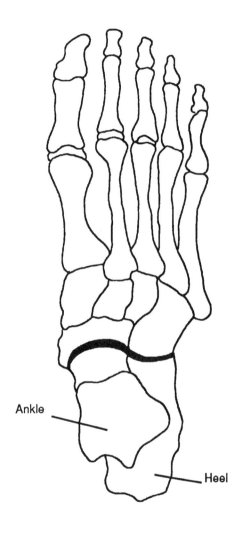

There are no muscles attached to the ankle bone. It keeps its place through the many joints with the heel bone below it, the ends of the lower leg bones above it, and the navicular bone in front of it. The ankle bone makes seven sockets with these bones; the many sockets are there for action. It may be hard to make an image for each of these seven sockets. Let's simplify our thinking by using a ball and cup image for the three most important socket connections at the front, top and bottom of the ankle. In each of these areas, one bone surface is molded like a ball, the other is hollowed out like a shallow cup.

The ball-like top of the ankle bone fits into the cup-like sockets formed by the ends of the two lower leg bones. Although the joint is too deep to be touched, we can get a sense of its shape in the following exercise.

Exercise 1: Remove your shoes and put your right foot on the edge of a chair placed in front of you. Run the fingertips of your right hand from the back of the heel along the outside of your right foot to the front end of your heel bone.

Notice in the illustration that the front of the heel and ankle bones end in a curved line. However, the ankle bone is placed on top of the heel and ends at a higher level. Place the middle fingertip of your right hand on the outer edge of the curved line at the front end of the heel bone. The end of your thumb will be on the inner edge of the line at the front end of the ankle bone. Draw the thumb and middle finger toward each other over the front of the ankle and heel a few times. Use the image of a ball for the ankle to sense the height of the top ankle joint behind your fingers. Place your left foot on the edge of the chair and use your left hand to repeat the exercise.

The heel is the largest bone in your foot. It is a long bone about one-third the length of the foot. The ankle bone is a little more than half the length of the heel and sits on its front end. On the bottom of the ankle bone is a shallow cup hollowed out to fit over a ball-like surface on the top of the heel. We can walk high on the ankle bone by sensing the sockets with the heel **underneath** the ankle bone. The feeling is of a cupping, deep in the sole of the foot.

Exercise 2: Sit on the floor or in a chair in a way that will bring one foot within reach of your hands. Let your fingers find the lower end of the large lower leg bone on the inside of the leg. Next find the bony projection or tiny shelf of bone just a bit beneath it. This is the "sustentaculum tali" or **supporter of the ankle** where the ankle bone centers itself on the inner top of the heel. The ball-like surface of the top of the heel articulates with the hollowed bottom of the ankle just beside and slightly in back of the sustentaculum tali.

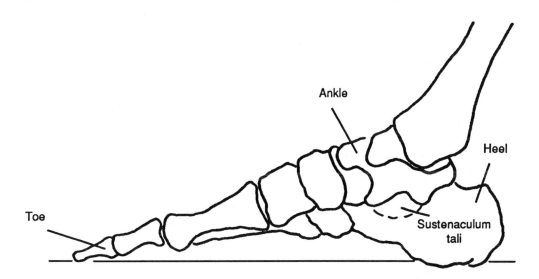

Exercise 3: Sit on the floor with your sitting bones resting on your heels. Point your large toes toward each other so they almost touch. Close your hands loosely and relax your knuckles. Place your right fist in the center of your right foot and your left fist in the center of your left foot. Begin to gently knead the soles of your feet with loose fists. Soften the foot thinking of space between the sockets. Hollow out the center of the long arch. Pause and loosen up your hands and repeat. Feel the length of the long arch from the base of the second toe to the front of the heel. The ankle bone is at the highest level of the long arch of the foot.

Exercise 4: The drawings on the next two pages can be copied onto cardboard and folded to make three dimensional models of the heel and ankle bones of the right foot. The numbers explained in the key will guide you in fitting the cubes together.

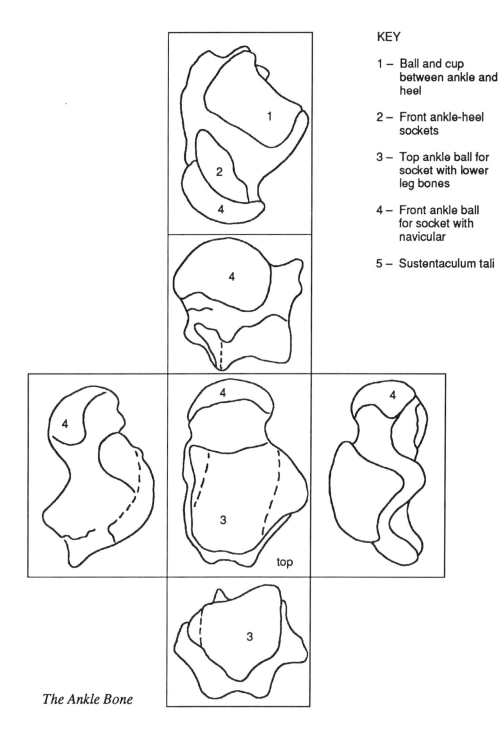

KEY

1 – Ball and cup
between ankle and
heel

2 – Front ankle-heel
sockets

3 – Top ankle ball for
socket with lower
leg bones

4 – Front ankle ball
for socket with
navicular

5 – Sustentaculum tali

The Ankle Bone

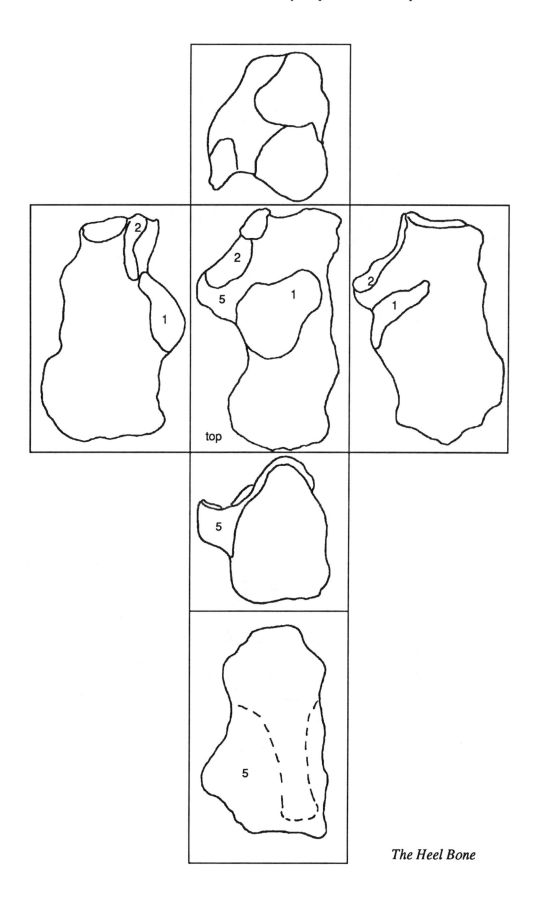

The Heel Bone

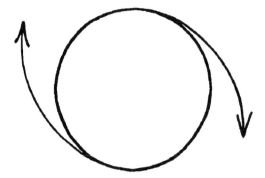

Rolling a Ball - The Back Goes Down as the Front Comes Up

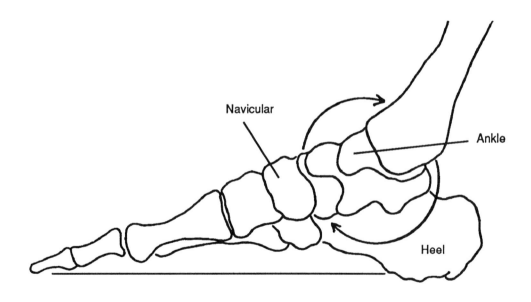

The Sockets Between Heel – Ankle – Navicular Work the Same Way

TOE TO HEEL – HEEL TO TOE ACTION

In the previous lesson, you learned that a shallow cavity, hollowed out underneath the ankle bone, fits over the ball-like surface on the top of the heel. Similarly, a shallow cavity in the back of the navicular fits over the ball-like surface on the front of the ankle bone. This socket arrangement gives toe to heel and heel to toe action to propel you in walking, jumping, running etc. Toe to heel, heel to toe action begins with the release of the heel in its socket. The navicular rolls up over the front ball head of the ankle as the heel drops its rear end.

In walking forward too rapidly, our tendency is to pull up on the back of the heel. If the achilles tendon in the back of the heel is too short, it pushes the ankle bone forward throwing it off balance as it meets the navicular bone. The circular pattern for the heel, ankle and navicular sockets in the illustration on the opposite page is an image for improving your balance at the ankle. As the **heel drops** down from the rear of the ankle bone, the navicular **rides up** in the front of the ankle bone. It is like a ball rolling—the back of the ball goes down as the front comes up.

Exercise 1: Sit on the floor or on a low seat. Place your right foot in front of you with the sole of the foot resting on the floor. Think of the ankle ball rolling down the back and up the front as you flex your ankle towards the front of your lower leg. When done easily, the back end of the heel will drop down and your toes will be relaxed in the folding action. Return to the starting position and repeat very slowly for a few times. Notice how the image makes your heel feel very long as it drops from under the ankle bone. This action is frequently half-done in our movement. Seldom do we take it slowly enough to achieve very much benefit. Deep ankle flexion done with a very slow rhythm strengthens your feet as well as your breathing. It increases the **depth** of the long arch and makes your ankle more flexible.

Exercise 2: Clear an empty space in the room so you can move backward without slipping or hitting anything. The image of circling the ankle bone will be used as you walk backward. Think of the direction of circling shown in the illustration as you move. Lift the left foot off the floor. The movement in walking backward begins with the touch of the toes to the floor a few inches behind. Think of flowing back through the long arch of the foot as the sole of the left foot settles back on the floor. Let the heel drop low enough so you can feel the circle rolling up over the front of the ankle bone and down the back of it. Repeat the action with the right foot and then change from side to side slowly and in rhythm.

This is the seesaw action of the foot. The ankle is the center, fulcrum or balance point. Practice this exercise frequently until you realize the control of the heel action lies in moving backward from the tips of the toes into the depth of the ankle.

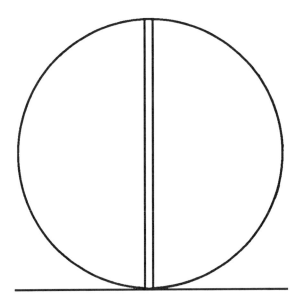

Foot Mound Viewed From Above

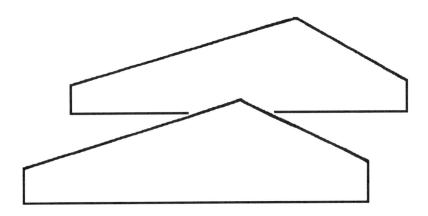

Foot Mound Viewed from the Side

A MOUND MAKES A BASE FOR THE BODY
AND HEIGHTENS THE LONG ARCHES

You can think of the feet making a small mound or hill, which is higher at its center than around its edges. The feet are two halves of a whole and make your base of support. This works best when the feet are in parallel. The reason for feet together is to place the height of the long arch under the center of the body.

Exercise 1: Sit on a low seat with your hands on your thighs. Think of the mounds made by your feet. What does this do? In sitting it helps you balance evenly through your legs so you may rest comfortably on your sitting bones. Place your hands in similar mounds over the middle of your thighs. Pick up your hands and loosely shape them into fists. Relax your wrists as the joints next to your fists. Now make fists of your feet toward your ankles by gently flexing the many joints of your feet in the same way. Making fists of the feet activates muscles in their soles so the navicular bone can ride up in the front of the ankle. Soon you will find yourself rocking back on your heels as you practice. What causes this reaction? Active muscles in the front and center of your leg allow your heels to drop down.

Exercise 2: Stand with the inner sides of your feet close together. Carefully pick up one foot and place it an inch away from the other, keeping the inner sides parallel. You now have two half mounds. Each half mound should keep the same height on their inner sides as when they were side by side, bracing each other. What does this do? It makes a secure base for the body.

Exercise 3: Try to keep the awareness of the mound in daily movement. The mound image can even be applied in the "turned out" movements for the dance. Remember the long arch of the foot is the highest at the ankle which is on top your heel. As you kneaded the inside of each foot, you felt the bottom of the platform that supports the ankle, the sustentaculum tali. The sockets between the top of the heel and the bottom of the ankle are at this level. The ball-like top of the ankle bone on the next higher level supports the center of the knees and also the thigh heads in the thigh sockets.

Improved balance of these many joints comes through the idea of heightening upward through the mound pattern. Take advantage of moments during the day as you stand to think of the feet making a mound. Think of the ball heads of the bone at the various levels pointing toward the center of the body. Notice the feeling of support this gives as you go into action.

Remembering the mound pattern for the feet as you rest or are active helps you toward good alignment throughout the body.

DON'T CROWD YOUR VERTEBRAE—
HOLD EACH BONE LOOSELY BETWEEN THE DISKS

The spine is our central core. It is frequently called a "backbone" which is partially wrong. We should not think of the spine as singular as the term backbone implies. Instead we should think of it as plural, because it contains so many separate bones. The bones of the spine are called vertebrae. There are disks between the vertebrae which are made of an elastic material. The disks give springiness to the spine, if the vertebrae are not crowded too closely together. Thinking of space between the vertebrae provides for the lengthening of the spinal muscles. Don't crowd your vertebrae, space them down.

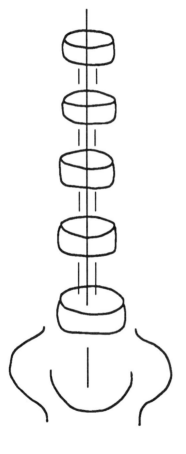

Exercise 1: Try this exercise in any position. Think of the breath weaving between the vertebrae—in and out and back to front—through the spaces occupied by the disks. You may do this naturally to a small degree during and after a yawn. As you yawn, notice how you lengthen up and down through your spine in the action. You are using the elasticity of the disks as well as the muscles while exhaling deeper. Think of weaving between the vertebrae as you exhale. Inhalation will follow a prolonged exhalation without effort on your part.

Exercise 2: While sitting or standing, think of the image of breathing between the vertebrae. When you feel you are doing this, very slowly lift an arm toward the ceiling in a line parallel to your center line. Work with gravity to lower the weight of the arm down the spine into the sacrum. This also gives better use of your muscles in breathing.

Breath weaves a pattern along the line of your deepest structure called the spine.
It spaces its threads both deep and high to put your feet on the ground and your head in the sky.
How else could it weave the elusive design to give you balance all sides of a line?

HOW ALIVE IS YOUR SPINAL COLUMN?
BEING ALIVE MEANS ACTION IN ITS JOINTS

Each vertebra is a strong reminder that nature intended us to **balance** through the spine, inch by inch, vertebra by vertebra. The animal balances through its spine into its tail. People will do well to imitate the animal by applying more leverage to the heel-like end (spinous process) of each vertebra. These "heels" of your vertebrae make an action row from your head to your sacrum.

Exercise 1: Stand and start walking backward, toes to heel. Picture the image of circling the ankle bone. After a little practice dropping the heels of your feet, imagine a vertebral heel at your waist level dropping also. As you imagine this action you may yawn, which lets the muscles lengthen around the spinal heel tips. Keep walking backward and imagine another vertebral heel a little lower down in your spine beginning to drop down also. Coax more action down the back of your spine by placing the back of your hand over the lower spine and gently sliding a knuckle down the heel line.

Exercise 2: In a position of rest or sitting, imagine a long center line. Think of an area in the spine where you need more flexibility, between your shoulders, for instance. Single out a vertebra in that area and think of it in the same way you are beginning to think of the center of your foot. The circling image you applied to the ankle can be used around the body of the vertebra.

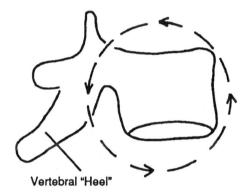

Vertebral "Heel"

The pattern for the imagery is up the front of the body of the vertebra, over the top, down the back by way of the vertebral heel, and underneath the vertebral body to the front where you started. Repeat the image **up the front, over the top, down the back** and **underneath**, several times. This will also allow the breath to be more effective. The diaphragm, as well as the arms and legs, uses the spinal levers for movement. As the pattern becomes more familiar, you may feel the effect in other joints along with those in your spine. Each joint, brought into better alignment, carries over into better joint patterning throughout the body.

THE THIGH HEADS SWING IN
AND UP AS THE KNEES BEND

Harmony for the joints of the legs begins by sensing the flow from the toe tips toward your ankle bone. This brings deeper flexion at the front of your ankle and signals the achilles tendon to lengthen and drop the heel. Centering your knee caps will get the front muscles of your legs into action as the knees bend for the climb ahead.

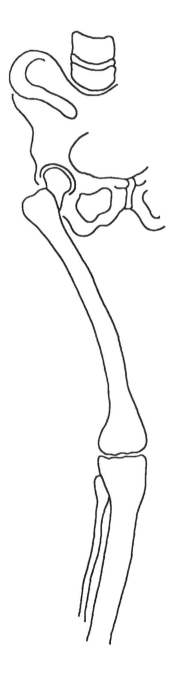

Exercise 1: Your kneecaps in front of your knees should glide easily upward as you move. Sit in a low chair. Place your right hand over the front of your right lower leg bone or tibia. Slide your fingertips up following the bony ridge along the mid-front of the tibia. Do this a few times taking your hand off each time and replacing it on the lower leg to begin again. Carry this upward line over the center of your knee and the top of the thigh toward your thigh socket. Change to your left side and repeat the directions.

Exercise 2: Review *Exercise 1*. As your right hand slides over your knee, let your right toes swing upward in the same rhythm. Notice how your thigh bone flexes deeper in its socket as you rock slightly backward on your sitting bones. Pause and readjust your foot on the floor. Your toes will enjoy taking their time centering in their line up. Change to your left side. As your left hand slides up the front of your left leg, let your toes swing upward. As you rock slightly backward on your sitting bones, your thigh head flexes deeper in its socket.

Exercise 3: Notice in the illustration that the thigh head points up toward the front of the spine. Review walking backward in a slow continuous rhythm. Let your heel drop quietly down on each step, down into gravity. Think of the reactionary force to gravity moving back through the long arch to its highest point in front of the ankle. **Let the floor work for you** —imagine the floor pushing backward from toes to ankle to heel. Pause to take a small plié by making the foot mound and folding slightly at the ankle, knee and thigh joints.

THE LITTLE TROCHANTERS ARE MORE IMPORTANT THAN THE LARGE

On the outside of the thigh is a large bone formation called the greater trochanter. On the opposite side, at the base of the neck of the femur, is a small bone formation called the lesser trochanter. We seem to think the large bone formations are important because we can see and feel them. The small area of bone along the axis of the thigh is really more important. Our deepest pair of abdominal muscles, the psoas muscles, use these centrally placed bony formations in lifting the thigh bones. Through the psoas muscles, the thigh bones can be lifted from above like the legs of a puppet. As one foot is placed to support your weight, the other goes into action up your front.

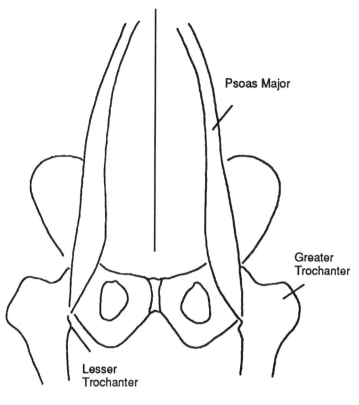

In the last lesson, you worked with the reactionary force to gravity through your feet from the toes to the center of your ankles. The reactionary force continues up the central axes of your legs into the middle of your body and then up the front of the spine. This idea will encourage the psoas and allied muscles to counteract the weight of your body dropping down the back of the central core.

Exercise 1: In a sitting position, place the feet side by side in a mound. Think of the knee caps gliding up the front of the knees. Imagine the little trochanters rotating backward and away from each other. This idea will strengthen your legs along their insides, from the ankles to the front of the pelvis. Then, imagine moving up the front of the spine. The imagery of letting down on the heels of the vertebrae while moving up the front of the vertebral bodies, sets the stage for this idea.

Exercise 2: Stand high on the tops of the ankle bones. Take a walk in the forward direction thinking of dropping your spinal heels and the heels of your feet. Then think up the front of your spine. The combined action of thinking up the front of your spine as you drop your heels will let your psoas muscles swing your thighs through your little trochanters. Taking easy short steps forward will help the psoas muscle lift the thigh bone toward the center of its socket.

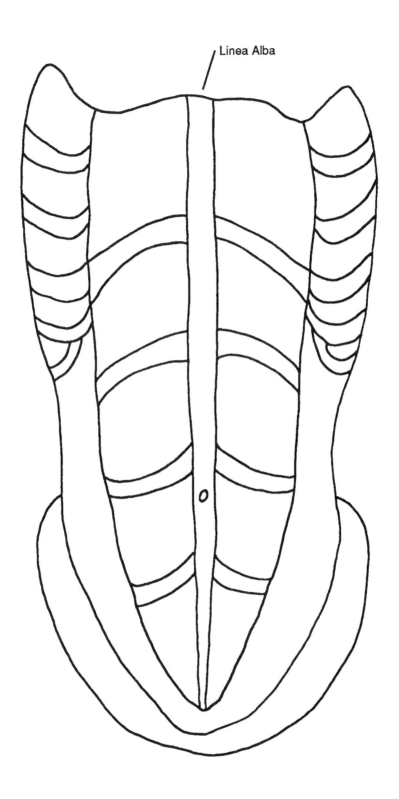

Rectus Abdominis Muscle Design

YOUR RECTUS ABDOMINIS MUSCLES NARROW
IN MOVING UP YOUR FRONT LINE

You have learned that part of the action of the psoas muscles is to pull your thigh bones alternately upward in walking. The other half of their action is to lower your rib case in your back by pulling down on your twelfth thoracic vertebra near the waistline. The rectus abdominis muscles should narrow in moving up your mid-front line. Your deep psoas muscles need this narrowing image for the surface of the body. Narrowing your rectus abdominis helps your psoas muscles to lower your rib cage in the back, support the pelvis in the front and move your legs in the walking pattern.

Look at the illustration. Notice the strong linea alba extending from the center front of your pelvis to your sternum. The rectus abdominis muscles on each side of the linea alba strengthen when their muscle fibers are kept narrow and long. Notice how the muscles are divided into sections. The third section is just above your umbilicus or navel. Less good alignment and overeating can cause the body to bulge in this area. Breath can help you to correct poor habits if you patiently work with it.

Exercise 1: Sit on a low seat to deeply flex your thighs. Begin by touching the left side of the third section of the rectus abdominis muscle with your right fingertips. Think of the fibers going inward toward the linea alba as you gently trace over the muscle. Visualize the breath moving a bit in the inward direction as well. Time the finger action and image with your inhalation. Think of breathing in and up on inhalation in the area of your finger touch. After a few minutes of inhaling and narrowing on your left side, change to your right side and repeat the directions. Use your left hand fingertips to indicate the direction in and up on the right side as you think of narrowing toward your center.

Exercise 2: Think of the image of tubular breathing. The tube is parallel to the spine and in back of the rectus abdominis muscles. Imagine the breath within a tube at the center of the body rather than along the surface of the ribs. After you have become familiar with the image of tubular breathing on inhalation, try letting your breath go very slowly down the center of your back on exhalation.

Exercise 3: To vary your practice, try applying the same directions to the fourth section of the rectus abdominis muscle just below the umbilicus. Time the action with your inhalation, in and up. Start slowly and easily. Why is this important? In building new habits, working slowly feels better and gives you confidence. You begin to yawn and release your tension. Eventually, you will wonder why you let the tension build up in the first place.

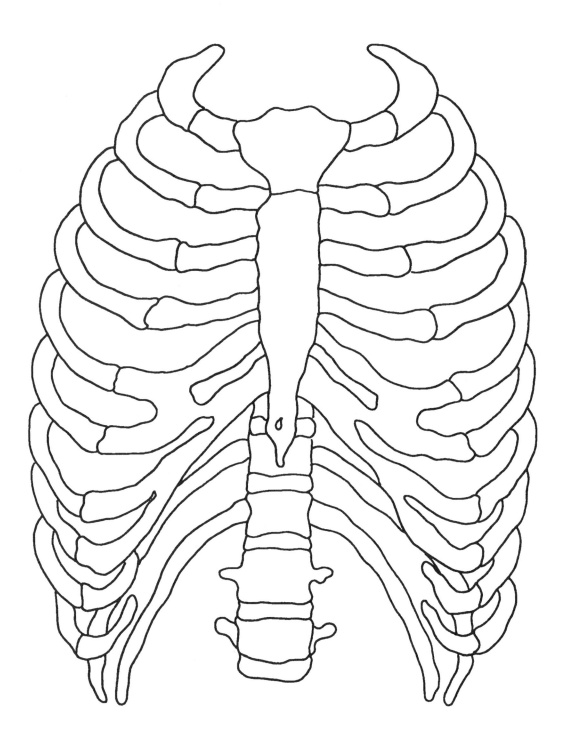

Your Sternum Leads Your Diaphragm Upward

YOUR STERNUM LEADS UP
IN YOUR MID-FRONT LINE

Your sternum leads the front ends of your ribs upward. Each of your upper seven pairs of ribs end in a socket with a bar of cartilage. It is the cartilage which then makes a socket with the sternum. This arrangement lets your chest wall expand and contract in breathing. There is no need to push out on the sides of the ribs. That is the wrong way to breath. The right way is through the flexible ends of the ribs in their sternal sockets. Tubular breathing—up the mid-front line in inhalation and down the mid-back line in exhalation—lets your diaphragm expand.

Exercise 1: In the illustration notice the cartilaginous areas between the front ends of the ribs and the sternum. Think of this area as softer and more like the diaphragm muscles underneath. Yawning is helpful in this. It releases tension in the muscles and ligaments around the central core of your body as well as the arms and legs. The yawn makes you aware of how easily breath can flow in and out, like the tide on the ocean beach.

Exercise 2: Thinking up on the rib ends in the front of the rib cage continues the action of the rectus abdominis muscles. Review the previous lesson thinking of the **in and up** action across the third section of the rectus abdominis muscle. Practice the same imagery as you work with the second section of the muscle and the first. As you reach the upper part of the rectus abdominis you are over the eighth, ninth and tenth ribs, which use the seventh rib socket as a fulcrum in their front ends. Narrowing the rectus at this level makes you more aware of the acute A-shaped angle between them. Narrowing the lower rib cage will help you lengthen it.

Exercise 3: You worked with dropping the vertebral heels in earlier lessons. If you can learn to get all the heels in the spinal row into the action, dropping down the back can become the power system for the whole body. Sit on a low seat so your thigh joints are well flexed. This will let your spine sink deep into your pelvis. Start a yawn as in *Exercise 1* and when you have finished the going up, take it down your back as far as you can. Allow the heels of your vertebrae to get into action. Remember that breath is a sequence in two parts:

Inhalation goes up the front of the spine,

exhalation goes down the back.

BALANCE YOUR BODY ON THE TOPS OF YOUR THIGH HEADS – WALK HIGH

In each foot you have the arches made by the tiny tarsal bones. In the pelvis you have the arches of your thigh sockets. You can think of the thigh socket arches as "ceilings." The thigh heads give an upward thrust to the ceilings of the thigh sockets. You started to work on these equal upward thrusts when you kneaded the arches of your feet. As you deepened the sockets in the bones in front of the heels, the thrusts carried you up into the space between the two lower leg bones. Cupping deep in the sole of the foot sent the upward thrust toward the thigh heads. Now you can learn to dig deeper into the pelvic bones through the thigh sockets to take the thrusts into the center of the body.

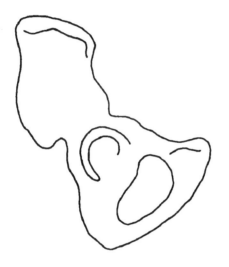

Pelvic Bone – Outside View

Exercise 1: The tendency of the thighs is toward outward rotation. This throws strain all through the body reaching as far as the eyes. Think of the thigh sockets as deep and of using the inner walls of the legs in rest as well as action. The animal does this in its crawl, where the rhythm of movement is always toward inward rotation. This maintains the axes of its legs as well as the axis of its spine. Thinking action along the inner walls of the thighs will help you raise the thigh socket ceilings.

Exercise 2: Instead of thinking forward as you walk, think up the front of your axis. The steady progression of weight falling down your back and flowing up your front will bring each foot alternately into place. Suck up a leg as you walk—suck up and swing. This lets the long muscles of your legs control two joints at once and gives rhythm to your gait.

Exercise 3: Thinking **up** as you walk will happen easily if you do not take too long a step. You can tell what is right for your height by walking slowly, to let each foot fall alternately into place. Do you balance your body easily and well in the fraction of a second that your weight is on only one leg? Too long a step makes you depend on momentum.

Exercise 4: Stand and review the movement of the plié. As you unfold the legs to come up, notice the action is similar to straightening the arms in the push-up exercise. Both use the support of the floor to push the weight of the body upward. In either case the action is in the center of the arm or the leg. Imagine the motion of the arms in the push-up exercise. Then, try thinking of push-ups through your legs into the ceilings of your thigh sockets as you practice the plié.

THE HEELS OF THE PELVIS ARE
BEHIND THE THIGH SOCKETS

Notice in the illustration that the spine of the ischia seems to point down the back. The heels of your pelvis (ischial spines) behind the thigh joints are like the heels of the feet behind the ankle joints. How are they alike? They both lead down your back. Dropping the heels of the pelvis also allows your internal obturator muscles to relax their hold on the large trochanters. Then the front of the pelvis can narrow in moving up the front line.

Exercise 1: Stand and begin walking backward, toes to heel. Review dropping the heel of a vertebra as you continue to walk backward. Pause, making the mound with your feet and begin a plié. Think of dropping the heels of your pelvis as you have the heels of your vertebrae and the heels of your feet.

Exercise 2: Think of the circling image you have used for the ankles and vertebrae as you work with the pelvic heels. First, on the left side, think of circling down the back of the spine of the ischia, underneath your sitting bone, up the front through the pubic symphysis and over the top of the thigh socket ceiling. Repeat the imagery on the right side.

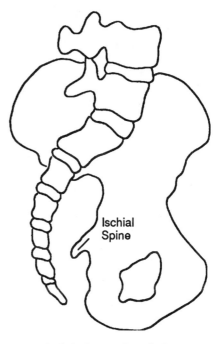

Pelvic Bone– Inside View

Exercise 3: Take the crawling position and balance your body over your hands and knees. Relax by lengthening your spine from the top of your head to the tip of your coccyx. This gives you a long row of vertebral heels. Now lower the front end of your body by dropping down to balance on your lower arms and elbows. Relax once again by exhaling down the back of the vertebral line. Begin crawling backward. Slowly drag your left elbow back and then go backward an inch or so with your right knee. Next drag your right elbow back and move slightly backward with your left knee. Continue left elbow to right knee, right elbow to left knee as you move backward. Think of the heels of your body leading down as you go. When you become more familiar with the crawling backward action, think of circling around the thigh socket as you did in *Exercise 2*.

When you are ready to end your practice, take some of your weight onto your hands. Bring your left foot forward toward your left hand, and then your right foot forward toward your right hand. Think up your front from your toes to the base of your head as you return to standing.

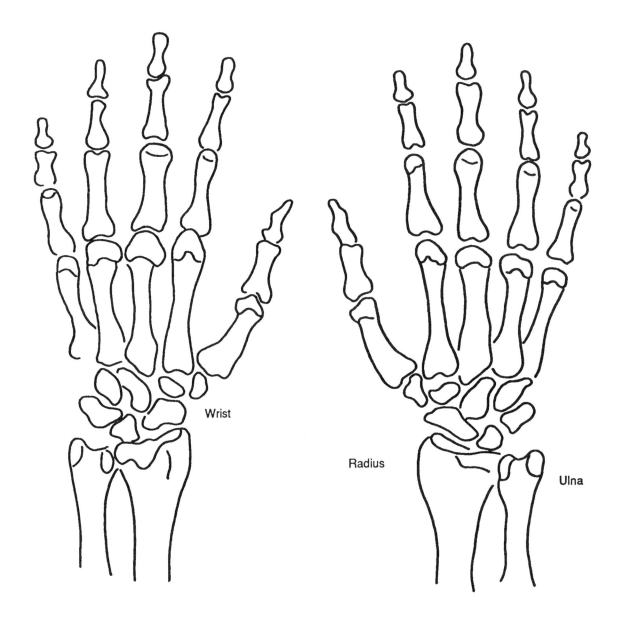

Back of the Hands

YOUR HAND BELONGS TO YOUR RADIAL BONE

The wrist is a group of tiny bones which center themselves in the end of the lower arm bone called the radius. In the illustration on the opposite page, notice that the hand balances in the center of the wrist. The thumb leads the fingers up the **inside** of the arm as the little finger drops down the **outside** of the hand.

Exercise 1: Twirling your thumb and fingers increases the space between the metacarpal (large knuckle) joints and gives flexibility to the hands and wrists. Let rhythm flow from the fingertips through the joints of the hand toward your wrist bones.

Sit and center yourself. Think of the heels supporting your ankles in the mound pattern. Hold the base of your right thumb with the thumb and fingertips of your left hand. Move your right thumb in a circle that goes counter-clockwise. Notice how easily your thumb sweeps out from under your second finger. Hold the base of your second finger and circle it counter-clockwise, sweeping it easily out from under the third finger.

Before beginning the action for the third finger, look at the illustration to see that it is your **balance** finger in the center of your hand. This means your middle finger will circle in both directions. First circle your middle finger counter-clockwise. Then circle the middle finger clockwise, sweeping it out from under your second finger several times.

Hold the base of your fourth finger and circle it clockwise several times. Finally, take the lower end of your fifth finger and circle it clockwise, letting it sweep out from under your fourth finger. Feel the freedom the little finger has at the end of the line. Think of it lengthening to balance your thumb.

Change to the other side. Hold the joint at the base of your left thumb with the thumb and fingertips of your right hand. Move your thumb in a circle that goes clockwise. Circle the second finger in a clockwise direction and sweep it easily out from under your third finger. Hold the base of the third finger and review its role as the balance finger. Circle the middle finger clockwise several times, and then let it sweep in the opposite direction, counter-clockwise. The fourth finger will circle counter-clockwise from under your third finger. The fifth finger will also circle counter-clockwise sweeping out from under your fourth finger. As you do this feel the freedom it has at the end of the line, and think of it lengthening to balance your thumb.

COME UP ON YOUR RADIAL JOINT –
GO DOWN ON YOUR ELBOW

The two lower arm bones (ulna and radius) meet the upper arm bone (humerus) at the hinge joint of the elbow. This hinge joint lets you fold the lower arm on the upper arm. There is another joint of the elbow which is the meeting place of the two lower arm bones. This is a rotating joint which allows the hand to face in many directions. When this joint moves in rhythm it allows space between the lower arm bones.

The elbow also has three bony projections. One is on the inside of the humerus. One is on the outside of the humerus. The large projection below and between the other two, you may think of as the point of the elbow. It is really the end of the ulna. The circle in the illustration represents the projection on the outside of the humerus. Notice it is near the joint between the humerus and the radius. The joint between the radius and ulna is also at this level.

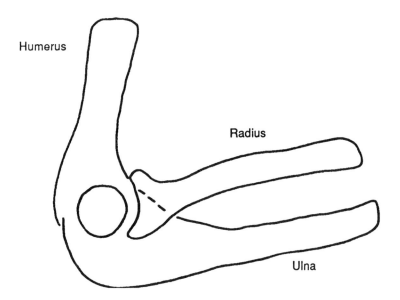

Exercise 1: You can add cross patterning to the twirling fingers exercise you began in the last lesson. First circle the thumb on the left side and then the other thumb on the right. Then the second finger on the left side followed by the second finger on the right. Then the third finger on the left side followed by the third finger on the right. Then the fourth finger on the left side followed by the fourth finger on the right. Then the fifth finger on the left side followed by the fifth finger on the right. If this seems a little awkward at first, your arm muscles may not be evenly developed around each arm or finger axis. A little **slow** practice will improve this and greatly benefit the use and appearance of your shoulders. Lengthening the spine as you practice increases the results.

Exercise 2: Take a sitting position and center yourself by thinking of narrowing your rectus abdominis muscles. Place your left lower arm easily in your lap with your elbow flexed. Lay your right lower arm over it. Feel the round projection on the outside of your left humerus with your right middle finger. Let your right hand fingertips circle clockwise around the point several times. Then slowly slide your right hand fingers along the outer edge of your left lower arm to your little finger. Think of lengthening the little finger line downward.

Change to placing your right lower arm easily in your lap with your elbow flexed. Then lay your left lower arm, with the elbow flexed, over the right lower arm. Feel the round projection on the outside of your right humerus with your left middle finger. Circle counter-clockwise around it a few times with your left fingertips. Slowly slide your left fingers along the outer edge of your right lower arm to your little finger. Think of lengthening the little finger line downward. As you practice, take time to breathe. Alternate the two arms in your practice.

Exercise 3: You can relax and separate the lower arm and wrist bones by clapping very slowly. First beat the rhythm with the hands only. Think of the hands as light as you clap, one-two, one-two, one-two and so on. Slowly begin to get the wrists involved in the rhythm, letting them loosen as you continue to clap slowly and evenly. Get the lower arms involved by allowing them to rotate as you clap. One hand will be the top hand for a few beats and then you can change, placing the other hand on top. Remember the hands are not flat like duck or seal flippers. Thinking of the center of your hand as hollow allows more space between the two lower arm bones.

Exercise 4: Sitting, place your right and left hands over the center fronts of your right and left lower legs just below the knees. Slide your hands upward toward your psoas muscle line. Make an easy action of it with your arms and hands. Your sliding action directs the thighs upward and slightly inward toward your thigh joints. It helps to release the deep muscle tension in the back of the knees and lower back.

Return your hands to the knee level. Find the heads of the fibulae on the outside of the lower legs just below the knees. On the left side, circle the head of the fibula with your left fingertips the way you circled the bony projection on the outside of the arm. Think **down the back, underneath, up the front, over the top,** and down the back again. Loosening the fibula bones will let the heel hang down more easily and the little toe lengthen in its line. Repeat the circling at the right fibula. Think of **space** between your lower leg bones, as you did between your lower arm bones.

CENTER YOUR ARMS IN THEIR SOCKETS
BY LETTING YOUR SHOULDER BLADES FLOAT

The socket for the arm is on the **outer** edge of the shoulder blade. Above this is a smaller socket where the collar bone meets the tip of the acromion. This arrangement forms a roof over the top of the arm. Another part of the shoulder blade juts out over the front of your body. This projection is called the coracoid process and is shaped somewhat like a curved finger. The pectoralis minor muscles between the coracoid process and your second, third, fourth and fifth ribs tend to hold your shoulder forward and down. These are very over-worked muscles. Let's begin to relax and lengthen them to allow your shoulder blades to float back and down.

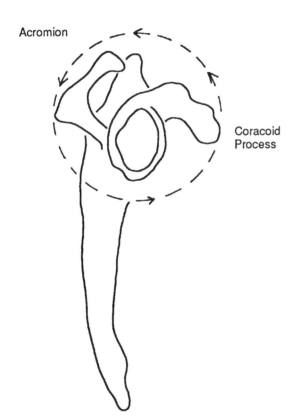

Acromion

Coracoid
Process

Exercise 1: Take a sitting position and feel a long spine with your head at its top. Place your right middle fingertip on the top of your left arm, toward its front. Move inward from there about an inch. Just below your collar bone you will find the round bony end of the coracoid process. Let your fingertip follow the circular pattern shown in the illustration. From the coracoid process, where your finger is resting, trace up the front and over the top of your shoulder. Continue down the back of your shoulder and underneath it. Repeat the action several times as you say the directions to yourself.

Change to your right shoulder and find the tip of your right coracoid process with your left fingertips. From the coracoid, circle up the front, over the top, down the back of your shoulder and underneath to where you started. Frequent repetition of the thought will help establish the action.

Circling around the arm socket can help you release the grip of tense muscles which pull the coracoid process down in front. Releasing these front muscles allows the shoulder blades to **float** down the sides of your spine. Balancing the shoulder blade places the arm socket in better alignment with the body and allows for more natural arm action.

YOUR FLOATING RIBS SLIDE DOWN TO WORK WITH YOUR 13TH RIBS

The inner circle of the pelvis is like a pair of ribs. To become aware of these "thirteenth ribs" you must forget about the outward flaring ilia on the sides of the pelvis. Look at the illustration and imagine the design of a thirteenth pair of ribs around the inner pelvic circle. These ribs come together at the pubic symphysis like the upper ribs meet at the sternum. The spinal ends of the pelvic ribs come together on each side of your sacrum the same way the upper ribs meet on each side of the vertebrae. Thinking of your inner pelvic circle as your thirteenth ribs helps to lengthen the body and strengthen the muscular connection to your floating ribs.

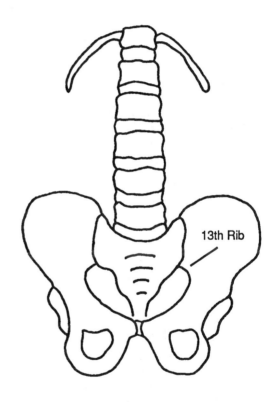

13th Rib

Exercise 1: The eleventh and twelfth pairs of ribs are called "floating ribs" because they have no sockets in the front of the body. They depend on you to direct their outer ends toward the center of the pelvis. Imagine the floating ribs sliding down through the waist area on exhalation. First, think of lowering the eleventh rib on the left side as you exhale. Then, think of lowering your right eleventh rib on exhalation. Continue by thinking of lowering the twelfth ribs, first on the left side and then on the right. Taking one rib at a time will help you gain better awareness and action.

Exercise 2: Stand and balance your body along your central axis or core. Begin to lower your body into a squatting position by folding through your thigh, knee and ankle joints. Let the vertebral heels lengthen down your back in a flowing line. The back of your shoulders will flow with the vertebral heel rhythm. Think of the eleventh and twelfth pairs of ribs sliding down as well. Forget the front of the body, just flow down your back as you flex your folding joints.

Exercise 3: In a sitting position, try shrugging your shoulders. This is an excellent exercise if it is also done through the lower ribs. Shrugging the lower ribs up and down uses the muscles in the lower back and abdomen and allows the shoulders to relax. Finish the exercise by thinking of the seventh rib along with the eighth, ninth and tenth moving up and in with inhalation. The eleventh and twelfth pairs of ribs **reach down** to work with the thirteenth ribs on exhalation.

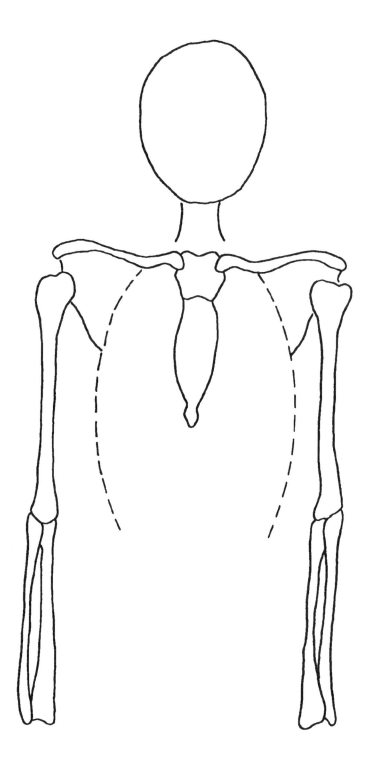

Shoulder Structure and Thorax - Front View

ALLOW SPACE BETWEEN YOUR
SHOULDER FRAME AND RIBS

In body imagery, it is helpful to have some idea of the relation of one body part to another. The sternum is an unknown bone until you begin to think of its connection with your collarbone, arm and rib action. Look at the illustration and notice that your collarbone joints are on the **top** edge of the sternum. Your rib cartilage sockets are below them and on the sides of the sternum. The higher level of the collarbone helps separate shoulder and arm action from the rib action below it. You should feel space between the two.

Exercise 1: Take a sitting position and feel a long spine by narrowing in and up on your rectus abdominis muscles. You may also experience other front muscles lengthening upward. Think of the curving design of the collarbones. The inner ends of the collarbones tie in with the sternum and front muscles. The outer ends tie in with the shoulder blades and back muscles. Imagine your arms hanging from the outer ends of your collarbones one side at a time. Notice how this frees your sternum to raise its head a notch higher. This will allow the inner end of your collarbone to be on the same level as the outer end. It gives freedom and strength to your arms and helps relieve strain in your lower back and neck.

Exercise 2: In a sitting position begin to do **push-ups** toward the ceiling with the heel of your hand. Start with your left arm as your right arm rests in your lap. Trace up the center front of your body as you think up the front of the spine. Unfold your left elbow loosely as you extend your arm up toward the ceiling. Let your fingers fall back as you imagine pressing on the ceiling with the heel of the hand. Pause for a moment and let your arm come down slowly. Feel the action move down the side of your spine through the latissimus dorsi muscles.

Change to your right arm. Let your left arm rest in your lap as you unfold your right elbow loosely and extend your right arm up toward the ceiling. Let your fingers fall back as you imagine pressing on the ceiling with the heel of the hand. Pause for a moment and let your arm come down slowly. Feel the action along the side of your spine in your back. Alternate the arms in your practice.

Exercise 3: Begin to think of alternating your right and left shoulders, arms, hands and fingers in daily action. One side should balance the other. Use your weaker side more in activities such as brushing your teeth, combing your hair, carrying a purse or other articles. Practice using the two sides more equally in sports and dance, as you can. This will help your whole body become better aligned. How can this happen? Through an unconscious rearrangement of muscles affecting many joints.

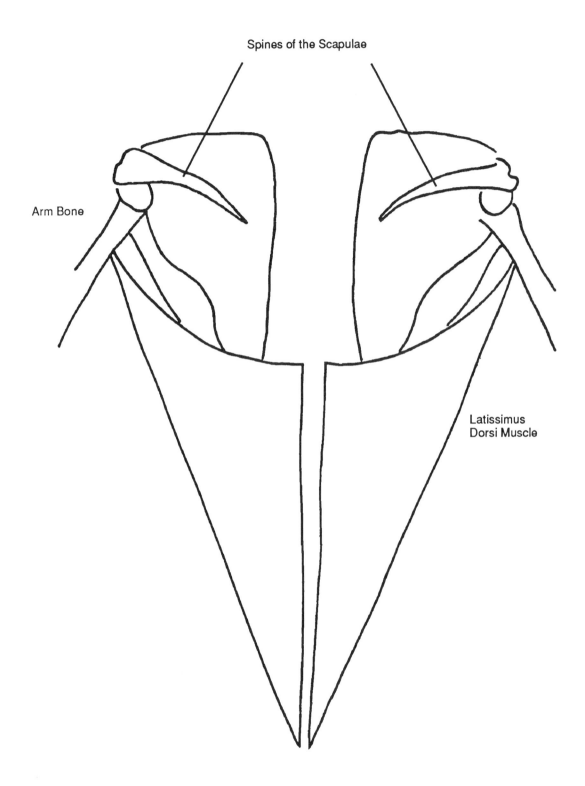

The Spine of the Scapula is a "Heel" for the Shoulder Girdle

THE BONE AND MUSCLE DESIGN IN YOUR BACK FLOATS YOUR SHOULDER BLADES BACK AND DOWN

The shoulder blades or scapulae slant inward and down from your arms to the sides of your spine. The large shoulder and arm muscles of your back follow this same pattern. Notice in the illustration that the latissimus dorsi muscles combine with the bones to work in rhythm down the back of your body. Letting your collarbones lengthen outward at the top of your body begins the pattern. This allows the inner edge of each shoulder blade to rest parallel to the spine, when the arms are at the sides of your body. Think of connecting the action of the arms to the spine through the latissimus dorsi muscles. Because the muscle design tapers down into your mid and lower back, it helps lower your shoulder blades **and** your vertebral heels.

Exercise 1: Sit or stand and place your right hand over the top of your left collarbone. Your hand should be relaxed and almost open. Notice that the base of your thumb lies over the forward curve of the collarbone and your fingers are over the backward curve in the area of the shoulder joint. Think of the collar bone lengthening at its outer end as you exhale. Change to placing your left hand over the top of your right collarbone with your hand relaxed and open. Notice that the base of your thumb lies over the forward curve of the collarbone and your fingers are over the backward curve. See the lengthening of the outer end of the collarbone on exhalation. Then let the inner edges of the shoulder blades fall toward each other on inhalation.

Exercise 2: The collarbones should be more on the **top** of the shoulder girdle than the average person allows them to be. The pectoralis minor muscle often takes the collarbone off balance by pulling the coracoid process forward and down. You have practiced lengthening this muscle and letting the coracoid process rise up in the front with the image of circling the arm socket. This begins the feeling of depth in your shoulder girdle. Think of the spines of the scapula as **heels** dropping down to aid your awareness of depth.

Exercise 3: Review your practice of push-ups on the ceilings of the thigh sockets. Follow a line starting with the second toe through the long arch of the foot into the ankle. Push-up from the tops of the ankle bones through the axes of the legs into the ceilings of the thigh sockets. From there think of a push, **up the front** of the spine. Your lumbar curve will stay long if you think up the front of it. Then your shoulders can stay relaxed, allowing the weight to gravitate down the back.

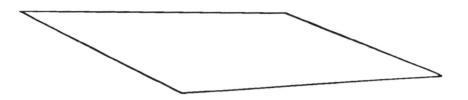

Line Up the Top of the Head
with the Ceiling

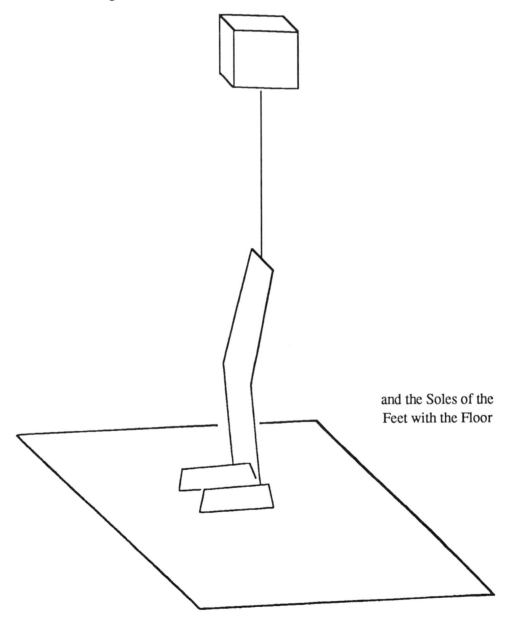

and the Soles of the
Feet with the Floor

YOUR HEAD IS A PART OF YOUR VERTEBRAL COLUMN

The balance of your head depends on the support of your vertebrae. The image of the head as the **top** vertebra helps in centering the weight of the head. The center of the base of the skull has two little bumps similar to the shape of the sitting bones on the lower end of the body. The first vertebra of the spinal column, called the "atlas," has two small hollows for the base of the head to rest on. The head sits on the top of the spine much like the way your body sits on a chair. Your awareness can take you from **lower level sitting** to **upper level sitting** when you begin to allow your head weight to rest in your center line.

Exercise 1: Many people believe the base of the head is at the same level as the chin. It may look that way from the outside but it doesn't work that way on the inside. Sit on a low seat and breath easily for a moment. Partially close your hands and place your thumb and fingertips over your ears. The sitting bones of the head rest on the atlas at this level. Close your eyes and imagine your head resting on the atlas, between the centers of your ears. Let your head rock slowly forward and back, testing the action at this socket between the head and the atlas. Pause a little at the forward end of the line as well as the backward end.

Exercise 2: The head pivots by using the next socket, between the atlas and axis. Place the fingertips of one hand over the bridge of your nose. Place the palm of your other hand at the same level on the back of your head. The "axis" for turning your head to the left and right is centered between your two hands. Turn your head slowly to the left and then slowly back to position. Repeat this action a few times. Then turn your head slowly to the right and back to position. Repeat this action to the right side a few times. Care should be taken to pause at the beginning and end of each turn to let the head come to rest at center. Alternate the two sides in your practice.

Exercise 3:   In standing, instead of lining up the back of the body with a wall, think of horizontal planes through the ends of the body. Think of the plane of the ceiling and then what would be the plane along the top of your head. Line up these planes in your imagination so they are parallel with each other. Then think of the plane of the floor and the bottom of your feet resting on the floor's plane. This helps lengthen your axis both up and down.

Exercise 4:   Think of the top of the shoulder structure as a shelf. The shelf tips neither forward nor back and is parallel with the planes of the ceiling and the floor. This allows a longer neck and spine all the way down the line. It will help you narrow your abdominal muscles and discover where your sternum belongs.

RHYTHM FLOWS EASILY AS YOU SLIDE
DOWN YOUR SPINAL HEELS ON EXHALATION

Our well being depends on combining the rhythm of movement with breathing. Babies and young children demonstrate this by breathing and moving so easily. Dancing, singing and other rhythmic activities help people blend movement and breathing in their work, rest and play. How has nature planned this? By working with gravity throughout the body's length.

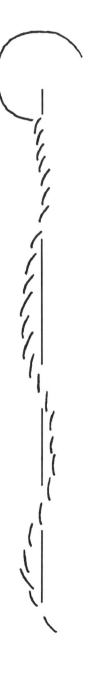

Exercise 1: Arrange the parts of the spine with your breathing action by stringing the vertebrae on a line. As you feel the inclination to straighten your spine, let your exhalation **press down** on the heels of the vertebrae in the back. Imagine that each spinous process is pressed downward in the same way a finger would lightly press down on a piano key. Continue to the next vertebra and the next vertebra and the next, making a phrase. Tip the vertebrae down as you exhale.

Tip the vertebrae up the front as you inhale. Since the front of the vertebrae cannot be touched, you will simply think of the front of the body of each vertebra. Tip the fronts of the vertebrae upward as you inhale.

Exercise 2: Yawning. As a yawn starts, slowly allow the lower jaw to soften and fall away. This begins the lengthening of the neck and upper back. Follow the line down through the spine into the lower back, pelvis, and thighs. The longer the line becomes, the longer the breath which follows it. Close the jaws as slowly and silently as possible. A prolonged yawn down the back of the center line should be followed by a slow release up in front of the line.

Breath is the activator
The bones are the keys
The disks are like air spaces
Can you sense all of these?

RHYTHM PLAYS THROUGH MUSCLE ACTIVITY
WHEN HARMONY PLAYS THROUGH ALL YOUR JOINTS

The heel pattern can be applied to many of the body joints. The heel end of the foot represents the force of gravity through the human body. You have learned to drop the weight down the back through the "heels" of the body at various levels. The front part of the foot in coming back towards the ankle can be thought of as the reactionary force to gravity. The idea of "push-ups" at various body levels is another way of thinking of this reactionary force.

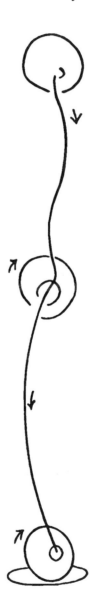

Walking backward from toe to heel may be our most important exercise in balancing gravity and the reactionary force to gravity. The force from the floor through the front of the foot pushes you back into balance where the ankle sits on top of the heel.

Walking forward is also achieved easily by remembering the heel pattern at the thigh joint level. See the thigh ball head rolling forward and up, back and down in the same way you imagined the ankle ball head. At both levels, as the back of the ball goes down, the front of the ball rolls up. Think of walking into yourself.

These ideas must be timed well with your breathing to allow a rhythmical walk. At first, the heel pattern will not work well if movement is too rapid. Rapid movement tends to be contracted and interferes with exhalation. If breath is slow on the outgo, it will be easy on the intake.

Let gravity work for you. If you can think of your bones as your framework to carry your weight, then the muscles can act as a flexible means for moving the bones. Balancing your joints through your bony framework helps your balance and movement including the breath.

Rhythm flows through muscle activity, when harmony plays through all the joints.

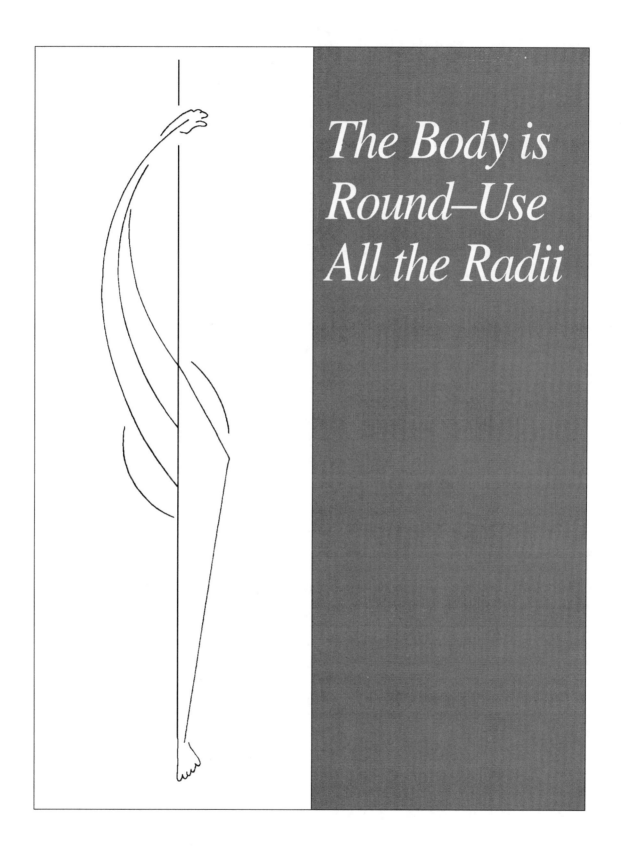

*The Body is
Round—Use
All the Radii*

INTRODUCTION

Nature has given us free movement by placing it under our unconscious control early in life. As the mind develops and matures, we can extend more conscious control to our bodies and the movements we make. You have probably already begun to notice your movement and relate it to your ideas about the body. This course in body balance and movement is intended to help you keep principles of body alignment in the background of your thinking throughout all your activity.

In explaining the process of exploring body balance, the use of the word "secrets" might be more appropriate than the idea of working with "principles." Education has not made this difference clear and has ignored our tendency to shrink away from too much information about movement. As a result, many people think learning to improve body alignment will be unpleasant and uncomfortable. For other people, learning to improve posture would seem to have little importance. Having established habits that seem workable, they hesitate to make a change. Your simple curiosity about the secrets of body balance can awaken impulses within you which can playfully transform the body and its movement. This makes posture study a pleasurable experience which greatly adds to the joy of living.

In this manual, we will explore the image of the body as round. Like a sphere, the body is built with height, width and depth. The body has spherical units like the vertebrae, ankle bones and wrist bones. There are spherical parts like the skull, pelvis and thorax. There are also spherical curves in the shape of the spine. Throughout the body we can think of the joints as parts of a sphere; bony sockets as rounded cups accepting ball-like bony ends.

Some individuals move as if they believed their bodies were flat just the way we once thought the world was. They have deleted the dimension of depth from their body concepts. Their tension may have also reduced the number of planes available for use in the movement of their joints. Perhaps, three-sided mirrors should be more generally used. Then we would become accustomed to looking at ourselves from all sides and more aware of our length, width and depth. However, a concept of the body based on an image of its surface could not convey the most important secret of body balance: a strong body has its strength at center.

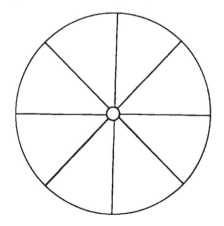

Through imagery, we can activate the infinite number of planes through the body's units, parts and curves. These ideas can help us develop the inner core of the body and release its perimeter.

> The body is round,
> hubs and spokes,
> centers and radii.

THE PELVIS IS THE HUB OF THE BODY WHEEL

There can be only one hub to a wheel. In a wheel each spoke balances its opposite in keeping the alignment of the whole. The movement of the wheel begins from within. It moves outward from the hub through the spokes to the rim. Good movement starts from within the body's hub. It moves out from the center within.

Animals know this secret unconsciously. They are careful to keep their weight supported at center in any movement. This is never overlooked. It is easy to see in the movement of the python because there are no legs or arms to confuse one's observation. The python gathers strength to raise its head or wave its tail by shortening into its middle. Other animals with arms or wings, legs and tails also realize the importance of centering. It allows the weight to flow through their bodies easily, and the bones to make soft contacts.

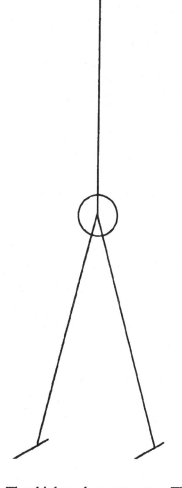

In the human body, the pelvis is the hub for body movement. It contains the center of gravity. The upper spoke for the pelvis is the spine; a flexible spoke. The lower ones are the legs; folding spokes. The thigh joints are closest to the center of gravity for the body as a whole. No joint in the body is the subject of more continuous movement. The thigh joints need development first.

Exercise 1: The pelvis is round like a basin or a drum. Give yourself depth in your pelvis by thinking of it as one of these round shapes. The sacrum curves **round** to form the back of the pelvis. It carries the body weight down. The front of the pelvis is also round. Here the thrusts from the folding levers of the legs ascend toward each other to give united support.

Exercise 2: The thigh heads are perfectly shaped half-balls. The thigh sockets are cups. The thigh sockets are deeper than other joints. The base of the cup of the thigh socket is in the back of the pelvis. You learned about the heel-like spine of the ischia in *Body Proportion Needs Depth*. Now you can think of it as the bottom of your thigh socket. In sitting or lying down, allow the weight of your legs to slide back into the pelvic basin. Picture the thigh sockets as funnel shaped, on the left and then on the right. Imagine the weight of the thighs dropping into the bottom of each funnel. Gravity falling to the bottoms of sockets leaves muscles free for expanding.

THE HEEL WHEELS THE ANKLE BONE HIGH IN WALKING

The floor, ground or pavement may be flat but your feet should not conform to that feeling. You walk at the ankle which is quite round. As the keystone for the foot arch, the ankle has no muscle attachments. It stays in place through the action between the heel sockets below and the lower leg sockets above. It depends on you to find its balance at center.

The ankle hinges in the sockets between the top of its ball surface and the ends of the two lower leg bones. The large bone (tibia) is on the inside and the small bone (fibula) is on the outside. The usual tendency is to slide forward over the top of the ball and backward under the ball as we move at this joint. In the last manual, you worked on reversing this pattern. The image of the navicular sliding up the front and over the top of the ankle ball starts the action. Then the heel can drop down in back, if the achilles tendon is sufficiently elastic.

Ideal ankle flexion and extension (hinging) begins with the tip of the axis of each toe. These axis ends should be sensitive to the feel of what they are contacting. The musician uses this sensitivity, as does the surgeon, the dentist and the sculptor. It comes into the emotional for everyone. Even a horse paws the ground for relief when hungry or cold or in need of exercise. It deepens the breathing and quiets the emotions.

Exercise 1: Review walking backward as you learned to do in *Body Proportion Needs Depth*. Think back from the tips of the toes toward the ankle with each step. Taking some easy short steps forward, think of the ankle bone riding high on the heel bone. This lets the heel roll back and down in the socket under the ankle bone. Much of the elastic spring of the foot depends upon good use of these sockets. The heel **wheels** the ankle bone **high** in walking forward and backward.

Exercise 2: There are also axes from the center of the ankle toward the rim of the heel. Look at the illustration. The circular shapes represent the centers of the ankles. The lines are the radii of the heels.

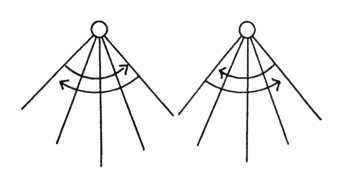

As you stand, think of these axes fanning open from the outside of the heel toward the inside. Then think from the inner heel toward the outer heel. Keeping this image in mind as you balance in standing will help you contact the floor softly and gently, rather than harshly.

FULL LENGTH OF AXIAL PARTICIPATION IS THE NORM FOR ANY BODY PART

The toe bones are so small it may be difficult to think of them having a long axis. Lack of this knowledge shows up throughout the body. In the illustration below notice that the foot is divided in two parts. The first, second and third toes join with the navicular to articulate with the front of the ankle bone. We can call this part of the foot the "ankle foot." The fourth and fifth toes join with the cuboid bone to articulate with the heel. We will call this part of the foot the "heel foot."

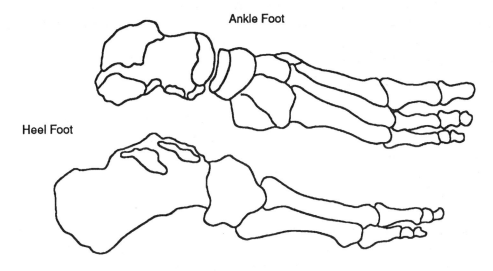

Side View of Heel Foot – Ankle Foot

Exercise 1: Sit on the floor with the sit bones resting on or between your heels. Point your large toes toward each other so they almost touch. As you arrange your feet on the floor, imagine sliding backward through the axes (center lines) of the large, second and third toes. Begin at the tips of the toes and go towards the center of your ankle bones. Place the centers of your fists in the hollows in front of your heels and gently knead these areas. Let your fists rotate your arms outward some of the time as you knead. This will help your shoulders too. To lengthen the outer toes (phalanges) of the heel foot, use your left thumb tip to rub your left toes outward in a line from your large toe to your little toe. You will be rubbing along your metatarsal area at the base of the toes. Then use your right thumb tip to rub an outward line from the base of your large toe to your little toe on the right foot.

Exercise 2: Sit on the sitting bones with the feet in front of you. Trace the directions shown in this illustration along the top of the foot. Trace **in** on the ankle foot lines toward the center of the foot. Trace **out** along the heel foot lines and see the fourth and fifth toes growing in length to equal the other toes.

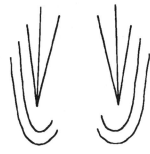

EXPAND THE AXIS PATH BETWEEN
YOUR FOOT AND KNEE CENTERS

You have thought of a path moving back from the tips of the toes to the ball-shaped top of the ankle. Now you can follow that path upward. Expanding up from the ankle through the center of the knee allows movement to flow freely toward the tops of the femur bones.

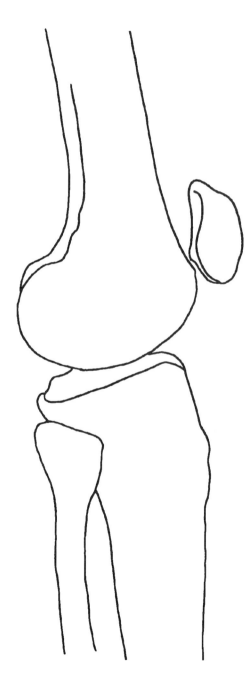

The muscle that fills the axis path between your two lower leg bones is the tibialis posterior muscle. Find the illustration of this muscle in the *Technique for Movement Lessons*. The tibialis posterior muscle stays close to the axis throughout its length. The feather-like spread of this long posture muscle acts as a long, slim cushion between the two bones. At its lower end, the muscle's tendon is like the quill of the feather. This quill end is flexible enough to follow closely along the inside of the ankle bone. It passes under the foot and then fans out into a tiny "hand" with many fingers. These fingers attach to the underside of the small bones of the foot (tarsals) as a rampart in front of the heel.

Exercise 1: The tendon of the tibialis posterior muscle is at the center of your foot. As you knead the soles of your feet use the tip of your thumb to find this area just forward of the heel. Let the center of your foot soften to your touch. Come to a standing position and imagine the tibialis posterior muscles supporting the arches of your feet. Allow space between the tibia and fibula for the length of the muscle. Think of its plume tip, beneath the knee, as very light and airy.

Exercise 2: Notice in the illustration that the knee joint does not include the kneecap (patella). The tibia and femur form a joint for flexion and extension. There is space between this hinge joint and the kneecap. Flexing the ankle deeply in the plié releases the knee cap to slide up the front. Think of the knee joint as round and the knee cap as thin.

CENTER THE PALMS OF THE HANDS AND SOLES OF THE FEET IN FRONT OF THEIR HEELS

The bones of your body interact with each other though the joint ends. One half of a joint has a ball-like end and the other half has a cup-like end. The cup-like surfaces of some joints are very deep and others are more shallow. However, all have something of this design. Why? So there is smooth and easy participation between the interacting ends at center.

Exercise 1: Sit, thinking of the mounds made by your feet. Let the knees approach each other and think of the little trochanters rotating backward and away from each other. Place your hands in the shape of mounds over the middle of your thighs. Let the rhythm flow through the fingertips toward your wrist bones. Hollow out the palms of your hands and relax the backs of them. Curve your fingers slightly and loosely. Notice how this relaxes the large knuckle joints between the palms and your fingers.

This simple action lets you breath deeper. Why? The inner ends of your arms and shoulders are associated with your diaphragm by way of your spine. If the inner ends of your arms are not active, your hands tend to be tense. Turn this idea around. Allow the hands to relax so the inner ends of your arms are more active.

Exercise 2: A similar hollowing action can take place in the foot. What is the action involved? The navicular bone in the front of the ankle slides up over the ankle as you flex the foot. The heel falls away and the toes hang loosely. It is like the hollowing of the hand deep through the wrist towards the space in the lower arm.

Exercise 3: Review tracing in on the **ankle** foot lines and out along the **heel** foot lines. Think of developing the outer edge of your foot and a longer little toe. The little toe has as many joints as the other toes. Develop the little toe by feeling out the joints with your fingers. See how large you can make each section. As you straighten your little toe, it will help your fourth toe lengthen. All the toes should be straight and long, not cramped or crooked. Crooked lines are the failure of the bones to meet evenly, one to the other.

THE HANDS AND FINGERS ARE ROUND

The feet communicate with the earth under you. The hands communicate with the world and its people. Do you have openness in your hands to help you in receiving ideas from the world? You can test yourself to see what you can do.

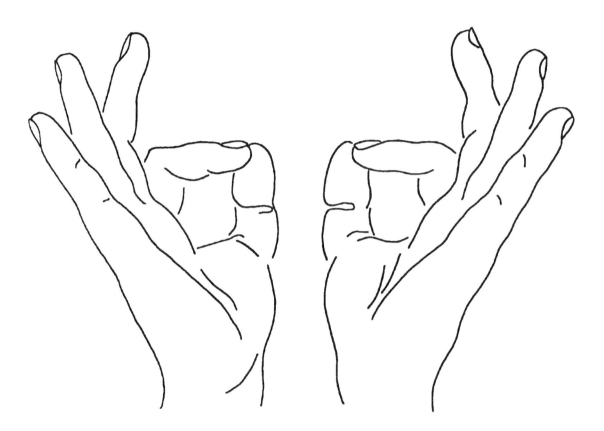

Here are your ten fingers. They are the doors to your world.

Exercise 1: Do you think of your fingertips as round or flat? To help in answering this, round the palms of your hands and point all ten fingertips toward you. Unless your work has been hard on them you will probably answer round. The fingertips should round well to keep a center.

Think of the fingernails as loose. Awareness should be in the flesh of the finger and you should have a sense of its shape as a circle and not a point. This releases tension in the joints of the hand. The human finger is not a claw. The axes of the bones of your fingers and toes should meet at the centers of the joints. The centers of the tips of the axes should **round** in communicating with your world.

Exercise 2: Sitting. Think of making a mound with your feet. Place your hands in the shape of a mounds over the centers of the thighs as you did in the last lesson. Bring your hands toward each other. Imagine holding a large rubber ball between your two hands. Arrange your hands as if they were holding the imaginary ball. The palms of your hands will be rounded and the fingers and thumbs will fan out.

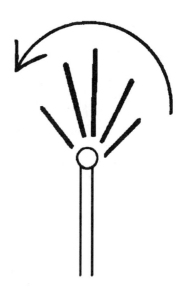

Exercise 3: Explore folding and unfolding (flexion and extension) the joints of the left fingers one at a time. Trace the axis line of the third finger toward the center (capitate bone) of the wrist. Think of the finger relaxing inward and then fold and unfold its joints. Take the second finger and trace its axis line toward the wrist, thinking inward. Then fold and unfold its joints. Repeat these directions for the fourth finger with the flexion and extension actions. The little finger needs extension only. It is frequently kept in a flexed position. The action in the other fingers will begin to take it into extension if you can release its tension down the line. Repeat the exercise on the right side.

Exercise 4: The action of the little finger on the outside of the hand is similar to the release down the back of the spine. The action of the thumb on the inner side of the hand is like moving up the front of the spine.

Think of planting your thumb in your wrist as you repeat the previous exercise. When you have repeated the exercise a few times, carry the impetus of the thumb up the front of the arm (inside) to the sternal socket. Relax down the back (outside) of the arm to the little finger and center at the wrist. The thumb leads the fingers into the wrist as the little finger drops down the outside of the hand.

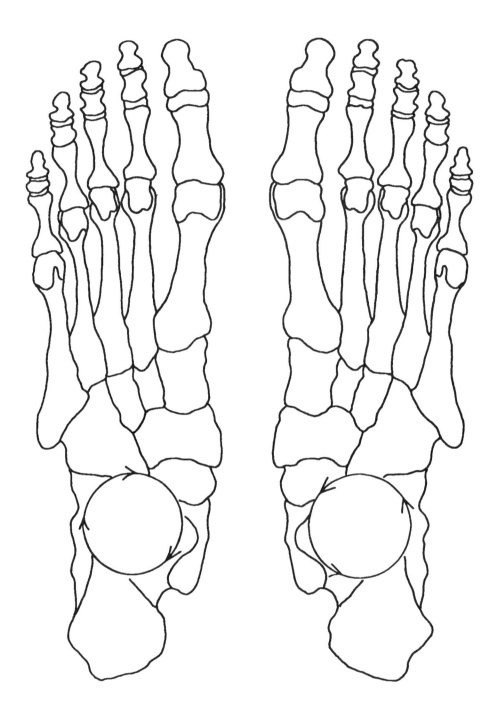

Plantar (Bottom) View — Circling the Soles of the Feet Horizontally

THE ANKLE SWIVELS ON THE TOP OF THE HEEL

The ball-shaped top of the ankle bone is between the two lower leg bones. Hinging (flexing and extending) the ankle takes place at this level. There are also sockets at a lower level, between the bottom of the ankle bone and the ball-shaped top of the heel. In *Body Proportion Needs Depth*, you explored these lower level sockets by hollowing out the long arch of the foot. As you kneaded the foot you felt the small platform (sustentaculum tali) on the inside of the arch that supports the ankle. On the top and to the side of this platform, are the two sockets where the ankle bone swivels on the top of the heel.

The ankle bone turns **in** and **out** in these sockets in a horizontal plane. Wrong ideas and poor shoes often encourage us to swivel the foot outward (eversion) more than inward (inversion). The action of circling the foot inward will help rebuild the long arch of the foot. This is similar to the inversion action the baby uses to build foot strength.

Exercise 1: This exercise can be practiced any time the weight of the body is not resting on the feet. The sitting position is the best one for learning the movement. Later you can practice lying down. In a sitting position, extend the left heel and let it rest on the floor in front of you. It will serve as a base for the circling action. Look at the illustration on the opposite page. The circling image is in the horizontal dimension at the centers of the soles of the feet, just forward of the heels.

The circle for the left foot will go clockwise around a circle about the size of a half dollar. Starting from the front, think of circling along the inside of the ankle bone, to the back of it. Continue around the outside to the front where you started. Take the foot into action following the image of the circular path at the center of the foot. Think of coming inward along the axis line from the tip of the first toe to the first cuneiform to begin the action. Repeat the circling on the left side several times, imagining the action deep in the center of the sole of the foot.

Change to the right side. Extend the right heel and let it rest on the floor. Think of the circle at the center of the sole of the foot just forward of the heel. The circle for the right foot will move counter-clockwise. Starting from the front, think of circling along the inside of the ankle bone, to the back of it. Continue around the outside of the ankle to the front where you started. Take the foot into action following your image of the circular path at the center of the foot. Think of the way the baby leads with the base of the first toe in this action.

Exercise 2: You can develop the outer line of the foot by using the image of striking an octave between your inner heels and your little toes. You do this in your hand by drawing in on your thumb as you move out and forward with your little finger. Slowly, let your feet begin to take similar action. Striking an octave as an image for the feet loosens the spaces around the cuboid. It also helps carry the large toe inward.

THE PELVIS WHEELS DOWN
THE BACK IN THE DANCE PLIÉ

The beginnings of dance movement can be found in the early history of man's physical development. The dance plié is used by the child in learning to balance on his feet. As the child progresses from rolling to crawling and then to standing and walking, he uses the plié for ease and pleasure in movement. This involves movement down the back of the axis and its counterbalance up the front of the axis.

The plié is similar to the crouch and spring pattern in the movement of many animals. The crouch lowers the body on its axis to gain leverage and strength for the spring that raises the body upward. The bird also lengthens its axis to go into flight. The axis lengthens down, the tail spreads wide and the thighs give their thrust for the push off.

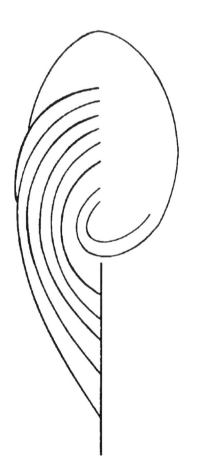

Exercise 1: As you begin to fold into the plié, lengthen downward through the back muscles. The superficial muscles, the trapezius and latissimus dorsi, make two V shapes leading down the back. They might be compared to the shape of a bird's wing. The gluteus maximus could be compared to an animal's tail.

To continue the down the back pattern, relax the lower part of the gluteus maximus muscle. Think through the gluteal lines pictured in the illustration to loosen your hold on the thigh bone from the rear. Then the thigh can fold more easily at the thigh socket. The gluteus maximus should be **long** enough to let the thigh move without strain.

Exercise 2: Dance combines the animal forms of movement with the bird forms such as flight. The bird soars upward but also descends to snatch its prey from the sea or ground. A wonderful image for breathing is the action of the sea gull as it wheels in circles. Inhale as you think of the bird soaring upward and then exhale as you think of it circling down.

THE ISCHIAL BRANCH OF YOUR SIT BONE BALANCES THE PUBIC BRANCH

Each of the sitting bones has two branches, a front or "pubic" branch and a back or "ischial" branch. The tilt of the pelvis is determined in part by the back-to-front balance between these two branches. Picture the front branch of your sit bone heightening upward toward your pubic arch where the two halves of the pelvis come together. The pubic arch, formed by the joining of the two pubic branches of the sitting bones, makes a brace for the front of your spinal column. This helps the rectus abdominis muscles narrow and stimulates action in your psoas muscles beneath them. Imagining the back branch lengthening down lengthens the sacrum too, taking the coccyx along.

Exercise 1: Stand with your back to the front of a low hard bench. Think of letting down on the ischial branch of the sit bone on each side of your body. One foot will step a little backward of the other as you lower your pelvis onto the bench seat. In *Body Proportion Needs Depth*, you learned that the "heel" of the thigh socket is the spine of the ischia. The spine of the ischia is in the middle of the ischial branch of the pelvis, behind the thigh socket. Allowing these heels to drop down brings better balance to the pelvic wheel in sitting. Then you can **scoop under** the sit bones to carry you high into the pubic arch in the front.

Exercise 2: Move to the back of the bench by inching each sit bone backward left-right, left-right. Then move to the front of the bench seat by lowering the back branches of your sit bones alternately and inching each sit bone forward.

Inching the sit bones alternately forward and back, encourages action down the back of the ischial branch and up the front of the pubic branch. As you rest for a moment, think of the art of a well-balanced rocking chair as an image for the pelvis. The front half of each rocker should balance the back half and the left rocker should equally balance the right.

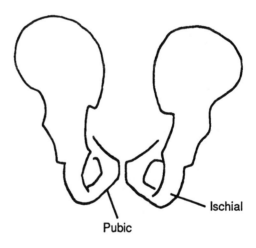

Back of Pelvis — Branches of Sit Bones

Exercise 3: Move toward the front of the bench. Place one foot a little forward of the other. Think of the push up from floor through the ankles to the thigh sockets as you come up to your feet. In standing, think **up** on your pubic branches in the front of the pelvis and **down** on the ischial branches in the back. This will help you arrange the support of the feet and thigh heads where balance can easily be maintained.

The Rectus Abdominis Narrows
the Abdominals

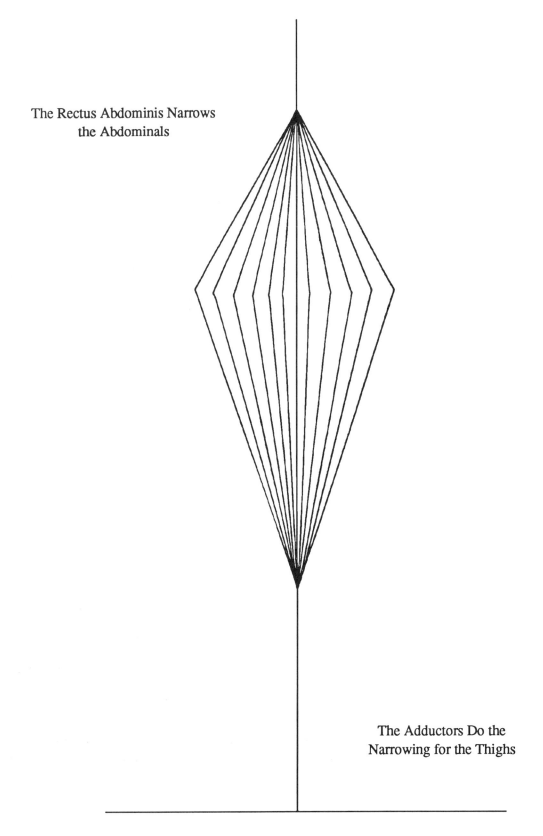

The Adductors Do the
Narrowing for the Thighs

THE ADDUCTORS ACT AS THE LOWER END OF THE PSOAS

The psoas major muscles are important radii for the pelvis as the **hub** for body movement. The child develops the psoas by kicking, rolling and crawling and builds its strength in vigorous play. Later in life, slumped sitting and fatigue in walking may create tension in these muscles. Then, the psoas muscles become contracted and upset the balance around the thigh sockets.

Exercise 1: Locate the action of the psoas muscle on the left side by thinking of its attachment at the little trochanter opposite the large trochanter. Repeat the imagery on the right side. As you walk, see the large trochanters rotating forward a bit and the little trochanters going backward to lengthen and free the psoas muscle. As you repeat the exercise and the spine lengthens, the psoas muscle will have more normal tone.

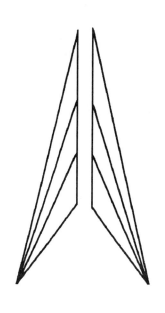

The adductor magnus aids the psoas in balancing the action around the thigh joint. The muscle is triangular which makes it very adjustable to a wide range of movement. The short upper side of the adductor triangle can be thought of as a continuation of the psoas muscle. They work together as radii around the thigh joint.

Exercise 2: Instead of bearing down on the upper short side of the adductor triangle, try thinking up on it. As you picture this action, the body can adjust to whatever direction in movement you choose to take. Thinking up on the short side of the triangle starts action in the psoas. It helps you center deeply in the thigh sockets resulting in freer movement of the thighs. The adductor action ascends upward in line with the thrust through the ankles and knees.

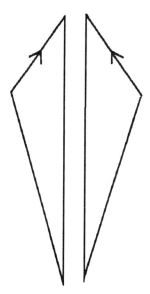

Exercise 3: The adductors are the beginning of psoas muscle action. In comparing their action to the foot pattern, you could say that the adductors act as "toes" in the pelvic foot pattern. The thigh head is the "ankle" and the ischial branch of the sitting bone acts as the "heel."

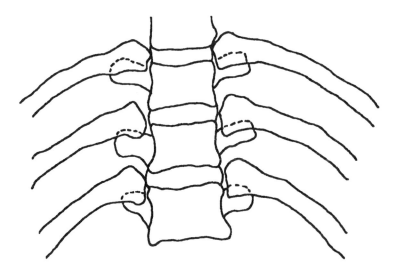

Vertebrae and Ribs – Front View

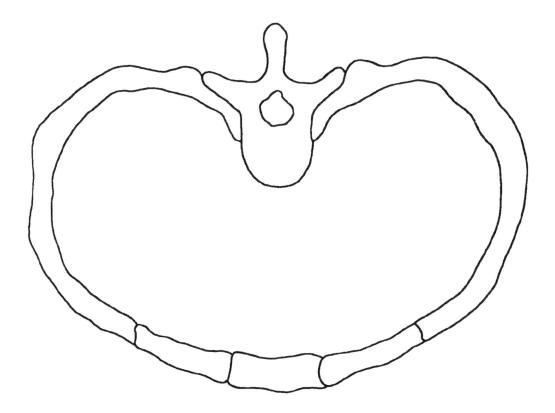

Vertebra and Rib – Top View

CENTERING THE RIBS IN THEIR SPINAL SOCKETS

Most people are unaware of the weight passing downward through the vertebrae. You developed a sense of this action in your study of the previous manuals. Perhaps you found that when weight passes easily through the vertebral centers to the sacrum, it is easy for the body to rest on the ischia. In *Body Proportion Needs Depth*, you were introduced to the depth of the spinal column and the play between the front and back of each vertebra. In this manual, you can begin to work with the idea of the vertebrae as **round.**

The vertebral bodies are round. The space for the spinal cord is round, and is as deep as it is wide. There are balls of elastic material within the disks (nucleus pulposa) between the vertebral bodies which act as cushions for the vertebrae. The disks make the lengthening or shortening of your spine possible in movement. The hard materials (bone) give your back its form. Softer materials (disks) give you action.

Exercise 1: The spine is not a rod, it has the qualities of a spring. The S-shaped curvature gives spring action to the length of the spine. The **spring factor** can be restored to the spine if you do not bear down on the disks continuously or unevenly. How can you ease up on the spine? By moving and breathing through your central axis. Lengthen your spine from the head level to the sitting bone level as you go into action.

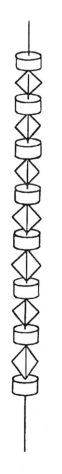
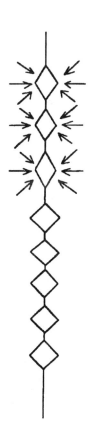

Exercise 2: Look at the illustrations on the opposite page. Notice that some of the rib joints are at the same level as the vertebral disks. This design allows the intercostal muscles to work with the elasticity of the disks.

Plumping up a pillow makes a good image for restoring elasticity to the disks. As you pat the pillow from its sides toward its center, the pillow grows a bit longer from top to bottom. This image applied to the spinal rib sockets deepens and heightens the disks. Try it out on the yawn. Allow each rib socket pair to thrust into the spine at its own level. This relaxes the thorax and lessens strain on the heart.

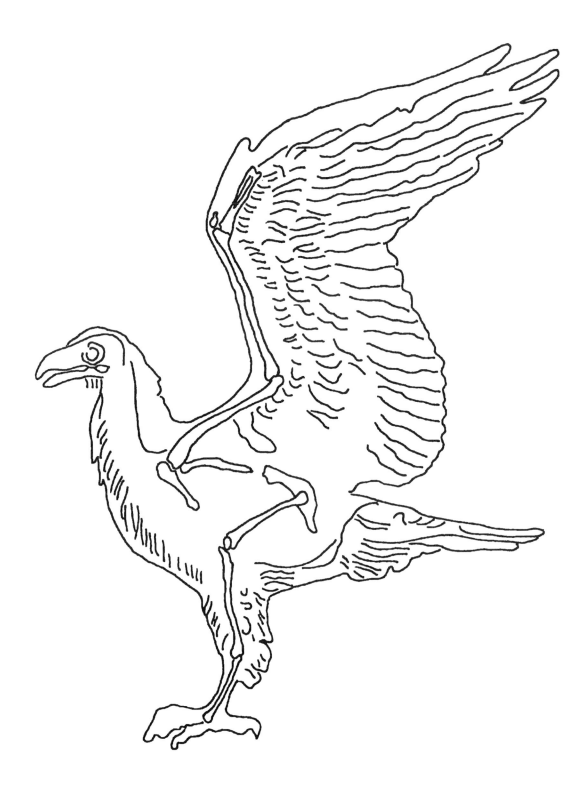

The Bird's Wing as an Image for Arm Action

THE WING PATTERN CENTERS ARM ACTION IN THE SPINE

You have worked with connecting arm action to the lower back and thighs through the latissimus dorsi muscles. The arm also connects to the spine through an extensive bony framework. Arm action moves inward from the arm socket on the side of the shoulder blade, through the collar bones to the top part of the sternum (manubrium). From the sternum, arm action travels in a circular path through the ribs into the spine.

Exercise 1: There are few joints on the sides of the body. Using the fingertips of the right hand, feel down the left side of your body from the armpit to the outside of your thigh. Using the left hand, feel down the right side of your body from the armpit to the outside of your thigh. As you brush along the ribs on the sides of the body, you are touching them midway between their articulating ends. The articulating ends of the ribs are in the spine or at the sternum. Thus, the greatest number of joints concentrate along the middle of your back and the middle of your front.

Exercise 2: Look at the illustration of the top view of the ribs and vertebra from the previous lesson. Notice the curving design of the rib in the back as it moves into the spine. This curve of bone is called the "costal angle." To get movement from the arms into the spine, you must center the ribs well in their spinal sockets. To do this, imagine a slight folding action between the costal angles and the spine. Lying on the right side, picture a folding action along the left side of the spine where the heads of the ribs center in their spinal fulcrums. Roll over to the left side. Repeat the image of a folding action along the right side of the spine where the heads of the ribs center in their spinal fulcrums. Imagining the weight of the ribs resting in the spine will help your awareness of the folding action. Think of the round shape of each pair of ribs and how they **bow** back behind the spine.

Exercise 3: The range of arm movement can be compared to the action of the bird's wing. Stand with elbows slightly flexed. Spiral the arms up over your head as you think a bird's wing opening. As you bring the arms down to your sides, think of the bird relaxing its wings into the back of its body after flight. As you try this you may begin to realize how static your body concept has been in the rib area.

Spiral the arms overhead once again. As your left arm returns to your side, visualize folding your ribs along the left side of your spine. This will let the left ribs settle deeper in their spinal sockets. Change to the right side of your thorax. Sense the folding along the right side of the spine as the right arm returns to your side.

As you become more familiar with the exercise, picture the dynamic action of feathers when you move your shoulders and arms. This will help the ribs settle deeper in their spinal sockets. Breathe easily and realize you have a **back** to your lungs.

THE RIBS ARE LIKE FINGERS

As you know, there are twelve pairs of ribs. In the last two lessons, you have been working with the vertebral beginnings of the ribs. These are spread along your thoracic spine from the base of your neck downward. The front ends of your ribs are spread along each side of your sternum from the seventh rib upward. The ribs are like fingers. Each has is own role to play in balancing the torso. You know each finger individually as the thumb, index, middle, ring and little fingers. Now, let's get to know each of the ribs.

Exercise 1: Feel your sternum in your mid-front line. It is about two to three inches wide and goes from the top of your diaphragm to the base of your neck. The ends of each of your top seven pairs of ribs have sockets on each side of the sternum. Slide your right hand fingertips from the outer end of your left collarbone towards its inner end to find the sternal socket. Then move down a bit to find the sternal socket of the left first rib. Think of a circle moving around the sternal socket of the first rib on the left side. The movement will go up the front of the rib, over the top, down the back and underneath. Circle the rib slowly three or four times.

Follow the round path of the first rib to the spinal socket in the back. Circle this deep sunken socket a few times in the same way; up the front, over the top, down the back and underneath. Change to the right side. Think of the circling the sternal socket of the right first rib. Then follow around to the back and repeat the circling around the vertebral end of the rib. Think **up the front, over the top, down the back** and **underneath** at each socket. This imagery will help lengthen the muscles at the base of your neck (scaleni) by drawing your attention to their lower ends.

Take the second pair of ribs an inch or so below the first rib pair. Work with the sternal and vertebral ends of the right and left ribs following the directions above. Then take the third rib and follow through in the same way. Repeating this exercise adjusts the top ribs in their sockets. It helps the ribs inch up a bit in the front and down a bit in the back. This gives you a longer neck by taking away your desire to hunch up in the back. The same method can be used to advantage with the fourth, fifth, sixth and seventh ribs.

Exercise 2: The eighth, ninth and tenth pairs of ribs use the seventh rib's sternal socket. Locate these ribs with your fingertips. Notice how they relax in rhythmical curves at the sides of the body and then come forward and up. Each of these ribs has an individual vertebral socket in the back. Add these to your practice when you can do so comfortably.

Exercise 3: The eleventh and twelfth pairs of ribs do not connect with the sternum. They float through the area of the waist toward the pelvis. Imagine the twelfth ribs encircling a ball. Combine this image with your exhalation. Repeat the exercise at the next highest level, thinking of eleventh ribs encircling the ball on exhalation.

YOUR STERNUM IS A MOBILE HANGING FROM THE BASE OF THE HEAD

The sternocleidomastoid muscles suspend the top of the sternum as well as the inner ends of the collar bones from above. The muscles begin behind your ears on the bumps of bone called the mastoid processes. You can see and feel these muscles as you turn the head from side to side.

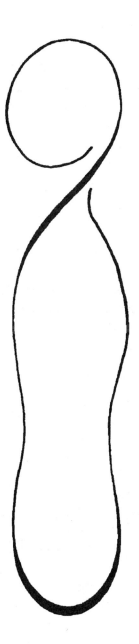

Exercise 1: Place the tip of the left second finger over the hole of your left ear. Your thumb tip will be touching your mastoid process behind your ear. You middle fingertip will be touching your jaw socket. Check by opening and closing the lower jaw. Feel out the right side in the same way. Next, using both hands, place your second and third fingertips over the mastoid processes. Get a good yawn started. As you do, let the sternocleidomastoid muscles lengthen as much as feels good to you. This can take place easily when the ligaments around your vertebral and spinal rib sockets are sufficiently flexible. You have begun this process through your practice of circling the rib sockets in the previous lesson. Repeat the circling imagery for the upper rib levels. Then swing the head from side to side and let the sternum go along as a mobile.

Exercise 2: Prolong an exhalation as you lengthen the spinal muscles down the back. Notice that each vertebral heel drops a little. Once the long row of heels drops down the line with a very comfortable feeling, you feel balanced and ready to tackle any job that is in front of you.

Exercise 3: Lengthen the spine as you flex the thigh, knee and ankle joints in a plié. Think of the sacrum as the back of a ball. Let the coccyx follow the curve in the ball underneath you. This idea will carry the pubis up the front of the ball. Extend the legs and walk forward taking these long curves with you. Balance the head as a ball on the top.

Exercise 4: Don't let your head tumble forward and down. Unroll the sternocleidomastoid muscles up the front. Roll them over the top of the atlas to go down the back with the shoulder and spinal muscles.

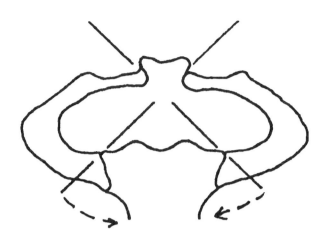

Cross Patterning at the First Rib Level

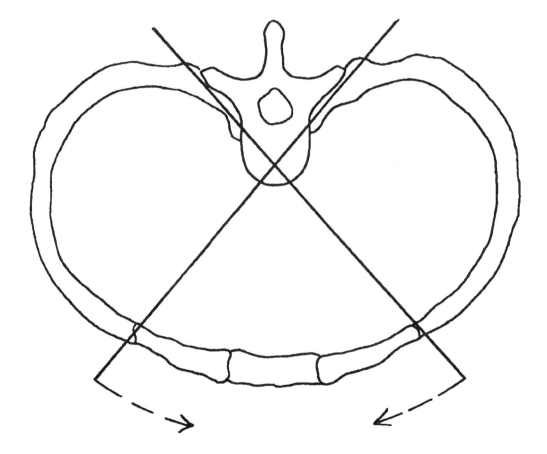

Cross Patterning at the Fourth Rib Level

THE RIBS CROSS PATTERN TO ROUND THE THORAX

The ribs cross pattern to round the thorax. Balancing the serratus anterior and serratus posterior muscles also helps bring the ribs around. The areas between the vertebral sockets for the ribs and the costal angles on either side of the spine can be thought of as "gutters" for the extensor muscles. The serratus posterior muscles in the middle of the back help keep the gutters narrow. An illustration of the serratus posterior in an anatomy book will show the **V shape** of these muscles. They begin on either side of the thorax near the costal angles of the lowest four ribs. They end over the spinous processes of four vertebrae at your waist level. The contraction of the serratus posterior pulls down and inward on the back of these ribs. This keeps the gutter from bulging outward in breathing or in movement of the legs and arms.

The serratus anterior muscle connects arm action to the sides of the ribs. Find the illustration of the serratus anterior in the *Technique for Movement Lessons* and study its design. Notice that it lies between the front of the shoulder blade and the sides of the ribs. You can imagine these muscles directing each rib forward into its sternal socket.

Exercise 1: Review the plumping pillows imagery for centering the ribs in their spinal sockets. Think of the serratus anterior muscle fanning open. Beginning in the armpit, think of lengthening each section of the muscle from under the scapula at its spinal margins, around and up toward the sternum. Later you can combine this action with the image of the little finger lengthening.

Exercise 2: Sit high on the sit bones with hands at rest in your lap. Look at the illustration representing a cross section of the fourth pair of ribs. The fourth pair of ribs is as high in the chest as the mid-shoulder blade level. Start by picturing the left fourth rib going into its spinal socket on the left side of the spine. Continue the thrust along a diagonal line toward the sternal end of the right rib in the front of the chest. Take the line inward toward the middle of the sternum and your chest will begin to expand in **depth**.

From the sternal end of the right fourth rib follow the curved line of bone back to its spinal socket on the right side of the spine. Continue the thrust along a diagonal line toward the sternal end of the left fourth rib in the front of the chest. Take the line inward toward the middle of the sternum. Follow back along the curved line of the left rib to its spinal socket. You have now completed the cross patterning of one pair of ribs.

Slowly, repeat the imagery at the fourth rib level. You are now ready to take the third rib level and proceed through the directions. Repeating the directions at least once at the third rib level, prepares you for doing the second pair of ribs. Finish by cross patterning the first ribs at the top of the thorax to deepen the chest front-to-back.

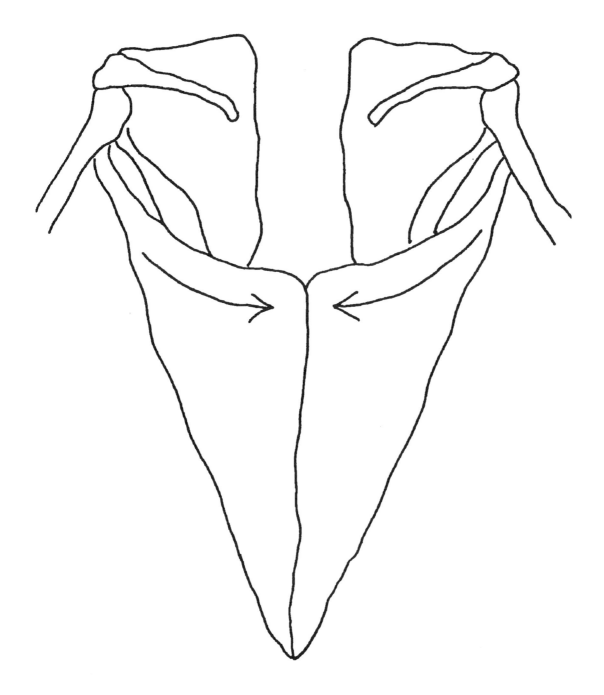

Latissimus Dorsi - Horizontal Lines

A STRUCTURE'S FOUNDATION DETERMINES THE SET OF THE ROOF

The foundation for the shoulders is the rib structure. Balancing the shoulders begins with balancing the body from beneath the shoulders. As you explored the spinal and sternal ends of the ribs in the previous lessons, you probably began to appreciate the cone shape of the upper thorax. This makes the neck seem very long and allows the shoulders to rest lightly on the top. The inner ends of the collar bones join the rib structure at the top of the sternum. The collar bones can ride **high** in the front, if the thorax is in balance.

Exercise 1: The sternum rides up on inhalation and pushes the collar bones up and out. This takes the weight of the shoulders and the strain of arm action off the rib cage. Imagining a thin inflated cushion between the top of the ribs and the shoulder structure is the way to begin. Trace up the front of the body with your fingertips on inhalation. As you move, think from the thumb along the inside of the arm to the sternoclavicular socket. This activates the muscles around the shoulder structure and lets the shoulder bones swim over the top of the thorax.

Exercise 2: Repeat *Exercise 1*. With the arm overhead, circle the outstretched arm in a figure-eight pattern. With the arm in motion, notice the outer end of the collar bone is drawing the figure-eight pattern as well. Continue to circle the arm as you think around the top ribs from the sternal sockets to the spinal sockets. Thinking of the rib thrusts moving front-to-back and back-to-front helps straighten the cervical spine.

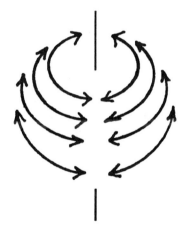

Exercise 3: Think of **hollowing out** the back side of the arm socket. This turns humeral bone outward and lets the shoulder blade drift back and down along the side of the spine. This image also gives the latissimus dorsi a better line. The illustration on the opposite page shows that the upper part of this muscle is horizontal. Think inward along these horizontal lines from the arms toward the spine.

Exercise 4: In walking, we throw ourselves off balance through the shoulders by continually thinking forward. Let's throw our shoulder action into reverse. Think down the back of the upper arm to the point of the elbow. Let the elbow swing to the back as you walk. Swing the elbow with the same push to the rear that you use habitually to the front. This will lower your shoulder blades in the back. It will help you gain more awareness of the ribs at their spinal sockets and ease up on the sternal ends of the ribs.

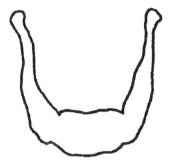 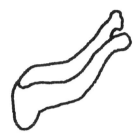

The Hyoid Bone — Front and Side Views

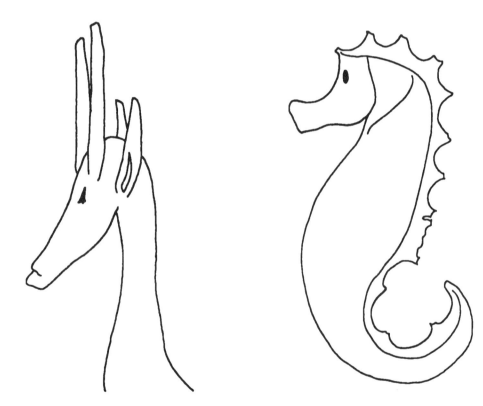

Natural Images of Hyoid Balance

THE HYOID BONE FLOATS HIGH IN YOUR NECK

Your hyoid bone lies deep in the neck crease, at the top of your throat and behind your jaw. The hyoid does not attach to other bones. It acts as a floating center for its many muscular attachments which you can think of as flexible radii. Find a picture of the hyoid and its many attachments in an anatomy book. Notice that some of the muscular radii of the hyoid assist the sternocleidomastoid in suspending the circular rib ladder in the front. These muscles pick up the rib weight on the front of the thorax and transfer it to the back of the ribs and the spine. Other muscles connect the shoulder structure to the hyoid. The hyoid bone also makes a floating base for the tongue.

You can balance your hyoid bone well if you remember that it floats high in your neck toward your atlas. Look at the illustration. Notice the **U shape** of the bone. In your thinking, the ends of the U shape should slant up and back toward the atlas. This frees the head to center on the atlas and turn on axis, the same as the ankle swivels on the heel.

Exercise 1: Sit or stand and gently place your hand around the crease of your neck in the front. The tip of your thumb will be on one side of your hyoid bone and your second fingertip will be on the other side of the bone. The width of the bone in the front is between two and three inches. Use the image of slanting the bone **up and back** toward the atlas. Your thumb and finger pressure should indicate the back and up direction.

Exercise 2: Sit or stand and center yourself. Exhale a few times and notice how exhaling helps you let your breath go down from your upper back into your lower back. Test this out by exhaling a few more times. You are now ready to add a further step.

Your tongue is long. The base of the tongue has its roots on the front end of your hyoid bone. Its tip is above your front upper teeth. We are apt to pull the hyoid bone forward with the tongue as we speak or chew. To correct this, use the image of a center line or axis through your tongue. Think back along this line from the tip of the tongue toward its roots on the hyoid bone.

Exercise 3: The throat forms a muscular circle one level higher than the top circle of ribs. Use the image of the depth for the throat circle. Think of a line from the front to the back of the circle. Let go of the tendency to widen the throat from side to side. As you go into a yawn, think of expanding the circle from front to back. This will help you balance your shoulders over the top of your structure.

FAN WIDE BEHIND THE ATLAS AND THE ANKLE BONES

The achilles tendons attach to the heels of the feet. The ligamentum nuchae attaches to the heels of the cervical vertebrae. They have a similar shape and similar spaces to fill.

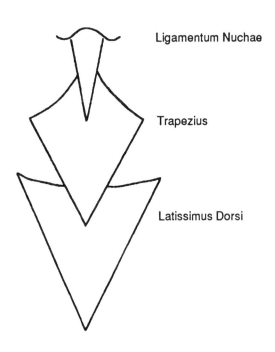

Ligamentum Nuchae

Trapezius

Latissimus Dorsi

The achilles tendon fills the space behind the lower leg bones and attaches to the back of the heel. The ligamentum nuchae fills the space behind the back of the cervical spine and attaches to the base of the head. You have seen the ligamentum nuchae used by mother dogs and cats in carrying their young from place to place. Find a picture of the ligamentum nuchae in a good anatomy book to study its back and side views. In this illustration, notice that it is triangular in design and points downward, much like the trapezius and latissimus dorsi muscles.

Both the ligamentum nuchae and achilles tendons should be more relaxed. Then they can help to give balance to the sphere-shaped ankle bones and the hyoid with its many radii.

Exercise 1: Sit and center your ankle bones over the tops of your heels. Think of the axes of the heels fanning open behind your ankle joints. Place the fingertips of both hands around the base of your head to meet in the top of your neck in the back. Using one hand at a time, gently outline the head's circular base. As you do, you may feel one of the three ridges of bone where your long spinal muscles attach. Let these muscles lengthen down from the base of the head, through the spinal curves to between your sitting bones. Relax your arms and place your hands in your lap. Think up the front from your toes to your thigh sockets. Climb the rib ladder in the front and slant up and back through the hyoid to the atlas. Pause to think of dropping your heels—your spinal heels, pelvic heels and the heels of your feet.

Exercise 2: The neck pattern is similar to the foot pattern. Come up the front of the neck through the sternocleidomastoid and the many radii of the hyoid bone. Round over the top of the atlas. Fan the back of the neck open as if it was a heel. Think of the ligamentum nuchae as longer, looser and wider. Extend the head as you extend the heels.

THE HEAD IS ROUND

Tension tends to collect in the spaces around the outer ends of the legs and arms, and at the upper end of the axis. These outer ends should relax so the weight can be felt around the inner ends of the extremities and near the center of gravity deep within the pelvis. Think of the head as round. Feel a line through the center of the sphere. Let the head find its balance **front-to-back** on the atlas and turn **side-to-side** on the axis.

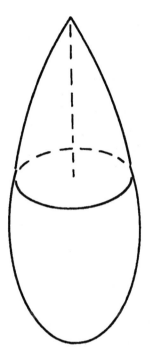

Exercise 1: Look at the drawing and think of capping your head with a cone. The tip of the cone points directly up to the ceiling. First, picture moving clockwise around the circle at the base of the cone. Then think of the action around the base of the cone moving counter-clockwise. Finally, think the line from the center of the top of your head through the middle of the cone to its axis tip. Drop down through the spinal heels as you direct the tip of the cone toward the ceiling. Both the circle around the base of the cone and thinking up to its axis tip can be used to locate the axis line through your head and neck. Try the first image for a while and then use the other.

Exercise 2: Awareness of balancing the head at the center of its depth gives you a sense of a round back of the head. The forehead is also round. To sense this shape, get **behind** the back of the forehead. Think of how it curves forward into a spherical shape. This allows the forehead to take the lead in movement as the chin and jaw soften downward. Then you will be able to feel the uplift of the brain and not its weight.

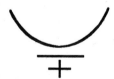

Exercise 3: The base of the head needs a gradual approach to centering on the pivot point (dens) of the axis. Think of narrowing inward from the base of the head, through the width of the atlas to the axis pivot. Then widen between the outer ears.

USE YOUR SENSES IN BALANCING THE HEAD

As they move in their daily lives, people pass through openings from one area into another. These openings outside the body are called doors or entrances. Ideas also pass through openings from the world outside your body to the mind within your body. These openings are called the senses. Your concept of these entrance places can affect you in many ways. Some people hold the sense openings of their faces quite rigidly set. Without their awareness, thoughts and emotions gather in the sense openings and rob them of their full movement. Imagery can bring your senses into fuller action and provide another way to balance the head.

Awareness of the depth of the eye may have been the purpose of the old exercise of focusing on a point of a pencil. The pencil was brought near the eyes and then moved back in the distance. However, for many people, the exercise was too conscious and created more tension. Imagery can do a better job in gradually reducing eyestrain and bringing the eyes into better balance. Think of your eye sockets as deep, following a path toward the front of your spine. This lets the eyes come to rest with the base of your head on your atlas.

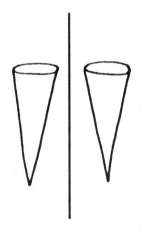

Exercise 1: A small cone is good imagery for the eye socket as it fits the bony space that your eye actually uses. The shape of the cone helps in expansion of the eye depth by reminding you that the eye socket is **long** as well as **round.** Think from the top of the cone (surface of the eye) to its inner tip deep within the center of the head. Use the inner walls of the cone-like eye socket, in your rest as well as your activity.

Let's start with your left eye. Visualize the space which is the inner or nose side of the cone. Think of the inner side of the cone having dots in a line. Follow the dots, one by one in your imagination, to the tip of the cone.

After a few minutes of practice on your left eye, change to the right one. Again think of the nose side of the cone and then follow the dots back toward its apex. Gradually, you will notice that the eyes tend to converge as you relax them. Bringing the inner walls of the cones into action helps release the tension in the outer walls and front surfaces of the eyes.

Exercise 2: As you walk or ride in a car, let the objects in the distance ahead come to you. We generally think of sound coming to us, and taste and smell coming to us. But, for some reason, we think we must reach out for sight by holding ourselves tense. We should let sight come to us also.

Exercise 3: When the first exercise becomes familiar to you, begin to circle the rim of the eye cone. Trace along the outer socket of the left eye with your fingertip in an inward direction. From the outer edge of the socket, just under the eyebrow, circle inward toward the bridge of the nose. Trace down along the side of the nose bridge to the inner cheek bone. Move along its edge to the outside of the eye socket and up to the eyebrow where you started. When this becomes easy, let the hands rest. Think of circling the eye socket as you circle the head in the same direction. Repeat the exercise on the right side.

As you continue your practice, think from the front of the eye socket back into the depth of the cone as you repeat the circling pattern. The circles spiral inward from the surface to the tip of the eye cone. This releases tension in the eyes and centers them in the depth of the head.

Exercise 4: The ears of animals are very active. You can observe them pricking up their ears and wheeling them forward and back in response to sounds. Let's use the action of circling the outer ear to free its action.

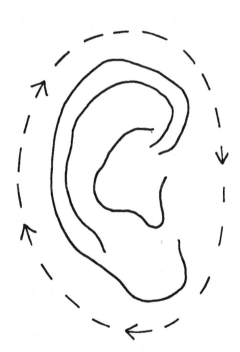

Place the fingertip of the left hand over the left ear lobe. Slowly begin to circle up the back of the outer rim of the left ear toward its upper front corner. Then slide your fingertip straight down along the front of the ear toward the ear lobe. The image can be repeated as you trace the circling design in the crease between the outer ear and the skull. The directions are the same, circling **up the back**, rounding **over the top**, and tracing **down the front**. Repeat the circling action on the right ear and then behind the rim, within its crease. The circling action centers the ears.

Exercise 5: In *Let's Enjoy Sitting – Standing – Walking*, you thought of softening the outer sides of the nostrils. This encourages the inflow of air to take a central path along the inner walls of the nose and strengthens the action of the diaphragm. Now you can think of the tip of the nose softening and rolling downward. Nod the head very slowly at the level of the atlas as you think of this. The ligamentum nuchae opens around the back of the neck in the action. Allow the head to return to position and take the breath down the back of the spine.

THE BODY'S ARCHES ROUND UPWARD

The human structure is arched and buttressed from within. The reactionary force or counter-thrust to gravity works up through the body arches.

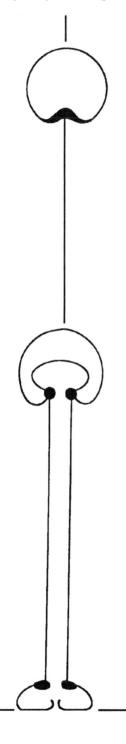

In *Body Proportion Needs Depth*, you placed the feet together in a mound. Thinking of the feet as two halves of a mound, higher at the center than around its edges, brings the foot arches into their best balance. The arch of the pelvis is also more easily remembered with the feet together. Holding tension around your great trochanters widens the pelvic arch. Thinking of psoas action on the insides of the thigh bones narrows and heightens the pelvic arch. This makes the thigh axes more vertical and centers their thrusts toward the sides of the sacrum.

Exercise 1: In *Body Proportion Needs Depth*, you also learned that the inner rim of the pelvis is like a pair of ribs. The spinal ends of this thirteenth rib pair meet on each side of the sacrum. The front of the rib pair meet at the pubic symphysis. Imagine as much space from the front to the back of your thirteenth rib as from the right side to left side. Then think of the two sides of the thirteenth rib bracing each other through the pubic symphysis at the center front.

Exercise 2: The mouth, at the center of the sense area, also uses the mound pattern. The roof of the mouth as an arch also rounds. There are two levels to the roof of the mouth. The tip of your tongue can easily feel the lower level. The upper level is higher where sight, smell, sound and taste come together in front of the atlas. Tension in any of the senses tends to stiffen and flatten the shape of the upper level. Think of raising the roof of the mouth whenever you yawn. Move from the front to the back of this arch as you think up, over and down.

Exercise 3: Look at the illustration. Feet together in a mound places the foot arch under the thigh head arch which is under the head arch. When you are familiar with this design, relax the outer edges of the diaphragm and heighten upward through its central tendon. Making mounds heightens all the body's arches.

USE IMAGERY AND SENSORY AWARENESS
TO CHECK A QUICK TEMPER

Perhaps you use the old formulas of thinking twice before you speak or counting to ten before sounding off. While these can be helpful, there is a more effective way that gives you enjoyment at the same time.

Exercise 1: In dealing with feelings we can benefit by watching animals. Everyone is familiar with smoothing down the muscles over the spine of a pet. The direction a cat or dog enjoys is toward the tail. The cat purrs its gratitude and the dog wags its tail for the same reason. It is the lengthening of the spinal muscles on the back of the vertebrae that feels so good. It allows the spines of the vertebrae, sacrum and coccyx to move down the back ever so slightly.

Your nervous system is present throughout your body. Instead of being wound up inside your head, let the nervous system **unwind** itself down the back. Think of a spiral stairway and go down through the neck as if descending the stairs. Continue the descent through the thorax and lumbar spine to the sacrum and coccyx. Move down the backs of the legs toward the heels. Pause and finish the exercise by moving up the stepping stones in the front of the central line, through the hyoid to the atlas at the top.

Exercise 2: A real smile is an indication of well being within. What does a smile do on the inside? It lifts the roof of the mouth and centers the eyes. A real laugh is a shimmy dance of the organs which makes it excellent internal medicine. Like the yawn it washes the eye surfaces. It opens the rib spaces and slips weight over the top from the pectorals to the trapezius lines.

The next time you go into the "ha-ha" state, focus some of your attention on your rib sockets. Let the laughter help you center the ribs in their spinal sockets in rhythm with your exhalation. If you have laughed heartily you may find you feel a bit weak and tired. This is because you laughed so well down into the lower rib sockets in the back.

Exercise 3: You can use your sensory awareness and the body alignment imagery to quiet the emotions. The spine is like a candle coming to rest in its holder. The mind is like a flame. It gives the most light when the candle is quiet and steady.

INTEGRATE BODY ACTION INCLUDING THE BREATH

Athletes crouch at the start of the race to wait for the starting signal. They know how to make use of the waiting period to find strength in dynamic balance. Integration of action including the breath is the center of their attention. The squatting position is excellent because it encourages the lowering of the spinal and pelvic heels. The psoas muscles can pull down on the ribs in the back and move forward through the center of the body to pull up on the legs. This is a key to the integration of the body the athlete uses; the ribs space down to pull the legs upward.

Exercise 1: You have two pair of floating ribs, the short twelfth set and the longer eleventh set. Narrow them at their lower ends. Just as the sternal rib thrusts narrow upward with the rectus abdominis as you inhale, the floating ribs should narrow as you think down on exhalation. Change from a horizontal pattern in the use of the ribs toward a more vertical one. Narrowing the floating ribs down the back as you get ready to go, prepares the psoas to lead the legs up the front at the starting signal.

Exercise 2: Repeat the first exercise in the standing position a few times. When you are ready, add a plié that backs down into the crouch position. The feet will be separated for this movement, one foot in front of the other, rather than in the mound position. From the crouch move into a crawling position on your knees, with the entire lower arms resting on the floor. Relax the elbows and spaces between the lower arm bones, along with the hands. Think of depth in the hollows of the thigh and arm creases. Begin sliding the left lower arm backward and then the right knee. Slide the right lower arm backward and then the left knee. Repeat the action and enjoy getting into the rhythm.

Focus your attention on the inner walls of the thighs as you move. Placing your attention there will help you get better use of the inner walls of the eyes. Change to using your hands to support your upper body when you desire to do so. Try getting up from the floor by backing up through the crouch to an erect position.

Exercise 3: In throwing a ball, remember the **down** of your motion takes you **up**. This happens along the spine and through the muscular radii which relate to your pelvis. In throwing a ball your strength comes from the lower back. As you prepare for throwing in the wind-up, follow through the inside of the arm from the radial socket to the shoulder socket. Extend the spine downward by thinking of the latissimus dorsi spreading out along its spinal length into the back of the pelvis and thighs. Then let the ball fly.

Exercise 4: To get ready to kick a ball, think up the front of the thigh from the center of the foot to the thigh socket. Continue up to the twelfth rib through the psoas muscle. Uncoil spinal action as you kick the ball, down the back of the leg and out your heel.

THE BODY CAN BE COMPARED TO A TREE

Think of a tree balancing in the wind. Movement begins with a slight stirring of the leaves. With a stronger breeze, there is more action of the twigs until the entire branch is involved. When the wind is very strong, the grip of the roots steadies the trunk as it sways in the current.

In the human body the upper ends of the thighs, lower ends of the shoulders and central ends of the diaphragm all need to **dig in** to the spine. The greater the struggle each puts up for its share of the axis the stronger the body becomes in every way. It is the source of their strength, as the root system is for the tree. If this is developed, order is maintained for organic functioning, smooth running of the nervous system and supple action of the skeletal system.

Exercise 1: Don't be reluctant to admit your fatigue. Human functioning takes place in rhythm, alternating activity and rest. Many people think they must maintain an upright position and rest in a chair rather than lying down. This is done at the expense of shortening the spine. A tired body tends to hold up the back. As a result, it dumps down the front.

In extreme emotion or mental effort, the organic system is inhibited and energy pours into the muscular system to prepare for maximum power and speed. When such efforts are over, you should rest and re-balance the skeletal system. Learn to use frequent rests during the day to center your body systems. Don't think of rests as a negative or inactive phase. They are an opportunity to let go of the ends of your branches and take hold of your roots.

Exercise 1: Think of how animals stretch the spine and extremities with the yawn as they complete a rest. In your next rest period on the floor, roll from one side to the other lengthening the leg and arm of the same side. Start by lying on the floor on your left side with your knees slightly flexed. Place your right arm up over your head with your hand resting on the floor. Turn slowly to your right by taking short steps sideways. Your right arm will move slowly along the floor like the arm of a windmill. As you reach your right side, your right arm will come to rest in front of your body. Then the left leg will open downward, straightening the knee and extending your heel to lengthen your Achilles tendon. To counterbalance the downward movement of your leg, your left arm reaches up over your head.

Let your left leg come back to a position of rest over the right. Pause for a few moments to center yourself. Then the left arm will slide slowly along the floor as your feet take tiny steps to your left. Your left arm will move very slowly with the rhythm of your moving body and legs. Bring your left arm down to rest in front of your body as your right arm slowly reaches up over your head. The right leg will open down straight to extend your heel. Let go of the Achilles tendon along with your ribs.

Move out to the ends of your radii – center them lightly into the hub.

THE RADIAL PATTERN CONTINUES
BETWEEN YOUR PELVIS AND RIBS

Continuity of extensor and flexor action unites the head, thorax and pelvis. You have begun to equalize front and back muscle action between the ribs. You have also become aware of balance through the musculature of the neck, between the thorax and head. Equalizing the ischial and pubic branches has helped you balance the muscles supporting the pelvis. Let's continue with the muscles between the thorax and pelvis.

In the back of the body, the quadratus lumborum muscle helps integrate the thorax and pelvis. Lying between the twelfth rib and the back of the pelvis, it provides "intercostal action" through the back of your waist. The transverse abdominis muscle serves a similar purpose in the front and sides of the body. The muscle begins in the back in an envelope-like covering surrounding the spinal muscles. In the front, the muscle moves through another envelope around the rectus abdominis.

The quadratus lumborum and transverse abdominis muscles surround your diaphragm. The diaphragm is placed in a circular pattern as a ceiling for the abdomen and a floor for the lungs. Having such a position between the digestive and circulatory systems means that its rhythm serves to integrate them. The muscle fibers of the diaphragm also radiate from its center to the skeletal system. They attach in a circular pattern to the ribs as well as the intercostal muscles between the ribs.

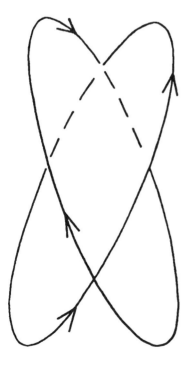

Exercise 1: The abdominal cavity is **round**. Think of the abdominal area as a ball. The diaphragm serves as the top of the ball. The pelvic floor is at the bottom, the quadratus lumborum is in the back, and the transverse abdominis is in the front. Go down the back of the ball on exhalation. Come up the front of the ball on inhalation.

Exercise 2: Stop pulling the front of the ball in toward the spine. This habit interferes with the action of the bones, muscles and your organic systems. The center of the body should be in action, not held rigidly.

Exercise 3: When you have become familiar with *Exercise 1*, try some cross patterning as you circle. The illustration provides directions for you to follow.

Use all the radii of your body center.

USE THE ESSENCE OF MOVEMENT
AS A BREATHING IMAGE

The diaphragm is the least understood of all the vital agents of human living. It is the time-keeper for all the changing rhythms of the various body systems. Breath and movement evolve together in the early weeks of life. As we grow older, lack of mind-body integration may lead us to hold on to our breath.

Exercise 1: One factor to be absorbed from observing babies and animals is to breathe as you go. Changing position frequently throughout the day automatically lets you breathe deeper. You stop holding your breath when you move out of a fixed position. Test this idea by rising from your chair to stand. As cramped muscles lengthen and relax, you can also let go of your breath.

Exercise 2: Our pattern for balance in movement, **down the back** and **up the front,** is followed by the breath. Exhalation is associated with weight. Inhalation is related to lightness. Think of the flight of the bird, swooping and soaring. Remember, the bird's lightest feathers are on its front.

Exercise 3: Breath is radial. It consists of many layers. Each rib layer supports itself on its own level radiating from center back to center front and back again. You can free breath action by imagining more rib layers between your rib cage and pelvis. There is room for five or more rib layers below the twelfth ribs. Think front-to- back and back-to-front through these levels as you have for your upper twelve pairs of ribs. Then exhale to the base of your imaginary rib cage at the **thirteenth rib.**

Exercise 4: Explore your breathing easily, without forcing it. Air moving through the leaves of a tree gently stirs them to move in many directions. Think of the breath circling through your body in a similar way. Let the breath drip through the tissues. Use your kinesthetic sense to enjoy the sway of your body fibers in rhythm with your breath.

Breath lies at the **heart** of all movement.

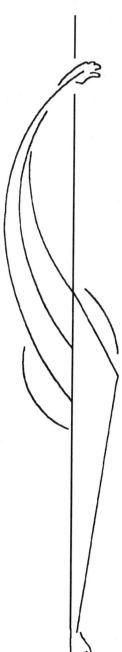

Appendix A
Lesson Notes from Todd's Boston Studio
1923–1924

SECTION I

October 22, 1923   **Miss Todd**

An atom is never in stagnation, there is always action. The body is constructed of atoms. Each is always free and in motion if allowed to live its natural life. Air is composed of gases—nitrogen, oxygen, carbon dioxide. Gases are not held in a chemical combination but exist more as a homogeneous mixture. Mechanical term—atom. Anatomical term—cell. A cell is a nucleated mass of protoplasm endowed with the attributes of life. Protoplasm is also a chemical compound. The body is changing constantly.

Relaxation is interpreted wrongly. We think of the term in respect to giving an order to relax to the body. This should not be done. Instead, think of softness. The nerve fibers will pick up the sensation, and this will spread into the tissues, releasing tension and stagnation. Do not let the mind give order to the body to relax. Think softness, separateness of atoms, floating suspended.

Venous circulation is near the surface of body. If surface muscles are tense, venous circulation is slowed and the heart muscle is forced to work harder to force the circulation onward. Respiration is the act of creating a vacuum inside the body, into which the air will enter of its own accord. We cannot keep air out of a vacuum, but man can regulate size of that vacuum. The force of the air on the outside of the body is equalized by pressure within the body. The diaphragm is the strongest muscle in breathing. Rib cage should be kept soft.

October 29, 1923   **Miss Todd**

The animal lives with motor forces always ready to spring into action. Man has lost that power and lives more in the sensory. The most improvement she saw in me from the last lesson, is in getting hold of the crouch muscles. The iliacus is on the inner surface of the pelvis. The leg is held up by all the little threads around the inner surface of the ilium gathering into one tendon.

Lengthening clavicle. I am inclined to get the thought of moving the arm in the humerus. Instead think of the clavicle and scapula sitting out over the humerus—illustration Holland Yoke. This releases the trapezius somewhat and allows the subclavius to act. Let the first rib, not all of the rib cage, go back into spine.

November 5, 1923   **Miss Todd**

Axial skeleton should include pelvis, otherwise the spinal column is divided into two parts. A very firm junction between sacrum and ilium, contrary to osteopathic view. Miss Todd says a green skeleton [recently deceased] has to be literally chiseled apart at these points. The legs and arms should swing perfectly free in their sockets.

Miss Todd classifies the shoulder girdle as an accessory structure to protect rib carriage. For instance, if arm were attached to rib carriage directly, the pull and strain would tear it to pieces. If the rib cage was firm enough to resist the strain, there would not be enough elasticity for the purposes it serves. In the rib cage, the liquids and gases need to have a structure that will expand as necessary.

In me, there is scarcely any pull in the clavicle and the levator scapulae and subclavius do practically no work. The trapezius and rhomboids are over-developed, tense and rigid, and take the pull from the clavicle and muscles attached to it.

Image Exercises

1. Think of spring block between heels and pressure by the heels on it. Heels should be active, Large toe feels drawn in. Inside of knees soft. With pressure by heels, the two ilia will be drawn toward each other in front.
2. Imagine a 5—10—15—25 pound weight at the end of the spine.
3. Think of the rib cage as cone-like with space between it and the clavicles. Think of the clavicles as two straight sticks in the front of the body and lengthening. Forget completely the whole back of the shoulder and back of the arm. Swing the front of the acromion forward from the inner ends of the sticks. Set the first rib back into the spine.
4. Think of weight of head slipping over scalp into forehead. The forehead, not the chin, should lead. Don't think at all about the legs—let them go.

November 10, 1923   Miss Todd

My right foot is not good, must work on it. Think of inner ankle, draw lines from each toe back to this point. This will fill out inner ankle and remove fullness in outer. The outer ankle is much too developed. I am exceedingly muscle bound in rib carriage. I think of it as a whole instead of many parts. I am much worse than the types who hold themselves rigid at times, systemic rigidity. Mine is structural rigidity. The fixed thought is the correct one in lumbar region. But the rib carriage should be flexible and moveable. Now, I must think of the many muscles of the rib cage and allow them movement.

Image Exercises

1. For the intercostals: wink eyes very rapidly and think of a child opening and closing shutters on a blind. Let this permeate into action of ribs and intercostal muscles.
2. Cradling [as if rocking a baby] from side to side. Let movement come in rib carriage not from hips or arms.
3. Python image: ribs inside of python—shoulder girdle on outside. Think of this during the week.

November 12, 1923   Miss Colwell

Work with psoas minor and iliacus. Shrink in front of sacrum to lumbar. Narrow across the front of the pelvis between ilia. Fold in ilia. Heels together not ankles. Point below knees together, not knees. Point above knees together, not knees.

November 19, 1923   **Miss Todd**

For the week, think about mass consciousness. Lower body is a living active mass. Holding to it two other masses—the legs. Resting on it another mass—upper body. Think of molecular freedom all through mass especially in upper dorsal [thoracic curve]. Think of sun shining through particles separating them. Get more separation between the particles. Mass consciousness instead of line consciousness.

The spine is the center of the body. Everything either sits on or hangs from the spine. Head sits on the spine. Pelvis hangs from the spine. Ribs hang from the spine. Review rack idea for clavicle. Think also of each rib as a rack and push towels to center of rack—spine.
Anterior of pelvis—superficial layer, mesenteric layer, deep structural layer—forms cuff holding spine in such a way that jars are not transmitted from walking, etc. Notice what is taught in anatomy about crura of diaphragm.

Concentration—this is my most important problem. Try not to force mind to stop at a fixed point. Train subconscious mind to hold firmly in pelvic area while thoughts travel around the vision or idea.

November 21, 1923   **Miss Galbraith**

Showed me picture of cross section of the body in pelvic region—the beefiness of the muscles. Should not think I must hold up the front of the pelvis. The normal position is what we want and the muscles will keep in that, if they are allowed their proper tonicity.

Image Exercises

1. Bisque [unglazed ceramic] doll, with legs which are separate from the body, but held up by elastic inside the body.
2. Cut large doughnut from one side of the hip, flip it over and slide up the spine. Cut on the other side and repeat the image, sliding the doughnut up the spine. Fit six doughnuts on the spine. Be careful not to crush doughnuts in back.
3. In breathing, can put little straw in front part of the doughnut holes and breathe through it. Think of diagonal as muscles draw through centers of doughnuts.

November 24, 1923   **Miss Colwell**

I must still walk with ilia thrown backward and the head of the femur outward. Change the idea to forward and inward. In upper body, after puckering the sternum upward, think of ropes passing from upper border of sternum to base of the head. This relieves tension at the sixth and seventh cervical vertebrae. Then ribs will slide down back. After two or three times, my middle ribs are apt to stiffen.

Image Exercises

1. Parallel lines of tibia and fibula at ankle.
2. Leg in the air [lying on back], "point" with the heel.
3. Pick up pencil or hairpin with the toes. Toes should move from center of foot near the heel.

November 26 and first week in December—ill.

December 8, 1923   **Miss Todd**

I must not work with idea of time limiting me. Watch myself change, don't work at it. Have a tremendous grip in the legs which I must lose. Can put teeth into my spine as much as I want to. Think of true pelvis [inner pelvic rim].

December 12, 1923   **Miss Galbraith**

Think of legs as severed from body and watch them grow on, granulation of tissue together. Shoulders slide off. Water trickling down the back—one drop running into another and other ones starting.

December 17, 1923   **Miss Todd**

Take pelvis and support with the hands as frequently as I have the opportunity. Do not try to wiggle spine and ribs down into the pelvis. If I work on the pelvis, that will work on the ribs. Miss Todd would like to have me snowshoe as that would help to get me into the pelvis.

January 22, 1924   **Miss Todd**

I am not in good condition. Todd could not give me a constructive lesson as outer muscles so tense, that she could not get at the others. In the toe exercise, corrected my false idea of big toe and thumb. The heel is akin to the thumb and the great toe to the forefinger. Toes should move straight up and down like a trip hammer. Showed me the bottom of the foot and the strongest and longest tendons. Thought should go from inside of heel to outer side of the ball of foot.

January 24, 1924   **Miss Galbraith**

I have not been sufficiently careful to carry and hold ribs in upper dorsal area well into spine. In tipping pelvis, I should separate the idea of spine from pelvis so as not to interfere with spinal curves. Follow the long lines down each side of the back, come to the pelvis and swoop down and under. Then, give just a little upward tilt to the front of the pelvis.

Image Exercises

1. Shoulder exercise: pricking through of the middle angle of scapulae. Releasing serratus and trapezius. Think of lower point of trapezius lengthening down like a kite tail.
2. Pucker at sternal ends of clavicle, then bring ribs into spine between scapulae using illustration of shortening a line or holding a snake by the neck.
3. Shirr [gathering material along two or more parallel lines of stitching] over the front of the pubis. Think of using needle and thread.
4. Toe exercise: big toe up and holding the others down, then reverse.

January 26, 1924   Miss Colwell

Miss Colwell says my body is in the best condition she has ever seen it since the start of lessons. Sacrum must be separated in my thought from the pelvic mass. Think of hole in the head of the femur [fovea of the head] held by ligament [teres] from there into the acetabulum. Then follow ridge of inner pelvic rim back to the sacrum.

Image Exercises

1. Shoulder exercise: holding ribs in upper dorsal area well into spine, wink first with one shoulder then the other.
2. Think of diagonals through ball and socket of hip joints. Release the long lines from the outer side of the thigh to the knee.

January 28, 1924   Miss Todd

Upper sternum [manubrium] must stay up and out. One hand placed across lower thoracic cage to keep it from elevating. Think upper sternum lifted about one-half inch and held up toward the chin. The upper rib cage holds firmly and the rest drops down. Smock [decorative shirring] the front surface of the body. Diagonals with line passing through sacroiliac. Be sure femurs are well into the sockets. Diagonals go through the torso. When finished, cross arms without depressing sternum.

Image Exercises

1. Image of stovepipe down into pelvis. Slip pelvis up over it without denting pipe.
2. Thought of living in the spine and swishing the tail.

February 2, 1924   Miss Colwell

In the chinning exercise, boy lets ribs slide down the back into the pelvis as he comes up with his body. Girl is more apt to hold herself stiff. Work out this idea and prepare the body. Think of boy pulling Union Suit [one piece underwear] up over one leg and then the other and squirming buttocks into it.

Image Exercises

1. Sewing: needle passes from weak spot in the spine to sternum.
2. Sew from the tip of the ilium to the tuberosity of the ischium as if through a cushion. Push needle back and forth, softening the cushion.

February 4, 1924   Miss Galbraith

Comparison of normal spinal curves with straight line. Straight line through center of body touches lumbar and cervical curves. Must not push backward on cervical curve. Think of Miss Chapin [another teacher] and widen between the ears, above the cervical curve. Don't strain hinges [costal angles] of the ribs. Points to keep soft and not allow ego consciousness to be in: acromion process, chin, sternum and knees.

February 9, 1924   **Miss Galbraith**

Lesson on standing. Soft at ankles and inside of knees. Spring block between the heels. Gird up [prepare oneself for action] loins. Clavicles like cat's whiskers. Ribs set into the spine. Crown head pulled up. Whole body suspended—then walk.

February 11, 1924   **Miss Colwell**

Body is torn to pieces by three processes: chemically, of which we know little; structurally, pull of legs and arms; and emotionally. Lowest floating rib has much importance attached to it. Lines through pelvis—ischium to front of the rim. Fastening up seventh, eighth and ninth ribs when working with twelfth.

SECTION II

General Principles

To most people inhibiting means doing nothing. There is action to contract and action to relax. Think of bones in a solution, bones moved by solution. Solution should not solidify. Greater power of solution in lumbar and thigh areas. Solution through the head, ribs, pelvis, between ribs, around leg bones, between toes, under shoulder girdle.

Image Exercises

1. Snugging the body together—then moving the extremities. At first, there would only be as much motion of the extremities as body could produce—small at first and growing stronger.
2. Think from each end of muscle towards the other to stimulate muscle action. Do not exert so much outward pressure. Body in air, like fish in water. Let the air push against sides of your ribs and thighs and soles of feet. On ischia when sitting—make upward push from below equivalent to downward pressure.
3. Body axis of weight is an imaginary line like the one called axis of the earth. Think of axis of motion and axis of support. Bring the two axes as close together as possible to release outer pulls of body.
4. Picture palm on the back—palm on the abdomen. Bring two points—two hands—toward the axis.

Lengthen Spine

Lying on the back. Spine touches table between sacrum and fifth lumbar. The ilia help in supporting this; tip of spinous process of the fifth lumbar would barely touch the table. If there is proper support in the pelvic muscles and those in front of sacrum, there will not be too much backward thrust of the spine at this point.

Avoid too straight a chair when lumbar spine is weak. Upper body over lower part, not upper body forward and lower body back. Coccyx into its fascia like finger into glove.

Image Exercises

1. Fascia below gluteus maximus snugged together. Space lower end of adductors.
2. Image of the sunken garden for pelvic floor. From the pubis going down the steps from the first to the second. Narrow and heighten the top step [pubic symphysis.] Broaden, widen and deepen the lower steps toward the front of the sacrum and coccyx. Releases gluteals.
3. Blow paper whistle down front of spine to the tip. See it roll back and blow down again. Hissing may be combined.

Pelvis

Spine should not be held upward. Leg thrust is toward center and upward. Spinal weight is toward center and downward. Pressure beneath feet to relieve drag at thighs. Make upward push from below equivalent to downward pressure from above. Bucket goes down into well and also comes up.

Psoas pushed up as much as diaphragm down. Diaphragm is a very thin muscle. It is logical that it could not be a supporting muscle. It is useless to carry the ribs down until they release from side to center. Greatest need of activity is in pelvis. A weak person is weak there. Relaxation of extremities brings centralization at center.

Image Exercises

1. Anterior superior [iliac] spine carries over to the opposite side of the pelvis. Like a leaf folding or curling over. Caution—ischia should not spread beyond the point of releasing. Should feel action between pubic arch and ischia. Feather waves from side to side.
2. Large ball within pelvis: roll upward in the front.
3. Pelvic floor, coccygeal area: think of flower opening—petals radiating outward. Center of flower goes in and out with breath.
4. Boat image for the pelvis: ischia—bottom of the boat, spine—the mast. Legs are controlled from inside the boat. Ribs are sails down the side of the mast. In walking leave the sails down.
5. Slip cover image for pelvis. Outer pelvic rim—arms of the chair. Inner pelvic rim—seat of the chair. Tuck slip cover between sides and cushion. Tuck slip cover in back of the cushion. Chair seat is open and soft.
6. Iliacus: think of fantail pigeons flaring tails. Psoas: a necklace around the spine holding femurs as pendants. Adjust the front pull—think of mobile or puppet.
7. Bran dolly—sew seam up the front of dolly, down the back. In lying on the side, one side seam is directly over the other on the opposite side.

Legs

Miss Todd always taught snugging along inside and front of thigh. Miss Colwell added lengthening back of thigh. Extremities like the elephant's trunk. Shrinking of the muscle into the body. Thinking from knee into thigh socket, releases outer hip.

Image Exercises

1. Wedge between ischia and little trochanter.
2. Bow legged feeling of trochanters and stuffing empty places.
3. Fascia on sides of thighs falls back on to table, put weight there and let it hang.
4. Soda straws through the centers of the legs.
5. Inner ankle back—outer ankle forward—pucker in front of ankle bone. Inner knee back—outer knee forward—soften above knee. Greater trochanter forward.

Feet

Correct feeling for foot is when all the fiber threads [through centers of the metatarsals] feel an even suction up a little pipe toward the center of the ankle. Radiating lines outward from heels of feet, as well as in toe area, relaxes tension. Heel substance can be more elastic. We hold at the tips of the toes because we think an end of a line. If we release it, it will be a more lovely line. There should be more action in walking, below ankle between heel and little toe. Relaxation of sides of the feet brings consciousness of center.

Image Exercises

1. Making the balls of the feet [heels, toes and metatarsal heads] into springs.
2. Snugging together at inner knee, snugging great toe into foot. Feet in a circle—lines from toes up into leg.
3. Small circle for great toe and large circle for little toe.
4. Set ball of each toe into foot and drag toes back over floor to straighten.

Rib case

Image Exercises

1. Ice cream cone inverted—head rests on peak—contents run down the back.
2. Rib carriage shaped like cucumber—narrowing side to side under the arms.
3. Ribs fit into sockets in spine like trains running into station with headlights leading the way. Carry tracks on the bias—a little upward—and not straight in, as we are apt to think.
4. Fish nets—hammocks slung from spine and sternum, heavy with sinkers and seaweed. Long ones into pelvis, shorter lines into lumbar area and mid rib area. Think of spine as the post. Nets flap in the breeze. Mesh can catch hold of the heads of the femurs and snug them in. Aid in correcting curvature tendencies and in shortening distance between ribs and pelvis.
5. Fitting ribs over inner pelvic rim—eleventh and twelfth pairs first and then the others.
6. Organ stops sliding in and out. First rib in and out, twelfth rib in and out—alternating and together. Ribs become elastic.
7. Working along and between the ribs, twisting and twirling them at their ends.
8. Windows to let the light shine at top of upper ribs, close to spine and under clavicle. Three upper pairs of ribs move upward as well as downward. This allows elasticity in the cervical muscles.
9. Tuck head into first rib like a tortoise. We have too large a head consciousness.

Breathing

Image Exercises

1. Squeeze water out of sponge in middle of body as you exhale.
2. Diaphragm like mushroom, strong stem and small, fragile top. Breath through the stem along front of the spine.
3. Teakettle lets off steam—hiss.
4. Eastern prayer position. Forearms on table parallel to spine—forehead touching—spine on an inclined plane. Draw back to sitting position letting ischia lead back. Do not spread ribs between shoulder blades. Hiss—relax vertebrae, empty lung sacs.
5. On inhalation expand dorsal vertebrae of the spine upward. Yawn like alligator—tongue stays on floor of mouth. Dog—"woof," pig—"ugh," cat—"meow."

Head

Image Exercises

1. Setting hyoid bone back and up.
2. Cervical spine like a stem. Blossom opens on front of the stem and on top.
3. Soften jaw. Tip the head to one side like a pot of gold and let the gold spill out that eye. Repeat with the other side. In manipulating the pupil, the pot of gold [head] rests on the hand under it as the gold spills. Head responds to light touch, not a harsh one.
4. Eyes look to right—back to center, look to left—back to center, look up—back to center, look down—back to center. Eyes should stay in sockets. Inner muscles should not contract and force eyes outward.
5. Sitting—mast [spine] secured at base. Psoas shortens as you turn upper mast to left or right. Loosen shoulder girdle—set ribs into spine. Standing like a stork, balancing with one knee flexed.
6. The lips are closed—jaw lets go. Pyramid up into the head.

SECTION III

Teaching Lesson   **Miss Todd**

Miss Todd has stressed in her teaching:

1. Flexibility of rib carriage in contrast to fixation.
2. Balance of weights through center of body.
3. Relationship between spine and heads of femurs.
4. Freedom of motion between the pelvic and shoulder girdles.
5. Freeing the muscles of the burden of holding body weights.

The first lesson to teach is the three masses—weight carried through the center of each. Think of equal distribution of weights. The nearer the base we carry our weight, the more stable it will be. In balancing weights, think bones first. Bones are the weight carriers and are grouped to serve the particular function of the organs they support. The three blocks must be so related that a plumb line could fall through the center of each. If these groups balance in a vertical line, the spine remains flexible but upright.

Action implies reaction. Power increases when tension is released, a basic principle. Muscles are reservoirs of energy. Tension is stagnation. Relaxation is perfect activity. Unlocking and loosening is energizing. Coordination produces rhythm. The more action you get on the inside, the more slack you will get on the outside.

The shoulders are suspended by tensile muscles and are only attached at the sternum. The weight of the shoulders is compression. The ribs must be free for action. Just as soon as you pull as hard on the inside of the ribs as you do on the outside, your legs will swing from the spine.

Teaching Lesson   Miss Galbraith

Watched Miss Galbraith teaching pupil. Felt feet—rigidity of outer lower leg and foot. Palm of hand under heel—coaxed muscles back into heel. Released muscles of the legs. Released muscles around ilia, directed head of femur into acetabulum. Released shoulders, narrowed upper thoracic, puckered upper sternal region, ribs into spine, pubic arch up.

After watching the lesson by Miss Galbraith, Miss Colwell comments about importance of firm easy touch that holds and makes the pupil work. Held the pupil at the lower thoracic, lifting up and then down. This released the tight spot in her left side. In a previous lesson, there was work on diagonals through the hip joint and releasing around the ilia. Holding across the lower abdomen to release transverse abdominal muscles. One hand at lower end of psoas, other hand at the upper end—press toward each other. Think of dough when working with body and take a large amount of flesh in hands. In this way, it does not hurt.

Teaching Lesson   Miss Colwell

Watched Miss Colwell working with a boy. Exercise of walking with hands on toes. On table taught much as to adult. Used idea of Indian spears for ribs. Pupil needs to vitalize nostrils, free diaphragm and breath. Think of high spirited horse. Has a very tight and hard spine. Must free the shoulder girdle.

Taught the idea of thigh revolving in. Worked on exercise of lifting head toward pubic arch, shoulders up. Explained that in upper dorsal area when the bodies of the vertebrae are forward we do not get the pull from the sternum. Story of the great trochanter. Related rib diagonals to the pelvis. In diagonals, if Miss Colwell takes thought outside, then follows with an inside thought.

Miss Todd comments on the lesson observed. Work with one fulcrum at a time. Don't do too much relaxing of a muscle. Strengthen its weak opponent. Relaxing is a negative factor, building strength is positive.

Teaching Lesson   Miss Colwell

Pupil is like Miss Danforth [studio secretary], locked in the upper dorsal vertebrae. One hand under back in that area, the other is on the other side of body. Work in circles, from one palm to the other. Hand working as a complete unit not in parts. Work on arm using same principle as with leg. Work on hand with same principles as with foot. Take up slack over the back of the hand beginning with middle finger with firm touch. Travel up the arm, more gentle touch near elbow cuff, turning in above elbow. Release over upper humerus and acromion, then snug arms toward spine.

For voice—placing voice in back of spine in the caverns of the head. To correct spine at eleventh and twelfth dorsal, narrow in front, folding thighs in. Shorten from ischia through the center of the body. Balances the parallel lines around spine reducing hump. Miss Colwell's comments after lesson: must not release one end of torso too rapidly. Start with little release at one point and then at the other end of the torso to balance. If ever you release a person too much, set him to work on himself with breathing. Get his mind off himself.

Teaching Lesson   Miss Galbraith

Lesson to boy of twelve. Told that dynamo of body should be strong muscles in lumbar area. Power for athletics should come from there. Where the inner leg muscles are hollow, think of filling out like filling a fountain pen. Instance of doctors examining students balanced on scales to show that blood flows to point of concentration. This is why this teaching comes through our minds too—what we think, we do. Image of palming inside of ilia—like hand prepared to catch a ball.

Don't roll pelvic bones backward—pushing back the spine. Get to the muscles at work—fastening the pelvis up into the spine. Think of pelvis as a basket with long handles—handles over body under shoulder girdle. The handles are broken in the front—bring the ends together.

The life current travels down the spine. Veteaux in France had a similar teaching to Miss Todd but not the structural side. Breathing: in inhalation lungs should deepen the cavity—the lower ribs enlarge. Think of two air shafts on each side of the lumbar vertebrae. Open the traps at the bottom of each side of the rib cage and let the air open down to the bottom of the shafts.

Teaching Lesson   Miss Colwell

Miss Colwell showed me the foot exercises and other exercises. She starts children right in on these and does the movements with them.

1. Great toe up, fingers making space—holding others down.
2. Other toes up and great toe down.
3. All toes up and down.
4. Pawing
5. Pawing with a bath towel—heel firm and rolling towel inward with the outer edge of the foot.

6. Walking crack [line on floor] on outer side of foot, keeping each foot exactly in front of the other.
7. Walking crack in crouched position, bringing one foot up and then the other.
8. Sitting have them feel the bottom of the foot with it crossed over the knee. The sole of the foot is like the palm of the hand. Action of the toes should come from near the heel.
9. On the back, arms around knees, hands grasping above the wrists. Rocking up and down. Sternum up in the up part of the rock—lower ribs down in the down part of the rock. Can also rock side to side. Do movement of walking on all fours. The hands holding the ankles in walking is very good but difficult for children and beginners.

Miss Colwell says, with adults in the first lesson, she explains that muscle tone is built up not by exercise but by blood supply carried to those parts. Silent exercises [visualization of images] does much toward directing this supply. Remember you could give a good lesson and the pupil might still not be released. Try to line up everything toward their weak spots. Calling their attention to the right points is where the focus should be, and getting away from tense points. Our biggest struggle in correcting faulty posture is the struggle to bring the pupil back to center. Balance the bones at center. Bony structure that is snugged together is well balanced. The muscular structure should have equal play all over the body. If it is unequal, it will be tense in some places, and over-relaxed in others. Sacroiliac case should not be put on all fours. Strain would come at this point. Should work snugging in the left femur and directing their attention around line of the inner pelvis to the sacrum.

Knee-chest position is not given until muscles over sacrum and ilia are sufficiently released so that pupil uses the right muscles. Arms can be folded under the chest or posteriorly down on the table. One or two pillows may be needed for chest depending on pupil.

Appendix B
Tom McEvoy Lessons

Lesson 1   **Date: June 10**

Name: Tom McEvoy   Age: 19 months

Birth Weight: 5 lbs. 9.5 oz.   Present Weight: 18 lbs. 2 oz.

Diet: Formula of evaporated milk and karo, one quart per 24 hours, one feeding at night. Refuses solid food by gagging. Ascorbic acid pill daily. Viosterol with navitol—15 drops.

Speech: Mummy, Daddy, no, hi-there, bye-bye and waves.

Physical Condition: Very pale, under-nourished, tiny child brought into the room in the mother's arms and held by grandmother while mother went to another room to give the history. Child fussed a little but was diverted by a rattle. Child manipulates toy well. Child is always put to bed at 6 p.m. It is now 8 p.m. Rolls over and can cover quite an area this way. Brings up the knees for the crawling position, but falls over on his face seemingly because of weakness of the arms. Stands when held, but the left leg turns outward at a right angle with the left foot pronated.

Therapy: Child placed on the table with the mother sitting in a chair beside him. Teacher worked inward and upward on the feet and legs for a few minutes. Then, with the child on his side, the teacher supported the pelvis from below the ischia, using a slow snugging action toward the center back. Child relaxed and expression brightened during this.

Advice: Watched mother as child sat in her lap waiting to go home. She was rubbing up and in on the outside of the thigh. Told her this was a good massage to continue on the left. Advised to keep child on a rug or blanket on the floor as much as possible to encourage rolling, crawling, kicking, squirming etc. Warned not to put him in the walker any more than is absolutely necessary.

Lesson 2   **Date: June 13**

Report: Child has not seemed happy on the floor but has slept for three nights without waking. This has never happened before. The child looks more rested and would seem to have more vitality.

Therapy: Child was laid on the rug before the lesson for a few minutes as he looked uncomfortable after sitting in his father's lap. He lacks the strength even for supported sitting. Laid with knees flexed and drew knees up to the chin some. Then, he rolled over. On the table, with the mother sitting beside him, a little work on the feet and legs. Turned child on the side to work on the mid-body. Teacher's palms nearly flat as child is so thin and tense. He relaxed and became so interested that I asked mother to move away from the table. He did not seem to miss her. She was very much impressed with the way he enjoyed and responded in the lesson. Intercostal action started, shoulder girdle loosened and lumbar area seemed stronger. Ischia support and snugging rhythm from beneath as in lesson before. Time of lesson: 20 minutes.

Advice: Give small pieces of cereal to eat with fingers or small pieces of toast.

Lesson 3   **Date: June 15**

Report: Mother has attempted to force the child in feeding resulting in gagging and vomiting. Child wakeful at night and extra feeding given (four ounce bottle). Child looks brighter to teacher.

Therapy: Child placed on blanket and rolled around some. On table child more relaxed in rib area than expected from the report. A little work here, then considerable on the thighs and feet and legs. Excellent response, child very interested in the touch and paid no attention to mother. Went to sleep on the table. Let him sleep for 20 minutes and wakened him to go home—very sound sleep. Time of lesson: 35 minutes.

Advice: Do not force feedings but be ready to respond to any increase of appetite from him. Suggested dark bread or oatmeal toast and small pieces of banana. Mother shown massage of feet.

Lesson 4   **Date: June 19**

Report: Child has slept through each night, once from 7 p.m. to 6:30 a.m. Would not touch zwieback, dry or moistened. Took a little piece of toast. Is taking five 8-ounce bottles. Sat in carriage for two hours watching children and cars and then did not want to be laid down.

Therapy: Work on back and shoulder girdle as in previous lessons, some on thighs and feet. Very good response. Placed on rug to check on actions. Came up on knees and hands twice. Was able to lower himself to prone position under muscular control fairly well. Time of lesson: 25 minutes.

Advice: Mother given samples of Multi-B to increase child's appetite— three drops. Do not put child in carriage for more than a few minutes at a time. Keep him on the floor and not many toys at present so that he will be more active. Mother shown massage of lower legs.

Lesson 5   **Date: June 24**

Report: Vitamin B given once with dropper then child refused. So mother gave it in two ounces of the milk at the first feeding.   Took three or four tiny bits of toast. Got into the sitting position and propped himself with arms for the first time; is very well pleased with himself and the commendation of parents.

Therapy: Same as in previous lesson. Active on rug with improvement in action.

Lesson 6   **Date: June 27**

Report: Parents are very pleased with child's progress. Each day brings new step. Child now sits up on the floor at will, which is often. Gets up and lies down quite easily from the prone position. Kept on the floor most of his waking time. Found a little bit of cookie on the floor and put it in his mouth. Showed surprise as he chewed it—later repeated the act. Chatters more as he plays.

Therapy: Placed on rug while mother was giving report. Child rolled around and sat up twice during that five minutes. As I carried him to the table noticed greater firmness in musculature. A harder and more tense feel than following lesson when I carried him back to the rug. After lesson the feel is of strength and compactness with relaxation. Sat up on the table twice during the lesson. Looked up in my face to see if I were going to praise him. Was pleased when mother and I did. Good response in lesson, but ready to stop in 25 minutes.

Advice: Told mother when he has not taken the full five bottles through the day, try to give him an extra bottle of milk when she goes to bed.

Lesson 7   **Date: July 2**

Report: He has taken five bottles of milk (eight ounces) through the hot weather when previously took less than the usual four. He has enjoyed his bath, sits up in the tub and kicks and splashes. Is putting things in his mouth—cloth, paper. Chatters much more than hitherto. Hearing seems very keen.

Therapy: Lesson as usual, 25 minutes.

Lesson 8   **Date: July 7**

Report: Took a sixth bottle of milk (four ounce).

Therapy: Mother doing very well in massage on feet and legs. I needed to spend very little time on them. Left shoulder rigid and sensitive to touch at beginning of lesson but it relaxed fairly well by the end. Worked over and around sternum and sides of ribs. Left side of the body responds better than the right. Mother noticed that the child sat up straighter when placed on the floor following the lesson.

Lesson 9   **Date: July 11**

Report: Child slept through the night July 7, 8, 9 and woke to take a sixth bottle of milk at 3 a.m., July 10.

Therapy: Lower back seems stronger. Work on upper back, neck and base of head for the first time. As child sat up on the table, spinal curvature was very noticeable.

Advice: Mother shown work on arms and hands. Child was tired and began to cry. Put on floor where he continued to cry. Put in crib with a bottle and four ounces was taken immediately. More appetite and strength in feeding than I had seen in him.

Lesson 10   **Date: July 16**

Report: Has slept through every night and taken five bottles each day. Weight taken while I was there at 18 lbs. 12 oz. Mother says child's cousin of five years practically lives on milk and is a strong child.

Therapy: Lesson as usual.

Lesson 11   **Date: July 21**

Report: Father watched lesson, standing all the time. Mother sitting in room very tired and discouraged because of lack of sleep the night previous. Child had extra sleep in the car on the previous day and was very wakeful during the night.

Therapy: Child did not relax as well in the lesson. Family will be going to the beach.

Lesson 12   **Date: July 30**

Report: Family back from the beach. Mother says child sucked his thumb. At beach he put stones in his mouth. When family started eating sandwiches, he wanted one. Put it in his mouth but did not bite any off.

Therapy: Child seems tired. Yawned two times which I had never seen him do. More muscular feel to the body. Worked on intercostal action to free the breath. In sitting child's back seems less hunched, shoulders nearer even and action freer. No drooling in the lesson.

No lessons until August 18. During vacation mother calls with following reports:

August 2: Baby has bad cold with cough. Took less milk but considerable water. Advised to give one half aspirin at night for a few nights.

August 12: Extreme heat—child took five bottles of milk and also water.

August 15: Weighs 19 lbs. Parents think he must have gained even more before his cold or wouldn't weigh as much now. When on floor watched kitten playing and then eating toast. Took toast himself and chewed it. Ever since has been eating 1/4 slice toast about two times a day. Mother spoke about how clear the baby's skin is now. Does not scratch himself anymore. Is sleeping very well and is not disturbed or wakened by noise during the evening. Sometimes has a bottle of milk in early a.m. but goes back to sleep.

Lesson 13   **Date: August 18**

Report: Grandfather says that child is more alert than he has ever seen him. Child stood up for a moment the previous day.

Therapy: Child sitting in stroller as I went into the room. Sits very well. Extremities somewhat rigid as the lesson began but very good response during it. Body seems more muscular with better tone. Chest area feels more normal. Chattered more than usual saying "papa" when father left room and "mama" in hearing mother's voice in next room. Child seems content and happy. At end of lesson took bottle with considerable interest—five ounces in five minutes. Lesson time: 30 minutes.

Lesson 14   **Date: August 23**

Report: Boy taken to beach on day previous. Enjoyed trip. Father seems very encouraged about his progress. Mother's brother who had not seen child for two months noticed improvement.

Therapy: Lesson as usual. Child seems a little tired but very happy. Observed child on floor going into crawling position. Moved the knees a little, hands almost. Takes toy to floor instead of playing with it on rug. Pushed toy and rolled himself.

Advice: Place child on bare floor during some play periods.

Lesson 15   **Date: August 27**

Report: Through very hot weather child has been set in large pan of water to play. Enjoys it very much. Stays in a while and then taken out and dried. Wants to go back right away.

Therapy: Best he has been in spite of the heat. Lesson as usual. Worked on thighs (especially the left) in thigh joint centering. Hungry at end and given six ounces, the third bottle that morning, besides toast.

Lesson 16   **Date: September 1**

Report: Mother has playpen in kitchen now and puts child in it when leaves apartment to hang out clothes etc. Child is starting to crawl, does not want to leave him free.

Therapy: Lesson as usual. Left leg and foot seem better, stronger. Asked mother to leave the room now during lessons. Child gives better attention without her.

Advice: Suggested to mother that a girl be found to care for the child occasionally and get him to know other people. It will mature him and give him new reactions, as well as relieve her. Let baby crawl on floor out of the pen some of the time.

Lesson 17   **Date: September 5**

Report: Child pulled up and walked around three sides of playpen previous day. Was interested in seeing the children from the window. Has crawled clear across rug at grandmother's house.

Therapy: Lesson as usual. Stood up straight on feet during the lesson. Left thigh straight, left foot only slightly pronated. Put in pen following lesson. Walked along two sides to his left but would not reverse to the other direction. Abdominal, thigh and lower leg muscles seem decidedly stronger. Less pronation.

Advice: Lessons no longer needed as often. Urge child to walk in pen in both directions. Most of time should be on floor. Try thin cream of wheat in his milk, drink from cup.

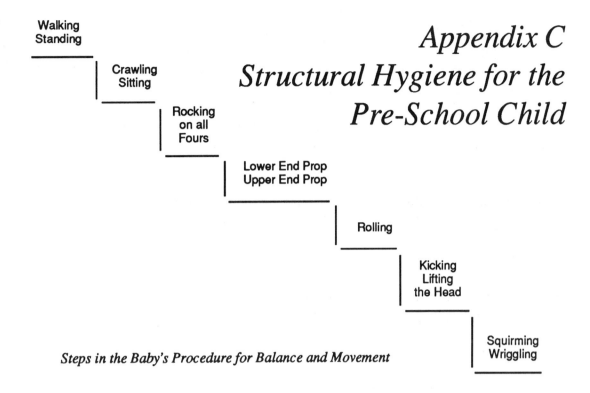

Walking
Standing

Crawling
Sitting

Rocking
on all
Fours

Lower End Prop
Upper End Prop

Rolling

Kicking
Lifting
the Head

Squirming
Wriggling

Steps in the Baby's Procedure for Balance and Movement

Appendix C
Structural Hygiene for the Pre-School Child

In earliest life, every child is involved in discovering the best way to balance and move his body. The child's structure increases so rapidly in size and weight that problems of balance are ever with him. Nature helps at the start by letting his body rest in the easiest way, in the horizontal plane.

Squirming and wriggling are the first steps the baby takes to discover balance and movement. Squirming and wriggling, while lying on the front or back of the body, develops the strength and flexibility of the spine. Since he knows nothing of movement for the purpose of going somewhere, the baby is content in the snake-like action. The rhythmic delight of the movement pleases him as he balances his structure around the central axis—the spinal column.

In the horizontal plane the baby also lifts his head, opens and shuts his hands and feet, waves his arms and legs in the air and kicks. He spends all of his time practicing coordination, showing such patience, perseverance and concentration. We would not interfere with the practice time of a musician and we should not interfere with the baby's.

The next step in the baby's development is rolling around his axis. The sides of the pelvis and the ribs provide a supporting framework for the spine as the baby rolls. The inner ends of the ilia support the sacrum at the sacroiliac joint. The inner ends of the ribs support the spine through their sockets on the sides of the vertebrae. The ribs make the spine doubly secure through their sockets with the sternum on the front of the body.

To help the baby accomplish rolling, dress the child in clothing that allows easy movement. Arrange the blankets of his bed so he may change position easily. Remember, soft mattresses cause the body to remain in only a few positions. An insecure surface or one with uneven support, will cause muscle tissues to become static to maintain security and balance.

The baby uses the horizontal resting surface until he has explored all the ways of balancing on that plane. Next, he comes to the semi-horizontal planes.

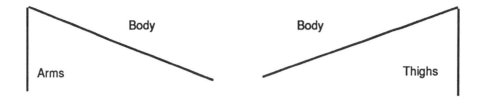

By propping himself up on his arms or his thighs, the baby becomes familiar with a new means of support for the body a little at a time. This leads to the simultaneous support of the body by the thighs and arms in the crawling position.

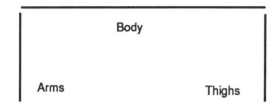

The strength of the arms and thighs are developed in the rocking balances which the child first practices in this position. Although he seems not to know where he is going, he is best left unhindered until he develops his coordination. Gradually, he reaches his next step, the ability to sit in the vertical plane without support. A little later, he achieves the ability to use the crawling action. In crawling, with the spine supported at both ends in the horizontal plane, the arms and thighs are free to move in their sockets. The baby needs a safe room to crawl in, not a play pen. He needs to move much more than the few steps a play pen will allow. Let him enjoy exploring his world, feeling the objects he may encounter and learning from all he experiences.

Standing and walking bring the child into the vertical plane, a more difficult one in which to balance and move the body. To make this developmental step easily requires familiarity with the art of balance on all the lower steps.

Let your baby direct his own movement development. Get your ideas from him about appropriate forms of play. If he takes the lead, he won't overstimulate himself. Let him decide when he wants to sit up. He won't try it too soon. Let him have free rein when ready to crawl and don't hold him back. Let him act when ready to stand, the urge comes from within. As the child grows older, encourage his return to the simpler planes of action during work and play. Help your child by giving him the privilege of natural body development. Use of all the steps for developing balance and movement, helps to build a beautifully balanced body.

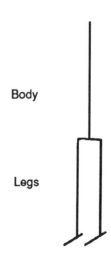

Appendix D
Balanced Movement and Relaxation

FILM STORY BOARD BY SHERMAN PRICE

Based on the Ideas of Mabel Elsworth Todd and Barbara Clark

PICTURE	SOUND
Main title superimposed over scenes which continue after titles:	Life is the alternating merger of movement into balance, and balance into movement.
Fish swimming, animals running, birds flying and other actions of animals, insects, etc.	Living creatures swim, run, fly . . . and in their balanced movements they radiate satisfaction and joy. When pursuing, or hard pressed their purpose and feeling are one with their movement.
Animals come to rest and relax . . . birds perch, crane balances on one foot and tucks head under wing, etc.	And then freed from the necessity for extreme activity . . . they relax, with such balance to their bodies that no muscular tension halts the quick restoration of their living energy.
Slow motion high dive of swimmer, children running, playing . . . people relaxing in the park.	Humans can find equal satisfaction and joy in movement and balanced relaxation . . .
Camera pans to park walk; pick up awkard details. See man sitting in tense position, reading . . . camera zooms to close-up of muscle tensing in jaw on side of face.	though sometimes we fall into awkward habits arising from our complex human circumstances, or from false or narrow pictures which seize control of our imaginations, which have so much power to guide our bodies.
Montage of the pictures we will be seeing later in the film, principally the diagrams and tactile imagery.	So let's get the pictures into our minds and imaginations which will balance our movement and relaxation so we can grow and glow in the vibrant flow of living energy.
FADE OUT.	

FADE IN: Rock and roll dance couple move around so that only one is visible facing the camera.

(Rock and roll music fades down under narrator.) Most of our body movements consist basically of . . .

DISSOLVE TO: Skeleton dancing in slow motion. Could be realistic or a simplified one used by artists and looking like puppet.

moving our bones against the downward pull of earth's gravity.

CLOSEUP: Arm of skeleton.

We move our bones by means of muscles.

DISSOLVE IN: Addition of muscle which lifts arm as it tightens.

DISSOLVE TO: Scenes of people performing common tasks and movements. (Some of the movements may be filmed in slow motion to show lack of conscious effort.)

But how do our muscles move our bones with such accuracy and skill, moving in just the right direction, with just the right amount of energy—no more, no less? Such precision, with so little or no conscious effort, is quite amazing, when you come to notice it.

DISSOLVE TO: Fish darting, jumping, bird flying to perch.

The answer lies deep in the reflex coordinating centers of our brains which, over millions of years, have evolved the automatic ability to translate our intentions for action into precise movements required to reach the goals we picture.

DISSOLVE TO: Bus driver quite casually taking change, shifting gears, watching the road as he drives.

MEDIUM CLOSEUP: Golfer looks down, preparing to hit golf ball.

You know how it works, too. When you have a mental picture of the action . . .

SUPERIMPOSE: White negative image of golfer in back swing. Golf hole flag appears on other side of screen.

and of the goal . . .

CAMERA PULLS BACK TO FULL VIEW: Golfer swings and hits the golf ball, watches its flight into the distance.

you seem able to perform the action automatically, once you've given the conscious decision to start it.

Select another action where the person merely "does it" without apparent conscious effort.

These are your unconscious reflexes coordinating your complex muscle and bone movements.

DISSOLVE TO: Cat resting in an obviously relaxed and balanced way.

We can use such pictures to activate our automatic reflexes correctly for action . . . and also to guide our muscles to position our bones, and the body weight they must support. Then the muscles themselves need not strain to keep them there. Balancing our bodies at rest, gets the maximum energy restoring relaxation to our muscles so they can serve us best when activity requires.

DISSOLVE TO: Cat in awkward position.

When our bones are placed in out-of-balance positions, our muscles must exert continuous tension to hold the bones from going further off balance.

DISSOLVE TO: Simple diagram of jointed figure.

Our bodies are supported by a bone structure made flexible by more than two hundred joints.

The upper section of the figure bends away from the vertical balance in both directions and comes to rest in balanced position.

These bone units are held in place by opposing muscles enabling us to move the unit back and forth.

Continue diagram of figure. First one, then the opposing muscles appear . . . in support of the balanced bone unit.

Bones are made to support and balance the weight.

The muscles move the bone back and forth showing exertion.

Muscles move the bones.

Muscles are balanced and each is relaxed.

When the bone unit, and the body weight it supports, is closest to balance in relation to gravity, the supporting muscles have the least amount of work to do to maintain that balance.

Bone is pulled off balance in one direction. Muscle is contracted.

But, naturally, when the unit of weight is positioned away from the axis of gravitational balance, one of the sets of supporting muscles has more work to do and the opposing set has less.

ZOOM to CLOSEUP of the contracted muscle. It throbs with increasing intensity (signaled by visible and audible effects.)

Muscles were made to be contracted and then relaxed to restore their vigor. Tension interrupts movement, dissipating energy and the pulsating rhythm of life. Continued for long, it renders muscles unable to respond when needed . . . and also . . . to pain.

DISSOLVE TO: Figure moving from activity to relaxation.

Thus, we can use good pictures to guide our reflexes for the range of living balance from extreme activity to energy restoring relaxation.

CLOSEUP: Actor's hand holding a picture of a character he is about to play.

The magical ability of our automatic reflexes to move our bodies in conformity with imagined ideas is illustrated when an actor visualizes the character he is about to "play."

CAMERA PANS up to his face and he "acts" the part (we see the characteristics in his pantomime.)

With a clear picture in mind . . . his reflexes take over and his actions become those of the idea he holds in his imagination.

MONTAGE: Quick flashes of military statues and figures.

This projection of the images in our imaginations into the reflex controlled behavior of our bodies, can reflect narrow or incorrect ideas such as the posture of pompous power often displayed by the military.

CLOSE UP: Young man (still photo with exaggerated military pose.) DISSOLVE TO: Underlying skeletal structure. ANIMATE: Throbbing muscles which must hold the bones in this awkward pose.

With shoulders held back tensely, chest elevated to force the back into an exaggerated arch, the body bone structure is thrust off balance, requiring undue muscular tension to hold it from falling further out of balance.

DISSOLVE TO: Painting of Degas ballet dancer, featuring ballet foot position.

Many special activities and cultural influences have created unnatural, unbalanced pictures which, when adopted into our regular posture, can only lead to muscular strain.

ZOOM from full shot to close up of person walking with feet toeing out.

Mistaken emulation of ballet foot positioning has caused innumerable people to outward rotate and toe out.

DEMONSTRATE imbalances and muscular strain resulting from continual toeing out with the feet. Develop anatomical detail.

This causes the imbalance of the normal construction of the foot bones . . . (explain in some detail the mechanism of fallen arches.)

DISSOLVE TO: Famous or typical religious painting or sculpture displaying "humility" or "reverence" with head bowed and shoulders dropped forward.

Even religious concepts of humility or prayerfulness have provided images of the roles some people wish to play in life . . . which have resulted in taking on an unnaturally balanced posture.

DISSOLVE TO: Flipping magazine pages to see high heel shoe fashions.

Some influences on posture have a purely physical source such as . . . the fashion for high heels . . .

DISSOLVE from foot in high heels to cross section of bones and muscles.

which certainly throws off the balance of body weight.

ANIMATE: Explanation of imbalance showing structure of foot in high and low heeled shoes.

(Continue to explain difficulties and why no heels are ideal.)

DISSOLVE TO: Person calmly going about his activity unconcerned.

Scene continues . . .

then person suddenly notices some pain and succumbs to feeling of fatigue.

In our natural tendencies toward psychological balance, we adjust our mental consciousness to bad physical habits so they feel perfectly natural . . . but then . . . we experience unaccountable tiredness or even pain. As we become aware of the cause and its correction we can minimize or eliminate discomfort from unnatural, unbalanced use of the body architecture.

DISSOLVE TO: Sitting skeleton.

If we base our ideas on factual knowledge of our body architecture and of our muscular system for moving and balancing it . . .

DISSOLVE TO: Bowling pin with center line.

we can arrive at simple pictures. Our imaginations can use these pictures to trigger our reflex control centers . . . to produce, automatically, the balanced relaxed arrangement of the skeletal and muscular systems.

DISSOLVE TO: Real person sitting balanced and relaxed. (Camera could move around to show body from side and back, as well as front.)	This will permit us to be active and restfully relaxed with a minimum of strain and a maximum of vibrant, free energy making the body a joyful place in which to live.
Person sits down adjusts feet, camera shows side view. ANIMATE: Center line from the knees to the feet.	Let's see how this works. Try sitting in a chair that allows you to rest the center of your feet on the floor directly under your knees.
Camera moves to back view. Back of chair DISSOLVES AWAY so we can see person's back. ANIMATE: The center line of the body in the back.	The spine forms a center line through which the body sits.
MATCHED DISSOLVE TO: Ten pin in the some position as the body. ANIMATE: Center line down the center of pin.	Now think of your body as the ten pin . . . with your center line going from the center of your head to the lower end of your spine.
Scene continues . . . semi-transparent "ghost" hands rub down sides of ten pin to feel/show that it has no shoulders. (Note— this is intended as a visual-tactile cue.)	Notice that the ten pin has no shoulders to weigh it down.
ZOOM FORWARD TO CLOSE VIEW of person's shoulders . . . each drops as narrator mentions it.	So free your shoulders from weight. Imagine you have no left shoulder weight and then imagine you have no right shoulder weight.
PULL BACK TO FULL VIEW: Person might elevate shoulders and let them drop.	See how you can rest more easily on your sitting bones when you allow your shoulders to relax.
MATCHED DISSOLVE to superimpose ten pin image over body. SUPERIMPOSED "ripple" flows down the center line.	Notice there is no obstruction in the smooth flow of weight down to the base of the pin. You should feel the same easy flow of weight down through your center line.
SIDE FULL VIEW: Ripple of weight flows back from knees through tops of thighs. RIGHT ANGLE SUPERIMPOSED over body center line and thigh line.	Your feet should feel light. The weight of your knees falls toward the body passing through the thighs, which are at a right angle or less to the body center line.

REAR VIEW: Person elevates shoulders and lets them drop again. Center line weight flow ripples downward.

When you stop trying to draw your weight up with your shoulders, you will begin to sense resting on your sitting bones. This starts a flow down the back of the center line.

MATCHED DISSOLVE: Superimpose diagram of ten pin with rounded points where the ischial tuberosities are. Person feels bones with fingertips.

Now with your fingertips feel the two rounded bones that touch the chair. You might rock gently side to side, to help you feel where these bones rest on the chair.

SIDE VIEW: Camera pulls back to full view as person stands up.

The interesting thing is that these parts do not change position when you stand. They do not need to.

DISSOLVE from pelvic area of clothed body to MEDIUM CLOSEUP of superimposed diagram, showing where body weight rests at the top of the thigh sockets.

The weight of the body is now focused on the tops of the thigh bones.

FULL SHOT 3/4 ANGLE: Person standing sits down. Runs fingers from knee centers to thigh creases.

Now let's sit down again, with our knees close to each other. Place your middle fingertips over the centers of your knees and run them straight back to your thigh area. This is were the weight of your upper body rests when you stand.

REAR MEDIUM VIEW of body trunk. Sway side to side on the sitting bones. SUPERIMPOSE ten pin diagram.

Now . . . relaxing your shoulders, sway from side to side to feel your sitting bones. This is where the weight rests when you sit.

ANIMATE: Downward flow of rippling weight through center line.

Feel the weight flowing down the back of your center line.

SIDE VIEW: Person stands up.

Now stand.

ANIMATE: Center line going down from middle of head through middle of trunk, through thighs and legs to heels.

And let the center line of your body go down through the center line of your thighs and lower legs to your heels.

REFERENCES

Brown, Beverly. "Training to Dance with Eric Hawkins." *Erick Hawkins: Theory and Training*. Edited by Richard Lorber. New York: American Dance Guild, Inc., 1979.

Clark, Barbara. *Structural Hygiene for the Preschool Child: Steps in the Baby's Procedure for Balance and Movement*. Cambridge, Massachusetts: By the Author, 1929.

_____. *Let's Enjoy Sitting—Standing—Walking*. Port Washington, New York: By the Author, 1963.

_____. *How to Live in Your Axis—Your Vertical Line*. New York: By the Author, 1968.

_____. *Body Proportion Needs Depth—Front to Back*. Champaign, Illinois: By the Author, 1975.

_____. Clark Papers. Clark Manuals Trust, Tempe, Arizona.

Gibson, James J. *The Senses Considered as Perceptual Systems*. Boston: Houghton Mifflin, 1966.

Martin, John. "Isadora and Basic Dance." *Isadora Duncan*. Edited by Paul Magriel. New York: Henry Holt and Company, 1947.

Moore, Sonia. *The Stanislavski Method: The Professional Training of an Actor*. New York: Viking Press, 1960.

Novak, Cynthia J. *Sharing the Dance: Contact Improvisation and American Culture*. Madison: The University of Wisconsin Press, 1990.

Oestrich, Harry G. *The Identification of Principles Related to the Education and Training of the Individual for More Efficient Neuromuscular Function*. Ed.D. Thesis, New York University, 1956.

Rollyson, Carl E. *Marilyn Monroe: A Life of the Actress*, No. 39 *Studies in Cinema*. Ann Arbor: UMI Research Press, 1986.

Rugg, Harold. *Imagination: An Inquiry into the Sources and Conditions that Stimulate Creativity*. New York: Harper and Row, 1963.

Spalteholz, Werner, Spanner, Rudolf. *Handatlas der Anatomie des Menchen (Atlas of Human Anatomy)* 16th edition. Houten, The Netherlands: Bohn Stafleu Van Loghum, 1967.

Sweigard, Lulu. *Human Movement Potential: Its Ideokinetic Facilitation*. New York: Dodd, Mead and Company, 1978.

Todd, Mabel Elsworth. "Principles of Posture." *The Boston Medical and Surgical Journal* 182 (1920): 645-9.

_____. "Principles of Posture with Special Reference to the Mechanics of the Hip Joint." *The Boston Medical and Surgical Journal* 184 (1921): 767-73.

_____. "Our Strains and Tensions." *Progressive Education* 7 (1931): 242-246.

_____. *Early Writings 1920-1934*. Reprint. New York: Dance Horizons, 1977.

_____. *The Thinking Body*. 1937. Reprint with preface by Lulu Sweigard. New York: Dance Horizons, 1972.

_____. *The Hidden You*. 1953. Reprint. New York: Dance Horizons, n.d.

Wheeler, Mark Fredrick. *Surface to Essence: Appropriation of the Orient by Modern Dance*. Ph.D. Thesis, The Ohio State University. Ann Arbor: University Microfilms International, 1984.

Williams, Jesse Feiring *The Principles of Physical Education*, 8th edition. Philadelphia: W.B. Saunders Company, 1964.